THE FUTURE OF
THE PUBLIC'S HEALTH
in the 21st Century

Committee on Assuring the Health of the Public in the
21st Century

Board on Health Promotion and Disease Prevention

INSTITUTE OF MEDICINE
OF THE NATIONAL ACADEMIES

THE NATIONAL ACADEMIES PRESS
Washington, D.C.
www.nap.edu

THE NATIONAL ACADEMIES PRESS • 500 Fifth Street, N.W. • Washington, DC 20001

NOTICE: The project that is the subject of this report was approved by the Governing Board of the National Research Council, whose members are drawn from the councils of the National Academy of Sciences, the National Academy of Engineering, and the Institute of Medicine. The members of the committee responsible for the report were chosen for their special competences and with regard for appropriate balance.

Support for this project was provided by the Centers for Disease Control and Prevention; the National Institutes of Health; the Health Resources and Services Administration; the Substance Abuse and Mental Health Services Administration; the Department of Health and Human Services, Office of the Secretary, Assistant Secretary for Planning and Evaluation; and the Department of Health and Human Services, Office of Disease Prevention and Health Promotion, Contract No. 200-2000-00629. The views presented in this report are those of the Institute of Medicine Committee on Assuring the Health of the Public in the 21st Century.

Library of Congress Cataloging-in-Publication Data

The future of the public's health in the 21st century / Committee on
Assuring the Health of the Public in the 21st Century, Board on Health
Promotion and Disease Prevention.
        p. ; cm.
Includes bibliographical references.
    ISBN 0-309-08622-1 (hardback) — ISBN 0-309-08704-X (pbk.) — ISBN
0-309-50655-7 (pdf)
    1. Public health—United States. 2. Medical policy—United States.
    [DNLM: 1. Public Health—trends—United States. WA 100 F9955 2003]
    I. Institute of Medicine (U.S.). Committee on Assuring the Health of the
Public in the 21st Century.
    RA445.F885 2003
    362.1'0973'0905—dc21
                                2003008322

Additional copies of this report are available from the National Academies Press, 500 Fifth Street, N.W., Lockbox 285, Washington, DC 20055; (800) 624-6242 or (202) 334-3313 (in the Washington metropolitan area); Internet, http://www.nap.edu.

For more information about the Institute of Medicine, visit the IOM home page at: **www.iom.edu.**

The serpent has been a symbol of long life, healing, and knowledge among almost all cultures and religions since the beginning of recorded history. The serpent adopted as a logotype by the Institute of Medicine is a relief carving from ancient Greece, now held by the Staatliche Museen in Berlin.

"Knowing is not enough; we must apply.
Willing is not enough; we must do."

—Goethe

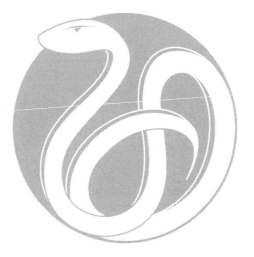

INSTITUTE OF MEDICINE
OF THE NATIONAL ACADEMIES

Shaping the Future for Health

THE NATIONAL ACADEMIES
Advisers to the Nation on Science, Engineering, and Medicine

The **National Academy of Sciences** is a private, nonprofit, self-perpetuating society of distinguished scholars engaged in scientific and engineering research, dedicated to the furtherance of science and technology and to their use for the general welfare. Upon the authority of the charter granted to it by the Congress in 1863, the Academy has a mandate that requires it to advise the federal government on scientific and technical matters. Dr. Bruce M. Alberts is president of the National Academy of Sciences.

The **National Academy of Engineering** was established in 1964, under the charter of the National Academy of Sciences, as a parallel organization of outstanding engineers. It is autonomous in its administration and in the selection of its members, sharing with the National Academy of Sciences the responsibility for advising the federal government. The National Academy of Engineering also sponsors engineering programs aimed at meeting national needs, encourages education and research, and recognizes the superior achievements of engineers. Dr. Wm. A. Wulf is president of the National Academy of Engineering.

The **Institute of Medicine** was established in 1970 by the National Academy of Sciences to secure the services of eminent members of appropriate professions in the examination of policy matters pertaining to the health of the public. The Institute acts under the responsibility given to the National Academy of Sciences by its congressional charter to be an adviser to the federal government and, upon its own initiative, to identify issues of medical care, research, and education. Dr. Harvey V. Fineberg is president of the Institute of Medicine.

The **National Research Council** was organized by the National Academy of Sciences in 1916 to associate the broad community of science and technology with the Academy's purposes of furthering knowledge and advising the federal government. Functioning in accordance with general policies determined by the Academy, the Council has become the principal operating agency of both the National Academy of Sciences and the National Academy of Engineering in providing services to the government, the public, and the scientific and engineering communities. The Council is administered jointly by both Academies and the Institute of Medicine. Dr. Bruce M. Alberts and Dr. Wm. A. Wulf are chair and vice chair, respectively, of the National Research Council.

www.national-academies.org

COMMITTEE ON ASSURING THE HEALTH OF THE PUBLIC IN THE 21ST CENTURY

JO IVEY BOUFFORD, M.D. *(co-chair)*, Professor of Health Policy and Public Service, Robert F. Wagner Graduate School of Public Service, New York University

CHRISTINE K. CASSEL, M.D. *(co-chair)*, Dean, School of Medicine, Oregon Health & Science University

KAYE W. BENDER, Ph.D., R.N., F.A.A.N., Deputy State Health Officer, Mississippi State Department of Health

LISA BERKMAN, Ph.D., Chair, Department of Health and Social Behavior, Thomas Cabot Professor of Public Policy and Epidemiology, School of Public Health, Harvard University

JUDYANN BIGBY, M.D., Associate Professor of Medicine and Director, Community Health Programs, School of Medicine, Harvard University

THOMAS A. BURKE, Ph.D., M.P.H., Associate Professor of Environmental Health Policy, Department of Health Policy and Management, Bloomberg School of Public Health, Johns Hopkins University

MARK FINUCANE, Principal, Leadership Development Solutions, Health Sciences Advisory Services, Ernst & Young LLP

GEORGE R. FLORES, M.D., M.P.H., Consultant, and Public Health Advisor to the California Endowment

LAWRENCE O. GOSTIN, J.D., Professor of Law, Georgetown University; Professor of Public Health, Johns Hopkins University; and Director, Center for Law and the Public's Health

PABLO HERNANDEZ, M.D., Administrator, Mental Health Division, Wyoming Department of Health

JUDITH R. LAVE, Ph.D., Professor of Health Economics, Department of Health Services Administration, Graduate School of Public Health, University of Pittsburgh

JOHN R. LUMPKIN, M.D., M.P.H., Director, Illinois Department of Public Health

PATRICIA A. PEYSER, Ph.D., Professor, Department of Epidemiology, University of Michigan School of Public Health

GEORGE STRAIT, Chief Executive Officer, MedComm Inc.

THOMAS W. VALENTE, Ph.D., Associate Professor, Preventive Medicine Director, Master of Public Health Program, Department of Preventive Medicine, University of Southern California School of Medicine

PATRICIA WAHL, Ph.D., Dean, School of Public Health and Community Medicine, University of Washington

LIAISONS FROM THE BOARD ON HEALTH PROMOTION AND DISEASE PREVENTION

GEORGE J. ISHAM, M.D., Medical Director and Chief Health Officer, HealthPartners, Inc., Minneapolis, MN

HUGH H. TILSON, M.D., Dr.P.H., Senior Advisor to the Dean of the School of Public Health, University of North Carolina at Chapel Hill

STAFF

MONICA S. RUIZ, Ph.D., M.P.H., Senior Program Officer, Study Director (until June 2002)

ALINA BACIU, M.P.H., Program Officer

LYLA HERNANDEZ, M.P.H., Senior Program Officer

ROSE MARIE MARTINEZ, Sc.D., Director, Board on Health Promotion and Disease Prevention

LORI YOUNG, Project Assistant

RITA GASKINS, Administrative Assistant, Board on Health Promotion and Disease Prevention

LIAISON PANEL ON ASSURING THE HEALTH OF THE PUBLIC IN THE 21ST CENTURY

MOHAMMAD N. AKHTER, M.D., M.P.H., Executive Director, American Public Health Association

HENRY ANDERSON, M.D., Chief Medical Officer, Wisconsin Department of Health and Family Services

EDWARD L. BAKER, M.D., M.P.H., Director, Public Health Practice Program Office, Centers for Disease Control and Prevention

JAMES BAKER, Executive Director, Institute for Public Strategies

WIL BAKER, Ed.D., Co-Project Director, Alabama Southern Rural Access Program

LEONARD BATES, Ph.D., Health Policy Fellow, Office of the Honorable Donna Christian-Christiansen, Congressional Black Caucus Health Braintrust

ERIC T. BAUMGARTNER, M.D., M.P.H., Former Director, Community Access Program and State Planning Programs

SCOTT BECKER, Executive Director, Association of Public Health Laboratories

BOBBIE BERKOWITZ, Ph.D., Director, Turning Point National Program Office

RONALD BIALEK, M.P.P., Executive Director, Public Health Foundation

BARBARA CALKINS, M.A., Executive Director, Association of Teachers of Preventive Medicine

WILLIAM CALVERT, M.S., M.B.A., M.P.H., Chairman, Department of Defense Sexually Transmitted Diseases Prevention Committee, and Program Manager, Sexual Health and Responsibility Program, Navy Environmental Health Center, Department of Navy

ANN CARY, Ph.D., M.P.H., A-CCC, Director, Institute for Research, Education and Consultation, American Nurses Credentialing Center

MARY CHUNG, MBA, President, National Asian Women's Health Organization

NATHANIEL COBB, M.D., Indian Health Service

DEBORAH DAMERON, M.P.S.H., President, Association of State and Territorial Directors of Health Promotion and Public Health Education

NILS DAULAIRE, M.D., M.P.H., President and Chief Executive Officer, Global Health Council

GEM DAVIS, M.A., Legislative and Governmental Affairs Coordinator, Policy Division, National Advocates for Asian and Pacific Islander Health

MORGAN DOWNEY, Executive Director, American Obesity Association

CLYDE H. EVANS, Ph.D., Vice President, Director of American Network of Health Promoting Universities, Association of Academic Health Centers

PATRICIA EVANS, Executive Director, Council on Education for Public Health

ADOLPH P. FALCON, M.P.P., Vice President, Science and Policy, National Alliance for Hispanic Health

MARIE FALLON, Executive Director, National Association of Local Boards of Health

MARY E. FOLEY, R.N., M.S., President, American Nurses Association

MARIANNE FOO, M.P.H., Director, Orange County Asian and Pacific Islander Community Alliance

MARILYN H. GASTON, M.D., Former Director, Health Resources and Services Administration

MARY J. R. GILCHRIST, Ph.D. President, Association of Public Health Laboratories

JESSIE C. GRUMAN, Ph.D., Executive Director, Center for the Advancement of Health

GEORGE HARDY, M.D., M.P.H, Executive Vice-President, Association of State and Territorial Health Officials

RUTH HARRELL, R.N., M.P.H., Co-Project Director, Alabama Southern Rural Access Program

BARBARA J. HATCHER, Ph.D., M.P.H., R.N., Director of Scientific and Professional Affairs, American Public Health Association

TRACEY HOOKER, Program Director, Prevention Project Programs, National Conference of State Legislatures

MARY JUE, P.H.N., M.S.N., Coordinator, Statewide Public Health Nurse Advocacy Group

STEPHEN KALER, M.D., M.P.H., Deputy Associate Director for Disease Prevention, National Institutes of Health

MIMI KISER, M.P.H., C.H.E.S., Health Program Coordinator, Interfaith Health Program, Emory University

DONNA KNUTSON, Executive Director, Council of State and Territorial Epidemiologists

CHARLES KONIGSBERG, Health Director, Alexandria Health Department

CHRISTINE MAKRIS, Executive Assistant, Global Health Council

LUCY MARION, Ph.D., R.N., C.S., F.A.A.N., Immediate Past President, National Organization of Nurse Practitioners

KAY McVAY, R.N., President, California Nurses Association

TOM MILNE, Executive Director, National Association of County and City Health Officials

SHARON MOFFATT, R.N., M.S.N., Vermont Department of Health, Association of State and Territorial Directors of Nursing

PEARL MOORE, R.N., M.N., F.A.A.N., Chief Executive Officer, Oncology Nursing Society

ANTHONY MOULTON, Associate Director for Policy and Programs, Public Health Practice Program Office, Centers for Disease Control and Prevention

ELLEN MURRAY, R.N., Consultant, National TB Nurse Consultant, Corrections Committee, Florida Department of Health, Bureau of TB and Refugee Health

MICHAEL O'DONNELL, Ph.D., M.B.A., M.P.H., Editor in Chief and President, *American Journal of Health Promotion*

ELIZABETH SAFRAN, M.D., M.P.H., Assistant Professor of Medicine and Community Health, Morehouse School of Medicine, Association of American Public Health Physicians

SARENA SEIFER, M.D., Executive Director, Community-Campus Partnerships for Health

BRUCE SIMONS-MORTON, Ed.D., M.P.H., Chief, Prevention Branch, National Institute of Child Health and Development, and Society for Public Health Education

HARRISON C. SPENCER, M.D., Ph.D., President, Association of Schools of Public Health

MELISSA STIGLER, President, Public Health Student Caucus

JESSICA TOWNSEND, Ph.D. Senior Fellow, Health Resources and Services Administration

KATE TREANOR, Program Associate, Grantmakers in Health

JONATHAN B. VANGEEST, Ph.D., Director, Section of Medicine and Public Health, American Medical Association

JIMMY VOLMINK, M.D., Ph.D., M.P.H., Director of Research and Evaluation, Global Health Council

ABRAHAM WANDERSMAN, Ph.D., Department of Psychology, University of South Carolina

RANDOLPH F. WYKOFF, M.D., M.P.H, T.M., Deputy Assistant Secretary, Director, Office of Disease and Health Promotion

Preface

Without health there is no happiness.

Thomas Jefferson

In 1988, the Institute of Medicine (IOM) report *The Future of Public Health* presented strong evidence to indicate that the governmental public health infrastructure was in disarray. The report provided a common language for national discussion about the role of public health (what we as a society do collectively to assure the conditions in which people can be healthy) and about the steps necessary to strengthen the capacity, especially of governmental public health agencies (e.g., local and state health departments and federal agencies), to fulfill that role. Moreover, the 1988 report prompted significant actions by policy makers, public health agencies, and educational institutions, including some remarkably successful efforts in several states to increase investment in governmental public health activities and to define more clearly the desired outcomes of such activities and the resources necessary for governmental agencies, such as health departments, to perform essential public health functions.

Much has changed in public health practice since 1988. Many of these changes reflect progress in the science of improving health at the population level, the emergence of innovative public–private partnerships in communities, and the development of new ways to dialogue and act on health. The Public Health Functions Steering Committee, as representatives of the national public health community,[1] developed a broad consensus definition

---

[1] The committee comprised the American Public Health Association, the Association of Schools of Public Health, the Association of State and Territorial Health Officials, the Environmental Council of the States, the National Association of County and City Health Offi-

of the essential public health services in 1994 (see Chapter 1, Box 1-1). Moreover, a national plan has been developed as part of *Healthy People 2010* to strengthen the public health infrastructure; significant progress has been made in describing the nation's public health workforce and its shortcomings, and the framework for a National Health Information Infrastructure has been defined.

At the same time, the broader context of public health practice has been undergoing a radical transformation, as evidenced by the demographic change in the age and diversity of the population, the shifting epidemiology of disease from acute to chronic illness, the explosion in technology, and the importance of global health to our national health. Further, state- and especially federal-level investment in governmental public health infrastructure—workforce, information systems, laboratories, and other organizational capacity—has been uneven and unsystematic. Recently, substantial appropriations to this infrastructure have been directed to address bioterrorism in the wake of the events of October 2001. However, concerns remain about the adequacy and sustainability of funding needed to assure the balanced capability of this infrastructure to act effectively across the spectrum of public health activities, not only in response to crises. These and other factors place unprecedented stress on governmental public health agencies as they struggle to carry out their mandates in an evolving microbiological, political, and social environment.

Given existing and anticipated challenges to assuring the health of the public, the Centers for Disease Control and Prevention (CDC); the National Institutes of Health (NIH); the Health Resources and Services Administration (HRSA); the Substance Abuse and Mental Health Services Administration (SAMHSA); the Department of Health and Human Services (DHHS), Office of the Secretary, Assistant Secretary for Planning and Evaluation (DHHS/OS/ASPE); and the DHHS Office of Disease Prevention and Health Promotion (ODPHP) entered into an interagency agreement to support an Institute of Medicine study. The Committee on Assuring the Health of the Public in the 21st Century was convened with the charge to create a framework for assuring population health[2] in the United States that would

---

cials, the National Association of State Alcohol and Drug Abuse Directors, the National Association of State Mental Health Program Directors, the Public Health Foundation, and several agencies of the U.S. Public Health Service (Agency for Health Care Policy and Research, Centers for Disease Control and Prevention, Food and Drug Administration, Health Resources and Services Administration, Indian Health Service, National Institutes of Health, Office of the Assistant Secretary for Health, and Substance Abuse and Mental Health Services Administration).

[2] Population health (also referred to in this report as *the health of the population* or *the public's health*) is the focus of public health efforts. It refers to "the health of a population as measured by health status indicators and as influenced by social, economic and physical

be more inclusive than that of the 1988 report and that could be effectively communicated to and acted upon by diverse communities. In support of that overall goal, the study sought to:

- enhance understanding of the core purposes, functions, and roles of governmental public health agencies and other entities engaged in public health action in improving health outcomes for all;
- crystallize knowledge about the conditions under which improvements in population health occur and how to affect those conditions (Chapter 2);
- set an agenda for scientifically credible research that informs efforts to improve population health outcomes and that also fits the complex, adaptive systems in which population health occurs (Chapter 8);
- provide evidence-based recommendations for improving the practices and the broader conditions that affect population health outcomes (Chapters 3, 4, and 5);
- address the capacity and workforce needed to support improvements in population health (Chapters 3 and 4);
- inform more strategic investments by grantmakers for population health improvement (Chapter 4); and
- promote engagement in the civic work of building healthier communities by a broad array of sectors, organizations, and people (Chapters 3 through 8).

To complete the report, entitled *The Future of the Public's Health*, in acknowledgment of the 1988 report but to suggest the broader scope, the committee met nine times over a 19-month period between January 2001 and July 2002. During this time, four workshops were held with representatives from a variety of federal agencies, state and local nongovernmental public health entities, private companies, and researchers in the field of public health. The committee also engaged in a visioning activity to forecast alternative scenarios for the status of population health in the United States in the coming decade and to assist with the development of recommendations that would appropriately address future challenges to public health and health care. Additional data collection activities provided input regarding the current status of the public health system and examples of how challenges to population health and health care delivery are being addressed at the state and local levels. Members of the committee also conducted site visits to two Turning Point projects (New Orleans, Louisiana; Franklin,

---

environments, personal health practices, individual capacity and coping skills, human biology, early childhood development and health services" (Federal, Provincial and Territorial Advisory Committee on Population Health, 1999).

New Hampshire) and three Community Voices projects (Baltimore, Maryland; Denver, Colorado; Oakland, California).[3,4] Additionally, multiple requests were made for public comment. The committee also reviewed the current literature on a wide range of subjects and received information from its liaison panel of representatives from federal, state, and local agencies, as well as advocacy and nongovernmental organizations (see the Acknowledgments for a complete listing).

Based on a consideration of this evidence, the committee decided against crafting a new vision statement. Instead, the committee embraced the vision articulated by *Healthy People 2010, healthy people in healthy communities*, and turned its attention to developing recommendations for the priority actions necessary to attain that vision.

Given the immensity of the charge, the committee struggled to select these priorities from the vast array of areas in need of consideration and response. Several broad themes emerged from the committee's discussion, including the need for a policy focus on population health; the need for greater understanding and emphasis on the broad determinants of health; and the importance of strengthening the public health infrastructure, building partnerships, developing systems of accountability, emphasizing evidence, and enhancing communication. These are the areas of action and change needed to improve our ability to protect and promote health.

The concept of a "public health system"—a complex network of individuals and organizations that, when working together, can represent "what we as a society do collectively to assure the conditions in which people can be healthy" (IOM, 1988: 1)—occurred early in committee deliberations. The committee also found that many entities and sectors are needed to act on the multiple factors that shape population health, and focused on several key partners who can have a particularly significant impact on health by working individually and as potential actors in a public health system. In addition to the governmental public health infrastructure, the committee examined the community, the health care delivery system, employers and business, the media, and academia.

---

[3] Turning Point is a grant program of the W. K. Kellogg and Robert Wood Johnson foundations that began in 1996 and that ended in 2002. The goal of Turning Point has been to "transform and strengthen the public health infrastructure in the United States" by supporting states and local communities to "improve the performance of their public health functions through strategic development and implementation processes" (ww.wkkf.org).

[4] Community Voices is a 5-year initiative launched by the W. K. Kellogg Foundation in 1998 in 13 U.S. communities. The goal of Community Voices is to improve health care for the uninsured and underinsured by strengthening and securing the safety net and community support services.

The broad themes outlined above are discussed in more detail in Chapter 1, which also provides a discussion about the status of the health of Americans at the beginning of the twenty-first century, with a special focus on the mismatch of health spending and health outcomes, the nation's shortcomings in health status (especially disparities in health among population groups), and the potential future challenges and threats to population health.

Chapter 2 presents a framework to illustrate the well-supported hypothesis that the health of populations and individuals is shaped by a wide range of factors in the social, economic, natural, built, and political environments. These factors interact in complex ways with each other and with innate individual traits such as race, sex, and genetics. The chapter then focuses specifically on several social determinants of health most robustly supported by the evidence. Approaching health from a broad perspective takes into account the potential effects of social connectedness, economic inequality, social norms, and public policies on health-related behaviors and health status. The chapter discusses seat belt and tobacco control policies as examples of public policies that have had considerable positive impacts on health status because they acknowledge the population-level and ecological factors involved in producing good or ill health.

The chapters that follow provide evidence of the positive impacts that key potential participants can have acting individually or in partnership, as appropriate, in a public health system working for the health of the public in the twenty-first century.

When most people think of public health, they think of state and local health departments, which have traditionally been responsible for public health services. Chapter 3 discusses the role of **the governmental public health agencies** at the federal, state, tribal, and local levels as the backbone of the public health system. In particular, the chapter examines the unique role and responsibility that governmental public health agencies have in promoting and protecting the public's health by facilitating, supporting, and empowering other potential participants in a public health system. This chapter also discusses the importance of political will to support and finance the development and maintenance of a strong governmental public health infrastructure that can ensure that all communities have access to the essential public health services.

Chapter 4 discusses **the community**, defined as narrowly as a neighborhood or as broadly as the nation. The community is both a setting—the place where health is supported and protected by social connections and healthy social, built, economic, and natural environments or risked and damaged by detrimental environments and social norms—and a potential partner in the public health system through its organizations, associations, and networks. Communities have the knowledge and resources that are necessary ingredients in assuring population health, and Chapter 4 illustrates clearly the significance of authentic community engagement in the public health system.

The health care delivery system and the role that it can play in maintaining both individual and community health are discussed in Chapter 5. Particular attention is given to this system's current fragility and the implications of this fragility for the effectiveness of governmental public health agencies and the broader public health system. The chapter makes note of the historic gap in priorities for investment between public health and health care. Also, it proposes ways for the health care delivery system to refocus its efforts in health improvement and strengthen its collaboration with governmental public health agencies to ensure the best possible disease surveillance, the promotion of healthier communities as well as healthier individuals, and preparedness for any emergencies.

Chapter 6 highlights the current and potential contributions of **employers and businesses** (private and public) to the health of their workforces and to the communities in which they are located. Although employers do not typically see themselves as partners in the public health system, their potential contribution to assuring population health cannot be underestimated. Most people spend at least a third of their days on the job; and the workplace may supply their health care insurance, may offer messages or activities that support or undermine health, and may also shape their health with occupational and environmental exposures and psychosocial stresses. Businesses and employers are also significant members of communities everywhere, and in recent years, many have acknowledged and acted upon their role as corporate citizens by fostering improvement in the economic and physical health of communities.

The role of the **media** in promoting health is the subject of Chapter 7. That chapter explores the unique potential of the news and entertainment media in communicating and informing the public about health risks and benefits, health policy, and related matters. Although their approaches and end goals are somewhat different, the news media's mandate coincides with that of the public health system: to serve and be accountable to the public. It is imperative for its own objectives and those of the public that the media "get it right." Also, a continuous dialogue among public health officials and educators and reporters, media leaders, and educators can play a crucial role in facilitating the development of media expertise in public health and public health expertise in providing timely, accurate, and understandable health information.

Chapter 8 highlights the responsibilities of **academia** in training the individuals who work in public health and health care professions and in building the science base for health promotion, disease prevention, and community health action. Assuring the health of the public depends in part on the efforts of well-trained professionals who are supported by an adequately funded research infrastructure.

The Future of the Public's Health began with an extensive charge. The committee thus endeavored to (1) examine and (2) explain the nation's health status, as well as (3) describe the key individuals and organizations needed to work individually or together as a public health system to create the conditions in which people can be healthy and (4) recommend the evidence-based actions necessary to make this system an effective force in attaining the vision of healthy people in healthy communities, and, ultimately, a healthier nation and a healthier world.

Achieving this vision will be a dynamic process as our knowledge about the factors that create the conditions for health increases. The sophistication of our actions must evolve to shape forces in the global, national, and local environments that can act for or against health. Finally, we must sustain our commitment to a healthier nation through education, investment, and political will.

> Jo Ivey Boufford, Committee co-chair
> Christine K. Cassel, Committee co-chair

REFERENCES

Federal, Provincial and Territorial Advisory Committee on Population Health. 1999. Toward a healthy future: second report on the health of Canadians. Ottawa: Minister of Public Works and Government Services Canada.
IOM (Institute of Medicine). 1988. The Future of Public Health. Washington, DC: National Academy Press.

Acknowledgments

This report represents the collaborative efforts of many organizations and individuals, without whom this study would not have been possible. The committee extends its most sincere gratitude to the organizations and individuals mentioned below.

Numerous individuals and organizations generously shared their knowledge and expertise with the committee through their active participation in workshops that were held on February 8–9, April 4–6, June 4–5, and July 31–August 1, 2001. These sessions were intended to gather information related to relevant issues to the future of population health and ongoing public health activities and initiatives, and helped to inform the committee's vision for assuring the health of the public in the twenty-first century. Members of the study's liaison panel contributed valuable information and suggestions that were helpful in preparing this report. These organizations and their representatives to the liaison panel are listed on pp. vii–ix. Additionally, the committee is grateful to all of the individuals who shared their experiences via their responses to the committee's request for public comment.

The committee is most grateful to Barbara and Jerome Grossman for sponsorship of the committee's visioning workshop. The workshop, held early in the process, helped focus the committee's thinking about the public health system and its actors. Also, the committee would like to thank Katherine Haynes-Sanstad from the Institute for the Future for her work in guiding the committee through the visioning workshop. Christina Merkley also assisted in facilitating the visioning workshop and provided lovely graphic representations of the future scenarios created during that workshop.

The committee is most grateful to the Henrie Treadwell and Barbara Sabol and the W. K. Kellogg Foundation for sponsorship of site visits to select Community Voices and Turning Point projects. Special appreciation goes to the directors and staff of the projects who graciously hosted committee members and project staff during site visits and enthusiastically shared their projects:

The Men's Health Center, Baltimore, Maryland: Jayne Mathews, Hakim Farrakhan, and project staff

Healthy New Orleans, New Orleans, Louisiana: Shelia Webb, Patrice Lee

Denver Health, Denver, Colorado: Patricia Gabow, Elizabeth Whitley, Raylene Taylor

Asian Health Center/Clinica de la Raza, Oakland, California: Tomiko Conner and project staff

Caring Community Network of Twin Rivers, Twin Rivers, New Hampshire: Rick Silverberg and Network members

We are also grateful to William B. Walker and the Bay Area Health Officials for hosting a very informative data-gathering meeting for the Oakland site visit by committee members and staff.

Additionally, the committee would like to thank all of the individuals who, at various points in the study, assisted the committee and project staff by providing insight and information pertaining to the many various population health and public health issues upon which the committee was deliberating.

Raymond Baxter, The Lewin Group
Ronald Bialek, Public Health Foundation
M. Gregg Bloche, Georgetown University
Julie Carlson, Research!America
Lori Cooper, Research!America
Kristine Gebbie, Columbia University School of Nursing
Dana Goldman, RAND
Robert Goodman, Tulane University Health Sciences Center
Bethney Gundersen, Economic Policy Institute
Shelley Hearne, Trust for America's Health
James G. Hodge, Jr., Center for Law & the Public's Health, Johns Hopkins University School of Public Health
Bruce Jennings, The Hastings Center
Laura Marie Kidd, Georgetown University Law Center and Johns Hopkins University School of Public Health
Vincent LaFronza, National Association of County and City Health Officials

Tom Milne, National Association of County and City Health Officials
Eugene Seskin, Bureau of Economic Affairs
Barney Turnock, University of Illinois, Chicago
Abraham Wandersman, American Psychological Association

The committee would like to thank the numerous staff members of the Institute of Medicine (IOM), the National Research Council, and the National Academies Press who contributed to the development, production, and dissemination of this report. The committee is most grateful to Monica Ruiz, who did a remarkable job of directing the study until June 2002, and to Alina Baciu, who stepped up courageously to shepherd the report through the internal and external review process and to bring the study to successful completion. A special thanks to Lyla Hernandez, who participated fully in the study process and contributed significantly to the development of the chapter on academia (Chapter 8). Carolyn Fulco, Carrie Szlyk, Mark Smolinski, and Rick Erdtman also deserve special thanks for their writing contributions. Margaret Gallogly, Sylvia Martinez, Gretchen Opper, and Marc Ehman provided outstanding research support to the project staff. Lori Young and Rita Gaskins provided excellent administrative support through the study and coordinated committee meetings, organized site visits, and maintained project records and files. Judy Estep competently prepared the report for publication. Rose Marie Martinez and Susanne Stoiber provided guidance and assistance above and beyond the call of duty, including research and writing. Melissa French handled the financial accounting of the study until June 2002, and James Banihashemi handled the financial accounting from June through project completion. Jennifer Bitticks provided editorial assistance. Jennifer Otten, Hallie Willfert, Christine Stencel, and Barbara Rice provided assistance with report dissemination. We are especially grateful to Bronwyn Schrecker, Clyde Behney, and Janice Mehler for cheerfully and skillfully guiding the staff through the report review process.

In addition to IOM staff, we are most grateful to Katrina Abuabara for her assistance in preparing the data needed for the determinants of health discussion in Chapter 2 and to Ron Goetzel from Medstat, Inc., for his assistance in preparing the background paper for Chapter 5. Special thanks go to Stephen Fawcett, Irving Rootman, and Barney Turnock for their noteworthy contributions to Chapters 4 (Fawcett and Rootman) and 8 (Turnock). Great appreciation goes to Patricia Peacock for her editorial assistance with Chapter 6 and to Jane Durch for her invaluable assistance in editing the report as a whole.

This project was jointly sponsored by six Department of Health and Human Services agencies—the Centers for Disease Control and Prevention (CDC), the National Institutes of Health (NIH), the Health Resources and

Services Administration (HRSA), the Substance Abuse and Mental Health Service Administration (SAMHSA), the Department of Health and Human Services (DHHS) Office of the Secretary, Assistant Secretary for Planning and Evaluation (DHHS/OS/ASPE), and the DHHS Office of Disease Prevention and Health Promotion (ODPHP)—which generously provided funding and lent support to this project. Our project liaisons—Edward Baker and Anthony Moulton (CDC)—were extraordinarily helpful in providing data, information, and support throughout the course of the study. Their encouragement and support are gratefully acknowledged.

REVIEWERS

The report was reviewed by individuals chosen for their diverse perspectives and technical expertise in accordance with procedures approved by the National Research Council's Report Review Committee. The purpose of this independent review is to provide candid and critical comments to assist the authors and the Institute of Medicine in making the report as sound as possible and to ensure that the report meets institutional standards for objectivity, evidence, and responsiveness to the study charge. The content of the review comments and the draft manuscript remain confidential to protect the integrity of the deliberative process. The committee wishes to thank the following individuals for their participation in the report review process:

Bobbie Berkowitz, Ph.D., R.N., Turning Point National Program Office

Haile T. Debas, M.D., School of Medicine, University of California at San Francisco

Gordon DeFriese, Ph.D., School of Medicine, University of North Carolina at Chapel Hill

Lori Dorfman, Dr.P.H., Berkely Media Study Group

David P. Fidler, J.D., University of Indiana School of Law

Claude Earl Fox, M.D., M.P.H., Johns Hopkins Urban Health Institute

Fernando A. Guerra, M.D., M.P.H., San Antonio Metropolitan Health District

Andrew Holtz, independent media consultant

LaVohn E. Josten, Ph.D., R.N., F.A.A.N., Center for Child and Family Health Promotion Research, School of Nursing, University of Minnesota

Jeffrey Milyo, Ph.D., The Harris School, University of Chicago

William L. Roper, M.D., M.P.H., School of Public Health, University of North Carolina at Chapel Hill

Mark A. Rothstein, J.D., Health Law and Policy Institute, University of Houston
Douglas Scutchfield, M.D., University of Kentucky Medical Center
Mary Selecky, Department of Health, Washington State
John D. Stobo, M.D., The University of Texas Medical Branch
S. Leonard Syme, Ph.D., School of Public Health, University of California at Berkeley

Although the reviewers listed above provided many constructive comments and suggestions, they were not asked to endorse the conclusions or recommendations, nor did they see the final draft of the report before its release. The review of this report was overseen by R. Don Blim, M.D., appointed by the Institute of Medicine, and Henry W. Riecken, Ph.D., appointed by the National Research Council's Report Review Committee, who were responsible for making certain that an independent examination of this report was carried out in accordance with institutional procedures and that all review comments were carefully considered. Responsibility for the final content of this report rests entirely with the authoring committee and the Institute of Medicine.

Contents

APPENDIXES

Executive Summary

The beginning of the twenty-first century provided an early preview of the health challenges that the United States will face in the coming decades. The systems and entities that protect and promote the public's health, already challenged by problems like obesity, toxic environments, a large uninsured population, and health disparities, must also confront emerging threats, such as antimicrobial resistance and bioterrorism. The social, cultural, and global contexts of the nation's health are also undergoing rapid and dramatic change. Scientific and technological advances, such as genomics and informatics, extend the limits of knowledge and human potential more rapidly than their implications can be absorbed and acted upon. At the same time, people, products, and germs migrate and the nation's demographics are shifting in ways that challenge public and private resources. Against this background, the Committee on Assuring the Health of the Public in the 21st Century was charged with describing a framework for assuring the public's health in the new century.

The report reviews national health achievements in recent decades, but also examines the hidden vulnerabilities that undercut current health potential, and that, if not addressed, could produce a decline in the future health status of the American people. The concept of health as a public good is discussed, as is the fundamental duty of government to promote and protect the health of the public. The report describes the rationale for multisectoral engagement in partnership with government and the roles that different actors can play to support a healthy future for the American people. Finally, it describes major trends that are likely to influence the nation's health in the coming decades.

The committee's work began with a vision—*healthy people in healthy communities*. This is not a new idea, but it is the guiding vision of *Healthy People 2010*, the health agenda for the nation. The committee embraced that vision and began discussing who should be responsible for assuring America's health at the beginning of the twenty-first century—a duty historically assigned to governmental public health agencies, through the work of national, state, tribal, and local departments of health. Current realities indicate that this is no longer sufficient. On the one hand, government has a unique responsibility to promote and protect the health of the people built on a constitutional, theoretical, and practical foundation. However, governmental public health agencies alone cannot assure the nation's health. First, public resources are finite, and the public's health is just one of many priorities. Second, democratic societies define and limit the types of actions that can be undertaken only by government and reserve other social choices for private institutions. Third, the determinants that interact to create good or ill health derive from various sources and sectors. Among other factors, health is shaped by laws and policies, employment and income, and social norms and influences (McGinnis et al., 2002). Fourth, there is a growing recognition that individuals, communities, and various social institutions can form powerful collaborative relationships to improve health that government alone cannot replicate.

Health is a primary public good because many aspects of human potential such as employment, social relationships, and political participation are contingent on it. In view of the value of health to employers, business, communities, and society in general, creating the conditions for people to be healthy should also be a shared social goal. The special role of government must be allied with the contributions of other sectors of society. This report builds on the foundation of the *Future of Public Health* report, which asserted that public health is "what we as a society do collectively to assure the conditions in which people can be healthy" (IOM, 1988). In addition to assessing the state and needs of the governmental public health infrastructure—the backbone of the public health system—this report also focuses on the roles and actions of other entities that could be potential partners within such a system.

The emphasis on an intersectoral public health system does not supersede the special duty of the governmental public health agencies but, rather, complements it with a call for the contributions of other sectors of society that have enormous power to influence health. A public health system would include the governmental public health agencies, the health care delivery system, and the public health and health sciences academia, sectors that are heavily engaged and more clearly identified with health activities. The committee has also identified communities and their many entities (e.g., schools, organizations, and religious congregations), businesses and employers, and the media as potential actors in the public health system. Businesses play important, often dual, roles in shaping population health. In the occupational setting, through environmental impacts, as members of communities, and as purveyors of products available for mass consumption, businesses may undermine health by polluting, spreading environmental toxicants, and producing or marketing products detrimental to health. However, businesses can and often do take steps to contribute to population health through efforts such as facilitating economic development and regional employment and workplace-specific contributions such as health promotion and the provision of health care benefits. The media is also featured because of its deeply influential role as a conduit for information and as a shaper of public opinion about health and related matters.

The events of the autumn of 2001 placed the governmental public health infrastructure under unprecedented public and political scrutiny. Although motivated by concern about its preparedness to respond to a potential crisis, this scrutiny offered an opportunity to assess the overall adequacy of the governmental public health infrastructure to promote and protect the public's health in the new century. This status check revealed facts that were well known to the public health community but that surprised many policy makers and much of the public. The governmental public health infrastructure has suffered from political neglect and from the pressure of political agendas and public opinion that frequently override empirical evidence. Under the glare of a national crisis, policy makers and the public became aware of vulnerable and outdated health information systems and technologies, an insufficient and inadequately trained public health workforce, antiquated laboratory capacity, a lack of real-time surveillance and epidemiological systems, ineffective and fragmented communications networks, incomplete domestic preparedness and emergency response capabilities, and communities without access to essential public health services. These problems leave the nation's health vulnerable—and not only to exotic germs and bioterrorism. The health of the public is also at risk when social and other environmental conditions undermine health, including toxic water, air, and housing; inaccurate and confusing health information; poverty; a lack of health care; and unequal opportunities for health. Government's partners, potential actors in the public health system, can contribute to assuring population health by helping to change the conditions for health in communities, at work, and through the media.

AREAS OF ACTION AND CHANGE

To address the present and future challenges faced by the nation's public health system—including potential actors in the private and nonprofit sectors—this report proposes six areas of action and change to be undertaken by all who work to assure population health. These areas include

1. Adopting a population health approach that considers the multiple determinants of health;
2. Strengthening the governmental public health infrastructure, which forms the backbone of the public health system;
3. Building a new generation of intersectoral partnerships that also draw on the perspectives and resources of diverse communities and actively engage them in health action;
4. Developing systems of accountability to assure the quality and availability of public health services;
5. Making evidence the foundation of decision making and the measure of success; and
6. Enhancing and facilitating communication within the public health system (e.g., among all levels of the governmental public health infrastructure and between public health professionals and community members).

FINDINGS AND RECOMMENDATIONS

Governmental Public Health Infrastructure

Finding: Public health law at the federal, state, and local levels is often outdated and internally inconsistent. This leads to inefficiency and a lack of coordination and may even pose a danger in a crisis requiring an immediate and effective public health response. Pioneering work at the national level has gone into developing models and guidance to assist states in reforming their public health laws as appropriate for their unique legal structures and public health preparedness needs, but a more comprehensive effort is needed.

1. **The Secretary of the Department of Health and Human Services (DHHS), in consultation with states, should appoint a national commission to develop a framework and recommendations for state public health law reform. In particular, the national commission would review all existing public health law as well as the Turning Point[1] Model State Public Health Act and the Model State**

---

[1] Turning Point, a program funded by the Robert Wood Johnson and the W. K. Kellogg foundations, works to strengthen the public health infrastructure at the local and state levels across the United States and spearheads the Turning Point National Collaborative on Public Health Statute Modernization.

Emergency Health Powers Act[2]; provide guidance and technical assistance to help states reform their laws to meet modern scientific and legal standards; and help foster greater consistency within and among states, especially in their approach to different health threats (Chapter 3).

Finding: The public health workforce must have appropriate education and training to perform its role. Today, a majority of governmental public health workers have little or no training in public health. Enhancing the knowledge and skills of governmental public health workers and nongovernmental workers who perform public health functions is necessary to ensure that essential public health services are competently delivered. Assessing and strengthening competence will help to ensure workforce preparedness, nurture leadership, and assure the quality of public health services.

2. All federal, state, and local governmental public health agencies should develop strategies to ensure that public health workers who are involved in the provision of essential public health services demonstrate mastery of the core public health competencies appropriate to their jobs. The Council on Linkages between Academia and Public Health Practice[3] should also encourage the competency development of public health professionals working in public health system roles in for-profit and nongovernmental entities (Chapter 3).

3. Congress should designate funds for the Centers for Disease Control and Prevention (CDC) and the Health Resources and Services Administration (HRSA) to periodically assess the preparedness of the public health workforce, to document the training necessary to meet basic competency expectations, and to advise on the funding necessary to provide such training (Chapter 3).

4. Leadership training, support, and development should be a high priority for governmental public health agencies and other organi-

---

[2] The Model State Emergency Health Powers Act (MSEHPA) provides states with the powers needed "to detect and contain bioterrorism or a naturally occurring disease outbreak. Legislative bills based on the MSEHPA have been introduced in 34 states" (Gostin et al., 2002).

[3] The Council on Linkages between Academia and Public Health Practice is comprised of leaders from national organizations representing the public health practice and academic communities. The Council grew out of the Public Health Faculty/Agency Forum, which developed recommendations for improving the relevance of public health education to the demands of public health in the practice sector. The Council and its partners have focused attention on the need for a public health practice research agenda.

zations in the public health system and for schools of public health that supply the public health infrastructure with its professionals and leaders (Chapter 3).

5. A formal national dialogue should be initiated to address the issue of public health workforce credentialing. The Secretary of DHHS should appoint a national commission on public health workforce credentialing to lead this dialogue. The commission should be charged to determine if a credentialing system would further the goal of creating a competent workforce and, if applicable, the manner and time frame for implementation by governmental public health agencies at all levels. The dialogue should include representatives from federal, state, and local public health agencies, academia, and public health professional organizations who can represent and discuss the various perspectives on the workforce credentialing debate (Chapter 3).

Finding: Developments in communication and information technologies present both opportunities and challenges to attaining the vision of healthy people in healthy communities. Harnessing the potential of these technologies will enable public health officials to collect and disseminate information more efficiently, improve the effectiveness of public health interventions, and enable the public to understand what services should be provided, and thus what they have the right to expect from their public officials.

6. All partners within the public health system should place special emphasis on communication as a critical core competency of public health practice. Governmental public health agencies at all levels should use existing and emerging tools (including information technologies) for effective management of public health information and for internal and external communication. To be effective, such communication must be culturally appropriate and suitable to the literacy levels of the individuals in the communities they serve (Chapter 3).

Finding: Existing information networks make it difficult, and sometimes impossible, for governmental public health agencies to exchange information and communicate effectively with the health care delivery system for the purposes of surveillance, reporting, and appropriately responding to threats to the public's health. Clear communication and enhanced information gathering, processing, and dissemination mechanisms will increase the accountability and effectiveness of governmental public health agencies and other public health system actors. Individuals and communities may also benefit by being able to contribute and collect information directly relevant to them.

7. The Secretary of DHHS should provide leadership to facilitate the development and implementation of the National Health Information Infrastructure (NHII). Implementation of NHII should take into account, where possible, the findings and recommendations of the National Committee on Vital and Health Statistics (NCVHS) working group on NHII. Congress should consider options for funding the development and deployment of NHII (e.g., in support of clinical care, health information for the public, and public health practice and research) through payment changes, tax credits, subsidized loans, or grants (Chapter 3).

Finding: At this time, DHHS lacks a system for conducting regular assessments of the adequacy and capacity of the governmental public health infrastructure. Such assessments are urgently needed to keep Congress and the public informed and would play an important role in supporting a regular process of assessment and evaluation at state and local public health agency levels.

8. DHHS should be accountable for assessing the state of the nation's governmental public health infrastructure and its capacity to provide the essential public health services to every community and for reporting that assessment annually to Congress and the nation. The assessment should include a thorough evaluation of federal, state, and local funding for the nation's governmental public health infrastructure and should be conducted in collaboration with state and local officials. The assessment should identify strengths and gaps and serve as the basis for plans to develop a funding and technical assistance plan to assure sustainability. The public availability of these reports will enable state and local public health agencies to use them for continual self-assessment and evaluation (Chapter 3).

Finding: The capacity of the nation's public health laboratories should be assessed. Every state has at least one state public health laboratory to support infectious disease surveillance and other public health activities. About 60 percent of the 3,000 local health departments provide some laboratory services. Enhanced funding has been provided to prepare states and some urban areas for bioterrorism and other emergencies. The adequacy of these funds and how effectively they are being used to address laboratory capacity problems are unknown. The appropriate funding levels to sustain current capacity and enable the laboratories to integrate new technologies as they emerge have not been determined and require investigation.

9. DHHS should evaluate the status of the nation's public health laboratory system, including an assessment of the impact of recent increased funding. The evaluation should identify remaining gaps, and funding should be allocated to close them. Working with the states, DHHS should agree on a base funding level that will maintain the enhanced laboratory system and allow the rapid deployment of newly developed technologies (Chapter 3).

Finding: After adequate funding levels are determined for the governmental public health infrastructure, the appropriate investment level is needed to assure that every community has access to the essential public health services.

10. DHHS should develop a comprehensive investment plan for a strong national governmental public health infrastructure with a timetable, clear performance measures, and regular progress reports to the public. State and local governments should also provide adequate, consistent, and sustainable funding for the governmental public health infrastructure (Chapter 3).

Finding: Current funding structures frequently burden the work of state and local public health jurisdictions with administrative requirements. "Stove-pipe" (i.e., categorical) funding is often inflexible, at times discouraging evidence-based planning and use of funds or the blending of resources in special circumstances.

11. The federal government and states should renew efforts to experiment with clustering or consolidation of categorical grants for the purpose of increasing local flexibility to address priority health concerns and enhance the efficient use of limited resources (Chapter 3).

Finding: Although the health care delivery system has several mechanisms for accreditation and quality assurance, the committee found that there are no such structures for the governmental public health infrastructure. Accreditation mechanisms may help to ensure the robustness and efficiency of the governmental public health infrastructure, assure the quality of public health services, and transparently provide information to the public about the quality of the services delivered.

12. The Secretary of DHHS should appoint a national commission to consider if an accreditation system would be useful for improving and building state and local public health agency capacities. If such a system is deemed useful, the commission should make recommendations on how it would be governed and develop mechanisms (e.g., incentives) to gain state and local government participation in the accreditation effort. Membership on this commission should include representatives from CDC, the Association of State and Territorial Health Officials, the National Association of County and City Health Officials, and nongovernmental organizations (Chapter 3).

Finding: Research is needed to guide policy decisions that shape public health practice. The committee had hoped to provide specific guidance elaborating on the types and levels of workforce, infrastructure, related resources, and financial investments necessary to ensure the availability of essential public health services to all of the nation's communities. However, such evidence is limited, and there is no agenda or support for this type of research, despite the critical need for such data to promote and protect the nation's health.

13. CDC, in collaboration with the Council on Linkages between Academia and Public Health Practice and other public health system partners, should develop a research agenda and estimate the funding needed to build the evidence base that will guide policy making for public health practice (Chapter 3).

Finding: Effective interagency collaboration on health issues at the federal level is crucial but difficult because of the specialized nature of agency structures and responsibilities. Furthermore, many agencies not traditionally associated with health issues make policy and manage programs with potential implications for health. More effective coordinating structures are needed to reduce obstacles to the effective use of federal regulatory and standard-setting powers in health. Mechanisms are needed to develop collaborative relationships and to harmonize regulations within DHHS, across federal agencies, and among federal state and local governments to assure effective action for protecting the population's health.

14. The Secretary of DHHS should review the regulatory authorities of DHHS agencies with health-related responsibilities to reduce overlap and inconsistencies, ensure that the department's management structure is best suited to coordinate among agencies within DHHS with health-related responsibilities, and, to the extent possible, sim-

plify relationships with state and local governmental public health agencies. Similar efforts should be made to improve coordination with other federal cabinet agencies performing important public health services, such as the Department of Agriculture and the Environmental Protection Agency (Chapter 3).

Finding: The success of the public health system depends in part on collaboration among all levels of government. Although noting the importance of preserving state autonomy and the ability to address local circumstances, the National Governors' Association (1997) acknowledged a need for a federal role in certain domestic issues—where issues are national in scope and where the national interest is at risk—and to help states meet the needs of special populations. Collaboration on such issues would also improve the alignment of policy across federal agencies. The committee believes that a more formal entity could facilitate the link between the Secretary of DHHS and state health officers for the purpose of improving communication, coordination, and collaborative action on a national health agenda.

15. Congress should mandate the establishment of a National Public Health Council. This National Public Health Council would bring together the Secretary of DHHS and state health commissioners at least annually to

- Provide a forum for communication and collaboration on action to achieve national health goals as articulated in *Healthy People 2010;*
- Advise the Secretary of DHHS on public health issues;
- Advise the Secretary of DHHS on financing and regulations that affect governmental public health capacity at the state and local levels;
- Provide a forum for overseeing the development of an incentive-based federal–state-funded system to sustain a governmental public health infrastructure that can assure the availability of essential public health services to every American community and can monitor progress toward this goal (e.g., through report cards);
- Review and evaluate the domestic policies of other cabinet agencies for their impact on national health outcomes (e.g., through health impact reports) and on the reduction and elimination of health disparities; and
- Submit an annual report on their deliberations and recommendations to Congress.

The Council should be chaired by the Secretary of DHHS and cochaired by a state health director on a rotating basis. An appropriately resourced secretariat should be established in the Office of the Secretary to ensure that the Council has access to the information and expertise of all DHHS agencies during its deliberations (Chapter 3).

Community

Finding: Community organizations are close to the populations they serve and are therefore a crucial part of the public health system for identifying needs and responses and evaluating results. Communication and collaboration between community organizations and health departments are often limited, leading to the duplication of effort and an inefficient use of resources. Moreover, foundation and governmental funding mechanisms are often not structured in ways that encourage broad community engagement and leadership at all stages. Communities are sometimes brought into the effort late, after planning has begun, or they are simply used as informants or subjects of research. The goal of achieving lasting change for health improvement should guide community groups and public and private funders.

16. Local governmental public health agencies should support community-led efforts to inventory resources, assess needs, formulate collaborative responses, and evaluate outcomes for community health improvement and the elimination of health disparities. Governmental public health agencies should provide community organizations and coalitions with technical assistance and support in identifying and securing resources as needed and at all phases of the process (Chapter 4).

17. Governmental and private-sector funders of community health initiatives should plan their investments with a focus on long-lasting change. Such a focus would include realistic time lines, an emphasis on ongoing community engagement and leadership, and a final goal of institutionalizing effective project components in the local community or public health system as appropriate (Chapter 4).

Health Care Delivery System

Finding: Health care is an important determinant of population and individual health. Although most Americans receive the health care services that they require, the approximately 41 million people who have no health insurance experience difficulty in accessing care and are often unable to obtain needed services. Furthermore, the services that they do receive may not be timely, appropriate, or well coordinated. Recent Institute of Medicine (IOM) reports have found that health insurance coverage is associated with better health outcomes for children and adults. It is also associated with having a regular source of care and with the greater and more appropriate use of health services. These factors, in turn, improve the likelihood of disease screening and early detection, the management of chronic illnesses, and the effective treatment of acute conditions. The ultimate result is better health for children, adults, and families. Increased health insurance coverage would likely reduce racial and ethnic disparities in the use of appropriate health care services and may also reduce disparities in morbidity and mortality among ethnic groups.

18. **Adequate population health cannot be achieved without making comprehensive and affordable health care available to every person residing in the United States. It is the responsibility of the federal government to lead a national effort to examine the options available to achieve stable health care coverage of individuals and families and to assure the implementation of plans to achieve that result (Chapter 5).**

Finding: In addition to a lack of health care coverage, many people are covered by health insurance plans that do not include coverage for preventive health care, mental health, substance abuse treatment, and dental health services or require copayments that lessen access (Allukian, 1999; King, 2000; Solanki et al., 2000). This causes many individuals to live with undiagnosed mental illness and others to go without treatment (DHHS, 1999). Many children and adults suffer from oral health conditions that may affect their overall health status (DHHS, 2000). These often-neglected services constitute gaps in efforts to assure the health of the population.

19. **All public and privately funded insurance plans should include age-appropriate preventive services as recommended by the U.S. Preventive Services Task Force and provide evidence-based coverage of oral health, mental health, and substance abuse treatment services (Chapter 5).**

Finding: As the public health system strains to meet the challenges posed by increasing costs, an aging population, and a range of threats to health, it will need a meaningful partnership with the health care delivery sector to attain their shared population health goals.

20. Bold, large-scale demonstrations should be funded by the federal government and other major investors in health care to test radical new approaches to increase the efficiency and effectiveness of health care financing and delivery systems. The experiments should effectively link delivery systems with other components of the public health system and focus on improving population health while eliminating disparities. The demonstrations should be supported by adequate resources to enable innovative ideas to be fairly tested (Chapter 5).

Businesses and Employers

Finding: Employers play a major role in the health of their employees and the population at large through their impacts on natural and built environments, through workplace conditions, and through their relationship with communities. For example, employers may be an important part of a region's economic development, which, in turn, may support health improvement. In addition, low unemployment rates and vibrant businesses are likely to mean better housing, higher incomes, and improved overall quality of life within communities. Furthermore, employers facilitate access to health care services by purchasing health care for their employees.

21. The federal government should develop programs to assist small employers and employers with low-wage workers to purchase health insurance at reasonable rates (Chapter 6).

22. The corporate community and public health agencies should initiate and enhance joint efforts to strengthen health promotion and disease and injury prevention programs for employees and their communities. As an early step, the corporate and governmental public health community should:

   a. Strengthen partnership and collaboration by

   - Developing direct linkages between local public health agencies and business leaders to forge a common language and understanding of employee and community health problems and to participate in setting community health goals and strategies for achieving them, and
   - Developing innovative ways for the corporate and governmental public health communities to gather, interpret, and exchange mutually meaningful data and information, such

as the translation of health information to support corporate health promotion and health care purchasing activities.

  b. Enhance communication by

  • Developing effective employer and community communication and education programs focused on the benefits of and options for health promotion and disease and injury prevention, and
  • Using proven marketing and social marketing techniques to promote individual behavioral and community change.

  c. Develop the evidence base for workplace and community interventions through greater public, private, and philanthropic investments in research to extend the science and improve the effectiveness of workplace and community interventions to promote health and prevent disease and injury.

  d. Recognize business leadership in employee and community health by elevating the level of recognition given to corporate investment in employee and community health. The Secretaries of DHHS and the Department of Commerce, along with business leaders (e.g., chambers of commerce and business roundtables), should jointly sponsor a Corporate Investment in Health Award. The award would recognize private-sector entities that have demonstrated exemplary civic and social responsibility for improving the health of their workers and the community (Chapter 6).

Media

Finding: Both the news and entertainment media shape public opinion and influence decision making, with potentially critical effects on population health. Moreover, public health efforts and especially the activities of governmental public health agencies often receive and attract little media attention, explaining in part the widespread lack of understanding about the concepts and content of public health activities (i.e., population-level health promotion and protection, as well as disease prevention). Editors and journalists and medical and public health officials generally do not understand each other's perspectives, methods, and objectives. This lack of understanding frequently leads to the provision of inaccurate or inadequate health information and missed opportunities to communicate effectively to the public. The journalism and public health communities have identified a clear need for training, research, and dialogue to improve their ability to accurately inform and communicate with the public, communities, and other actors in the public health system.

23. An ongoing dialogue should be maintained between medical and public health officials and editors and journalists at the local level and their representative associations nationally. Furthermore, foundations and governmental health agencies should provide opportunities to develop and evaluate educational and training programs that provide journalists with experiences that will deepen their knowledge of public health subject matter and provide public health workers with a foundation in communication theory, messaging, and application (Chapter 7).

24. The television networks, television stations, and cable providers should increase the amount of time they donate to public service announcements (PSAs) as partial fulfillment of the public service requirement in their Federal Communications Commission (FCC) licensing agreements (Chapter 7).

25. The FCC should review its regulations for PSA broadcasting on television and radio to ensure a more balanced broadcasting schedule that will reach a greater proportion of the viewing and listening audiences (Chapter 7).

26. Public health officials and local and national entertainment media should work together to facilitate the communication of accurate information about disease and about medical and health issues in the entertainment media (Chapter 7).

27. Public health and communication researchers should develop an evidence base on media influences on health knowledge and behavior, as well as on the promotion of healthy public policy (Chapter 7).

Academia

Finding: Academia provides degree and continuing education to a significant proportion of the public health workforce. Consistent with the previous recommendations to assess workforce competency and develop strategies to overcome deficits, changes are needed in both academic settings and curricula and in the financial support available to students training for careers in public health.

28. Academic institutions should increase integrated interdisciplinary learning opportunities for students in public health and other related health science professions. Such efforts should include not only multidisciplinary education but also interdisciplinary education and appropriate incentives for faculty to undertake such activities (Chapter 8).

29. Congress should increase funding for HRSA programs that provide financial support for students enrolled in public health degree programs through mechanisms such as training grants, loan repayments, and service obligation grants. Funding should also be provided to strengthen the Public Health Training Center program to effectively meet the educational needs of the existing public health workforce and to facilitate public health worker access to the centers. Support for leadership training of state and local health department directors and local community leaders should continue through funding of the National and Regional Public Health Leadership Institutes and distance-learning materials developed by HRSA and CDC (Chapter 8).

Finding: The committee finds that health-related research is disproportionately biomedical, focused on the health and health problems of individuals. Funding and incentives for population-level research and community-based prevention research are low, as these are not priority areas within academia or the governmental public health infrastructure.

30. Federal funders of research and academic institutions should recognize and reward faculty scholarship related to public health practice research (Chapter 8).

31. The committee recommends that Congress provide funds for CDC to enhance its investigator-initiated program for prevention research while maintaining a strong Centers, Institutes, and Offices (CIO)-generated research program. CDC should take steps that include

   • Expanding the external peer review mechanism for review of investigator-initiated research;
   • Allowing research to be conducted over the more generous time lines often required by prevention research; and
   • Establishing a central mechanism for coordination of investigator-initiated proposal submissions (Chapter 8).

32. CDC should authorize an analysis of the funding levels necessary for effective Prevention Research Center functioning, taking into account the levels authorized by P.L. 98–551 as well as the amount of prevention research occurring in other institutions and organizations (Chapter 8).

33. NIH should increase the portion of its budget allocated to population- and community-based prevention research that

   • Addresses population-level health problems;
   • Involves a definable population and operates at the level of the whole person;
   • Evaluates the application and impacts of new discoveries on the actual health of the population; and
   • Focuses on the behavioral and environmental (social, economic, cultural, physical) factors associated with primary and secondary prevention of disease and disability in populations.

Furthermore, the committee recommends that the Director of NIH report annually to the Secretary of DHHS on the scope of population- and community-based prevention research activities undertaken by the NIH centers and institutes (Chapter 8).

34. Academic institutions should develop criteria for recognizing and rewarding faculty scholarship related to service activities that strengthen public health practice (Chapter 8).

The findings and recommendations outlined above illustrate the areas of action and change that the committee believes should be emphasized by all potential actors in the public health system. Recommendations are directed to many parties, because in a society as diverse and decentralized as that of the United States, achieving population health requires contributions from all levels of government, the private business sector, and the variety of institutions and organizations that shape opportunities, attitudes, behaviors, and resources affecting health. Governmental public health agencies have the responsibility to facilitate and nurture the conditions conducive to good health. Without the active collaboration of other important institutions, however, they cannot produce the healthy people in healthy communities envisioned in *Healthy People 2010*.

REFERENCES

Allukian M. 1999. Dental insurance is essential, but not enough. In Closing the Gap, a newsletter. Office of Minority Health, Department of Health and Human Services, July, Washington, DC.

DHHS (Department of Health and Human Services). 1999. Mental Health: A Report of the Surgeon General. Rockville, MD: Substance Abuse and Mental Health Administration, National Institute of Mental Health, National Institutes of Health, DHHS.

DHHS. 2000. Oral Health in America: A Report of the Surgeon General. Rockville, MD: National Institute of Dental and Craniofacial Research, National Institutes of Health, DHHS.

Gostin LO, Sapsin JW, Teret SP, Burris S, Mair JS, Hodge JG Jr, Vernick JS. 2002. The Model State Emergency Health Powers Act: planning for and response to bioterrorism and naturally occurring infectious diseases. Journal of the American Medical Association 288(5):622–628.

IOM (Institute of Medicine). 1988. The Future of Public Health, p. 1. Washington, DC: National Academy Press.

King JS. 2000. Grant Results Report: Assessing insurance coverage of preventive services by private employers. Robert Wood Johnson Foundation. Available online at www.rwjf.org/app/rw_grant_results_ reports/rw_grr/029975s.htm. Accessed April 19, 2002.

McGinnis MJ, Williams-Russo P, Knickman JR. 2002. The case for more active policy attention to health promotion. To succeed, we need leadership that informs and motivates, economic incentives that encourage change, and science that moves the frontiers. Health Affairs 21(2):78–93.

NGA (National Governors Association). 1997. Policy positions. Washington, DC: National Governors Association.

Solanki G, Schauffler HH, Miller LS. 2000. The direct and indirect effects of cost-sharing on the use of preventive services. Health Services Research 34(6):1331–1350.

1

Assuring America's Health

The Committee on Assuring the Health of the Public in the 21st Century was charged with the task of proposing an inclusive framework for action to assure the health of the public in the twenty-first century. To guide this process, the Committee embraced the vision set forth by *Healthy People 2010* (DHHS, 2000)—*healthy people in healthy communities*—with its recognition of both individual and community dimensions. *Healthy People 2010* calls for a national effort to improve overall population health and, where possible, to eliminate disparities in health in the United States. This vision has been endorsed as national policy at the highest levels of government and by most states, many localities, and a large coalition of business and nonprofit organizations. What is needed now is action at a broad societal level to achieve this vision. This report provides a framework for action, identifies those who must be involved, and outlines priority steps to be taken. In this chapter, the committee outlines our approach and the rationale for it. We

    1.   Review the nation's health achievement in the past century, which is tempered by concerns about falling short in the present and being ill equipped to meet future challenges;

    2.   Explore the nature of health as a public good, the fundamental and statutory duty of government to assure the health of the public, and the need and rationale for multisectoral engagement in partnership with government;

    3.   Examine the reasons for the nation's deficient health status;

4.   Describe the system and actors who can work together to assure the nation's health;

5.   Propose action steps to help attain the vision; and

6.   Discuss national and global trends that may affect America's health in the coming decades.

ACHIEVEMENT AND DISAPPOINTMENT

The health of the American people at the beginning of the twenty-first century would astonish those living in 1900. By every measure, we are healthier, live longer, and enjoy lives that are less likely to be marked by injuries, ill health, or premature death. In the past century, infant mortality declined and life expectancy increased (DHHS, 2002). Vaccines and antibiotics made once life-threatening ailments preventable or less serious; and homes, workplaces, roads, and automobiles became safer. In addition to the many health achievements facilitated by public health[1] efforts such as sanitation and immunization, unparalleled medical advances and national investment in health care also have contributed to improvements in health outcomes. Roughly 13 percent of our gross domestic product—about $1.3 trillion in 2000, which represents a higher percentage than that of any other major industrialized nation—goes toward health-related expenditures (DHHS, 2001; Levit et al., 2002).

Despite the nation's wealth, expenditures for health care and research, and scientific and technical accomplishments, the United States is not fully meeting its potential in the area of population health (Kindig, 1997). For years, the life expectancies of both men and women in the United States have lagged behind those of their counterparts in most other industrialized nations (Starfield, 1998; Jee and Or, 1999). Life expectancy in the United States was slightly below the Organisation for Economic Cooperation and Development (OECD) median in 1999 (Reinhardt et al., 2002), and in 1998, the average life expectancy at birth for women was 79.5 years in the United States (73.9 for men), compared with 81.9 (76.9 for men) in Sweden and 84.0 (77.2 for men) in Japan (Anderson and Hussey, 2001). In 1998, the United States also ranked 28th in infant mortality among 39 industrialized nations (DHHS, 2002). In the area of chronic disease, reported inci-

---

[1] The definition of *public health* used throughout this report is "what we as a society do collectively to assure the conditions in which people can be healthy" (IOM, 1988: 1). Although government bears special legal responsibility (discussed elsewhere in this chapter), this and similar definitions extend to more than just the activities of government, broadly referring to the efforts, science, art, and approaches used by all sectors of society (public, private, and civil society) to assure, maintain, protect, promote, and improve the health of the people (IOM, 1988; Last, 1995; Petersen and Lupton, 1996; Acheson, 1998; ASPH, 1999; Kass, 2001; Turnock, 2001).

dence rates in 1990 for all cancers[2] in males and females were highest in the United States among a group of 30 industrialized nations (Jee and Or, 1999). Some birth defects that appear to have links to environmental factors are increasing (Pew Environmental Health Commission, 1999). The prevalence of obesity and chronic diseases like diabetes are increasing, and infectious disease constitutes a growing concern because of newly recognized or newly imported agents like West Nile virus, the emergence of drug-resistant pathogens, and the all-too-real threat of bioterrorism (DHHS, 2002).

Moreover, a focus on national averages often masks serious and persistent disparities in health status between racial and ethnic groups, men and women, and populations with lower and higher levels of income and education. For example, in 1999, the infant mortality rate for blacks was 14.6, a level 2.5 times higher than that for whites (Hoyert et al., 2001). Life expectancy is consistently higher for women than for men, with a difference of 5.5 years in 1999 (Hoyert et al., 2001). Additionally, people with less than 12 years of education are twice as likely to die from chronic disease than those with more than 12 years of education (DHHS, 2000).

Although data on the relationship between investments in health and health outcomes are not fully adequate at this time (Anderson and Hussey, 2001), several trends are worth noting because they may help explain why the nation seems to fall short of its potential. The vast majority of health spending, as much as 95 percent by some estimates (McGinnis et al., 2002), is directed toward medical care and biomedical research. However, there is strong evidence that behavior and environment are responsible for more than 70 percent of avoidable mortality (McGinnis and Foege, 1993), and health care is just one of several determinants of health (McGinnis et al., 2002). It then follows that the nation's heavy investment in the personal health care system[3] is a limited future strategy for promoting health. Social and environmental factors create unnecessary health risks for individuals and entire communities. Frequently, those who are most likely to be at social and economic disadvantage live in communities that are at higher risk of environmental contamination, face greater exposure to intentional and unintentional injuries, and are least likely to have access to good medical care. Moreover, although the benefits of our current investments permit American medicine to prevent, treat, and cure diseases, these benefits are

---

[2] Cancer incidences of 407 per 100,000 in males and 290 per 100,000 in females. Sources: International Agency for Research on Cancer and Australian Institute of Health and Wellness (as reported in Jee and Or, 1999).

[3] "Personal" refers to a characteristic of medical or health care services, which generally address the health of individuals on a one-by-one basis.

inaccessible to many because of a lack of insurance or access to services; about 14.6 percent of the population, or 41 million people, lacked health insurance in 2001 (Mills, 2002).

HEALTH AS A SOCIAL AND POLITICAL UNDERTAKING

It is hardly necessary to argue that good health is fundamental to a good society (Beauchamp, 1988). Without a certain level of health, people may not be able to fully participate in many of the goods of life, including family and community life, gainful employment, and participation in the political process. Ethicists point to the special role that health plays in the enjoyment of an active life, a thriving community, and a productive nation (Daniels, 1985). This view is also grounded in international codes and agreements to which the United States is party, from the World Health Organization's Constitution (WHO, 1946) to the United Nations' Universal Declaration of Human Rights, which ascribe intrinsic value to health.

Theories of democracy demonstrate that the public's health is an important collective good because public funds are expended to benefit all or most of the population (Walzer, 1983). The public's health can be supported only through collective action, not through individual endeavor. Acting alone, persons of means may procure personal medical services and many of the necessities of living. Yet no single individual or group can assure the conditions needed for health. Meaningful protection and assurance of the population's health require communal effort. The community as a whole has a stake in environmental protection, hygiene and sanitation, clean air, uncontaminated food and water, safe blood and pharmaceutical products, and the control of infectious diseases. These collective goods, and many more, are essential conditions for health, but these "public" goods can be secured only through organized action on behalf of the population (Gostin, 2000).

There are solid legal, theoretical, and practical grounds for government in its various forms to assume primary responsibility for the public's health (Duffy, 1990; Novak, 1996). Although governmental actions and agencies constitute the backbone of all efforts to assure the health of the public, government cannot assure population health alone; other sectors and parties have an interest and a civic role to help create the conditions that make health possible.

The actors selected by the committee to illustrate their potential individual power to promote health and the role they can play in an intersectoral public health system include the community, the health care delivery system, business, the media, and academic institutions. Some may question why the private sectors of society should act to produce "public" goods, such as the population's health. To be sure, these groups do not have a constitutional or statutory obligation to promote health, yet the private sector is affected by governmental actions. Government regulates private and nonprofit actors to ensure that they perform in ways that promote health (e.g., occupational health and safety rules, licenses, inspections, and nuisance abatements). Government provides economic incentives for engaging in health-promoting behavior (e.g., tax inducements to employers who provide health care benefits) and disincentives for engaging in risk behavior (e.g., taxes on cigarettes). Furthermore, the interest in and civic role for private- and nonprofit sector participation in health activities has been growing. For example, employers have recognized the benefits of making health and safety high priorities (WBGH, 2000). When businesses and voluntary organizations support the creation and maintenance of environments that are healthy and safe, they reap additional benefits from having healthy employees and satisfied consumers or clients and being good neighbors in communities (see Chapter 6).

This view of population health as an important social and political undertaking is justified by the importance of the natural (e.g., clean air and water), built (e.g., safe and livable cities), economic (e.g., reduced socioeconomic and racial disparities), and informational (e.g., accurate and accessible health information) environments in society (Gostin, 2002). "Healthy" public policy is an outcome of democratic and budgetary processes, and these political decisions should be informed by evidence, such as data showing the powerful influence of social and economic factors on the health of the population and the need to work with many partners to transform these factors. The collaboration of multiple actors in a public health system, broadly conceived, offers the best prospect for protecting and promoting the nation's health for the future.

ISSUES THAT MAY SHAPE THE NATION'S HEALTH STATUS

Societal Norms and Influences

Faced with a mixture of satisfaction and concern about the status of population health in the United States, the committee sought possible answers. Although many factors may contribute to the nation's less than stellar health, the committee believes some answers may be found in an examination of broad historical and cultural factors that have shaped health policy, planning and funding, and public perceptions and priorities about health.

Because health is the result of many interacting factors (see Chapter 2), it stands in the balance between economic, political, and social priorities and is caught in the middle of necessary and important tensions between rights and responsibilities—individual freedoms and community or social needs, regulation, and free enterprise (Brandt and Gardner, 2000). These tensions pose complicated questions. How can the public's health be maintained in the face of infectious disease threats without compromising individual privacy and confidentiality? Or how can a vibrant, prosperous economy be supported without sacrificing health to pollutants or to occupational hazards? How can society balance the individual desire to pursue the pleasures of life (e.g., food) with scientific evidence about health risk? Alternately, how are increased employment, better housing, health benefits, and an improved standard of living in a community achievable in the absence of economic development? In addition to securing the economic, environmental, and social elements that promote good health, how can more equitable access to them be ensured?

Moreover, health is part individual good served by medicine and part public good secured by public health activities. Instead of complementary and collaborating systems, the two disciplines, their institutional cultures, their agencies and organizations, and the public's opinion of them have often been deeply divergent; and the individual focus of one and population focus of the other have become further reinforced and polarized. Often it has been harder to motivate and accomplish the long-term changes needed in the broad environments that influence health status because of the potential of immediate "silver bullet" solutions that can address poor personal health once it occurs. These attitudes and social influences may in part explain three interrelated characteristics of health-related investment, policy, and practice in this country:

1. the disproportionate preeminence given to the individual over the population health approach;
2. the greater emphasis on biomedical over prevention research and on medical care over preventive services; and
3. neglect of the evidence (and of the need for more empirical research) about the multiple factors that shape individual and population health, from the political to the environmental and from the social to the behavioral.

The personal health and health care agenda has dominated the nation's health concerns and policy for quite some time. In fact, the majority of funding in the health care delivery system is public and there is a major public investment in biomedical research, yet the United States has failed to make the same level of commitment to population-based health promotion and disease prevention as it has to clinical care and research and biomedical technologies (Starfield, 2000). Medicine has thrived within the American economic system, and its remarkable advances in improving individual health have garnered understandable support from the public and from policy makers (Lasker and the Committee on Medicine and Public Health, 1997). The public health approaches undertaken by governmental agencies in fulfillment of their statutory obligation and with some support from partners consistently have been underfunded and their importance in keeping populations healthy have been overlooked. With the decline of infectious disease in the twentieth century, public perception of the usefulness and necessity of governmental public health services diminished. However, with the resurgence of infectious diseases and the escalation of chronic diseases, as well as the newfound awareness of the multiple determinants of population health and the potential impact of macro-level and even global threats to health, the necessity of population-oriented approaches has become clearer. It has also been recognized that the infrastructure and capacity for such approaches must be permanent and sustained by resources equitably distributed between the governmental public health agencies and their partners and the biomedical and personal health care system.

Health (or the lack thereof) is associated with a complex, and not entirely understood, interplay among innate individual factors (e.g., a person's sex, age, and genes), personal behavior, and a vast array of powerful environmental conditions[4]; investment and measures taken to address health needs do not give sufficient consideration to this issue. Because health is influenced by these complex interactions and because many threats to health (e.g., drug-resistant microbes or environmental contaminants) confront entire populations, protecting and assuring the population's health requires an organized communal effort.

Health care services and biomedical technologies can generally address only the immediate causes of disease—for example, controlling high blood pressure to prevent heart attacks—and do so on an individual basis. The fact that excellent health care exists in this country means little to millions who lack access to it or to those who are more likely to experience poor health because of their race, ethnicity, or socioeconomic status (IOM, 2002). Preventive approaches that focus on populations are based on the evidence, presented in this report and elsewhere, on the multiple factors that influence health (DHHS, 2000; IOM, 2001; McGinnis et al., 2002). These factors or determinants of health affect entire populations, and their impacts may occur long before the onset of disease or disability. Preventive approaches to address them may include policies that support education, adequate housing, a living wage, and clean air or that attempt to deal with

---

[4] *Environment* in this case denotes the broad context of health, which includes elements of the natural (e.g., air and water), built (e.g., houses, parks, and roads), social (e.g., connectedness and social capital), economic (e.g., income and employment), and political environments.

some of the pervasive social and economic inequities that appear to be associated with profound disparities in health status, access, and outcomes.

Furthermore, the nation has experienced deepening income disparities over the past three decades; the incomes of the poorest fifth of the population have remained static in absolute terms (Weinberg, 1996; Deaton, 2002). Because many citizens face the possibility of experiencing social and economic deprivation at some point in their lives and these problems are associated with poorer health, society stands to benefit from the enactment of social and economic policies that are founded on the principles of reducing inequity (Mechanic, 2002). A national- or community-level commitment to enact socially equitable policies is more likely to result in more equitable opportunities over a lifetime for personal and societal advancement and will ultimately lead to improved population health.

The preceding discussion underscores the necessity of complementary and collaborative health care and population health orientations (Brandt and Gardner, 2000). Investing in population-based health promotion and disease prevention, in concert with the attention already given to personal health care, can be expected to positively affect the general health status and health outcomes of the American people (McGinnis et al., 2002).

Systemic Issues

In addition to issues related to social norms and influences, there are a number of systemic problems that may provide additional explanations for the shortcomings of America's health attainment. In 1988, the Institute of Medicine (IOM) found that the governmental component of the nation's public health system was in disarray. The committee is seriously concerned that despite subsequent efforts for improvement, governmental public health agencies, the **backbone** of any public health system, still suffer from grave underfunding, political neglect, and continued exclusion from the very forums in which their expertise and leadership are most needed to assure an effective public health system (see Chapter 3). This calls for urgent action. The governmental public health infrastructure is built on a legal foundation replete with obsolete and inconsistent laws and regulations, and a great deal of public health law is not coordinated among states and territories. This state of affairs sometimes complicates rather than facilitates governmental contributions to the public health system. A similar fragmentation and lack of coordination is evident in the fact that responsibility for health issues is dispersed across several departments in the federal government and across federal, state, and local governments, with potentially dire consequences for the public's health. Although significant funding for the governmental public health infrastructure recently has been made available specifically to address the threat of bioterrorism, there is reason to be concerned about how it will be allocated, whether it is adequate to address the needs of the infrastructure, and whether it will be sustained in the long term, as funding decisions are often not based on evidence but, rather, on ideology or considerations of political expediency (Kinney, 2002). Additionally, the public health workforce is inadequate in terms of preparation for practice (CDC/ATSDR, 2001) as well as number, partly because of local budgetary restrictions (NACCHO, 2001).

Governmental public health agencies are plagued by deficiencies in the very tools and resources that are essential to assuring population health. Until recently, many agencies had limited or no access to the Internet and electronic mail (Fraser, 1999; Brewin, 2001) and had fragmented information systems that lacked optimal connectivity and technology. This has led to public health surveillance systems that provide little or no population-based data on chronic disease or health problems that may signal exposure to environmental toxins. Moreover, many state public health laboratories are unable to keep pace with the needs for the monitoring and tracking of known infectious agents and became overwhelmed in the wake of new health threats such as the anthrax attacks and the appearance of the West Nile virus. Governmental public health agencies constitute the backbone of the public health system and bear primary, legally mandated responsibility for assuring the delivery of essential public health services. Therefore, the role of government in assuring the nation's health is one that must be continued and sustained. Threats to the health of the population may evolve over time; but the facilities, information networks, workforce, and policies that form the infrastructure that protects the public's health must be supported by evidence and adequate resources. The resurgence of tuberculosis (TB) in the late 1980s offers a cautionary tale about what can happen when the public health infrastructure is not sustained (IOM, 2000). The success of TB prevention and treatment programs led to decreased funding and even dismantling of TB control as a routine public health activity. In the late 1980s, a resurgence of TB was beginning as a result of antimicrobial resistance, untreated immigrants, and the HIV/AIDS epidemic. The weakening of TB surveillance activities led to a massive spike in the prevalence of the disease and a renewed threat to the health of the public.

Efforts to assure the health of the public also face important challenges in the increasingly fragile health care sector, related, among other factors, to the high number of uninsured and underinsured people. The Medicare program, which provides health insurance for most adults aged 65 and older, provides little coverage for preventive services. People with mental health or substance abuse problems often remain untreated. Racial and ethnic minorities do not receive the same quality of care afforded to white Americans, even when socioeconomic differences and other factors affecting access to health care are considered (IOM, 2002). Furthermore, the resources within the health care delivery system are too poorly distributed to be able to address the complex health care demands of an aging population, absorb normal spikes in demand for urgent care, or manage a large-scale emergency such as that posed by a terrorist attack.

In Figure 1–1, the committee has outlined the logic framework for this report: from the problem statement and explanation, to the parties who are called to address the problem, and finally, to the strategies that should be employed to improve the current health status of the U.S. population and respond to the challenges and seize the opportunities that the future is expected to bring.

THE PUBLIC HEALTH SYSTEM AND ITS KEY ACTORS

In 1988, IOM, in its landmark report *The Future of Public Health,* defined public health as "what we as a society do collectively to assure the conditions in which people can be healthy" (IOM, 1988: 1), a definition that this committee supports and reiterates in this report. The organizational mechanism for achieving the best population health—the public health system—was defined as encompassing "activities undertaken within the formal structure of government and the associated efforts of private and voluntary organizations and individuals" (IOM, 1988: 42). While acknowledging the multiple participants in such an effort, the 1988 report focused specifically on ways to strengthen the performance of federal, state, and local governmental public health agencies—the governmental entities whose primary mission is to promote and protect the health of the public.

In the present report, the committee uses the term "public health system" in a manner that builds on the 1988 usage but that reflects present realities, including evidence about the determinants of health. The concept of a public health system describes a complex network of individuals and organizations that have the potential to play critical roles in creating the conditions for health. They can act for health individually, but when they work together toward a health goal, they act as a system—a public health system (see Figure 1–2). Furthermore, we must assure that our health and social policies facilitate their involvement in actions for health.

Actors in the Public Health System

The governmental public health infrastructure (e.g., local and state health departments and laboratories), the health care delivery system, and the public health and health sciences segments of academia are most heavily engaged in and identified with health-related activities and are obvious actors in a public health system. There are other, less obvious actors who can shape population health by influencing and even generating the multiple

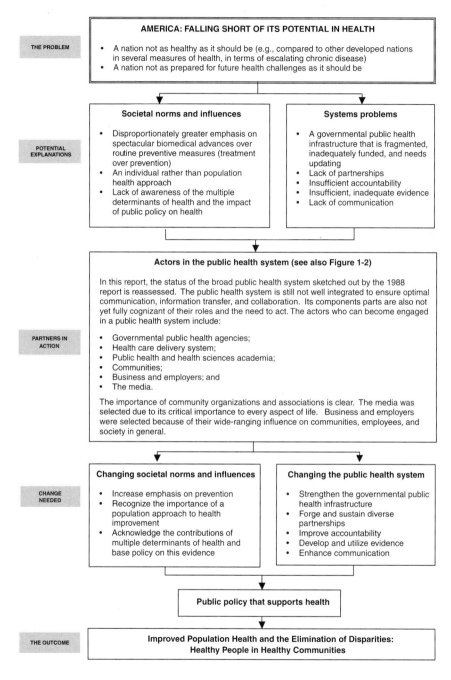

THE PROBLEM

AMERICA: FALLING SHORT OF ITS POTENTIAL IN HEALTH

- A nation not as healthy as it should be (e.g., compared to other developed nations in several measures of health, in terms of escalating chronic disease)
- A nation not as prepared for future health challenges as it should be

POTENTIAL EXPLANATIONS

Societal norms and influences

- Disproportionately greater emphasis on spectacular biomedical advances over routine preventive measures (treatment over prevention)
- An individual rather than population health approach
- Lack of awareness of the multiple determinants of health and the impact of public policy on health

Systems problems

- A governmental public health infrastructure that is fragmented, inadequately funded, and needs updating
- Lack of partnerships
- Insufficient accountability
- Insufficient, inadequate evidence
- Lack of communication

PARTNERS IN ACTION

Actors in the public health system (see also Figure 1-2)

In this report, the status of the broad public health system sketched out by the 1988 report is reassessed. The public health system is still not well integrated to ensure optimal communication, information transfer, and collaboration. Its components parts are also not yet fully cognizant of their roles and the need to act. The actors who can become engaged in a public health system include:

- Governmental public health agencies;
- Health care delivery system;
- Public health and health sciences academia;
- Communities;
- Business and employers; and
- The media.

The importance of community organizations and associations is clear. The media was selected due to its critical importance to every aspect of life. Business and employers were selected because of their wide-ranging influence on communities, employees, and society in general.

CHANGE NEEDED

Changing societal norms and influences

- Increase emphasis on prevention
- Recognize the importance of a population approach to health improvement
- Acknowledge the contributions of multiple determinants of health and base policy on this evidence

Changing the public health system

- Strengthen the governmental public health infrastructure
- Forge and sustain diverse partnerships
- Improve accountability
- Develop and utilize evidence
- Enhance communication

Public policy that supports health

THE OUTCOME

Improved Population Health and the Elimination of Disparities: Healthy People in Healthy Communities

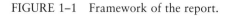

FIGURE 1–1   Framework of the report.

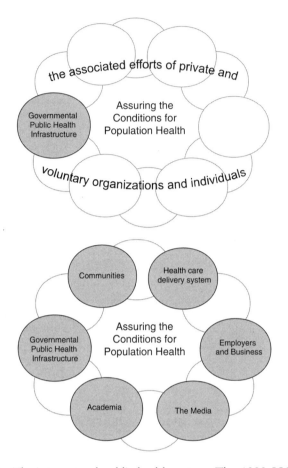

FIGURE 1–2 The intersectoral public health system. The 1988 IOM report described the public health system as the activities undertaken within the formal structure of government and the associated efforts of private and voluntary organizations and individuals" (IOM, 1988: 42). The report's primary focus was the governmental public health infrastructure. In the present report, the public–private nature of the public health system is further elucidated. Although the report examines the governmental public health infrastructure, some of its potential partners in an intersectoral public health system are also described. The committee has selected five actors who, together with the government public health agencies, are in a position to act powerfully for health. For the purpose of brevity, some sectors or potential partners have been subsumed under the category of community (e.g., schools, law enforcement). The shaded ovals represent actors who can work individually or together as part of a public health system to create the conditions necessary to assure the best possible health for the nation. The unshaded ovals signify other sectors and entities the committee did not single out for extensive discussion.

determinants of health (e.g., economic change, political will, knowledge, social connectedness, information, and language and cultural barriers).

A corporation may see itself solely as a manufacturer, for example, yet employers and businesses influence population health in many ways: through the provision of incomes to individuals and their influences on local economies, workplace conditions and health-related activities, the provision and type of employee health care benefits, environmental effects (industrial contaminants and other impacts), and the role they play in communities and neighborhoods. A television station may see itself as a source of news and entertainment, but the media may influence population health by shaping the relationships between individuals and the health care sector by conveying consumer information through broadcasts and online and between communities and governmental public health agencies by relaying breaking news and risk communication. The media also shapes public opinion, knowledge, and even behavior in the way in which it uses language and images and also through entertainment and advertising. Communities—schools, voluntary organizations, civic groups, local law enforcement and fire-fighting agencies, religious organizations, and others—play multiple roles in shaping health status, in terms of promoting a social connectedness that may support health instrumentally or psychologically, implementing organizational efforts and activism to attain policy change, and managing or engaging in population-level health interventions. By bringing communities, the media, and businesses and employers to the table, they can build the knowledge and capacity needed to channel some of their resources toward population health improvement. This benefits everyone. Businesses and employers will have healthier workforces and constructive relationships with the community, the media will better serve the public interest, and communities will be active participants and even leaders in their own health improvement process.

As these examples demonstrate, it is not just health departments that play a role in carrying out the 10 essential public health services (see Box 1–1). Other sectors of society can contribute by transforming their impacts on the public's health so that they are no longer the result of random and unintentional actions but are the result of informed, strategic, and deliberate efforts to positively affect health.

Roles of Public Health System Actors in Carrying Out Essential Public Health Services

Achieving the vision and reaching the goals set forth by *Healthy People 2010* will require the concerted and collaborative efforts of different components of society, whether it is the public sector, the private sector, state agencies, nongovernmental entities, learning institutions, or the community at large.

BOX 1–1
The Essential Public Health Services

1. Monitor health status to identify community health problems
2. Diagnose and investigate health problems and health hazards in the community
3. Inform, educate, and empower people about health issues
4. Mobilize community partnerships to identify and solve health problems
5. Develop policies and plans that support individual and community health efforts
6. Enforce laws and regulations that protect health and ensure safety
7. Link people to needed personal health services and assure the provision of health care when otherwise unavailable
8. Assure a competent public health and personal health care workforce
9. Evaluate effectiveness, accessibility, and quality of personal and population-based health services
10. Conduct research to attain new insights and innovative solutions to health problems

SOURCE: Public Health Functions Steering Committee (1994).

To attain the vision of *healthy people in healthy communities*, we must assure that all communities, no matter how small, have access to the essential public health services. All partners who can contribute to action as a public health system should be encouraged to assess their roles and responsibilities, consider changes, and devise ways to better collaborate with other partners. They can transform the way they "do business" to better act to achieve a healthy population on their own and position themselves to be part of an effective partnership in assuring the health of the population. Health policy should create incentives to make these partnerships easier.

Clearly, the health care delivery system already plays an important role in providing several of the Essential Public Health Services (ESs). For example, health care providers can contribute to public health surveillance and assessment of community health status (ESs 1 and 2), and they can employ their resources in health promotion and education activities (ES 3). The many entities that operate within communities can collaborate with other partners to monitor health and investigate health-related needs (ESs 1 and 2) and can play a dynamic role in education, empowerment, and mobilization for health improvement (ESs 3 and 4). Communities can also become involved in policy development (ES 5), either directly or indirectly through organizational efforts and advocacy. Academia informs, educates, and empowers people about health issues (ES 3) through partnerships with communities that provide practical and service-oriented learning opportunities for students. Academia also assures workforce competence by providing high-quality education and training (ES 8), in addition to its substantial roles in evaluation and research (ESs 9 and 10). America's businesses and employers have the opportunity to promote health and prevent disease and disability in their own workforces (ES 3). Employers are also a critical source of health care payment for personal health care services (ES 7). Furthermore, because businesses are closely involved with communities, they can collaborate in partnerships that monitor, identify, and address community health problems (ESs 1 and 4). Finally, the mass media can educate, inform, and thus empower (ES 3) communities with accurate and timely health communications.

PRESENT AND FUTURE CHANGES NEEDED
FOR A HEALTHY NATION

The committee's findings call attention to the fact that achieving the vision of *healthy people in healthy communities* is a difficult and complex task that cannot be accomplished through a single plan of action or by a single governmental agency or nongovernmental entity. Rather, broad societal action is required at every level; and such action needs to be better coordinated by all individuals, families and community members, businesses and workers, and health care providers and policy makers. Furthermore, responding to this vision requires a long-term public and political commitment to ensure that the policies, financial and organizational resources, and political and public wills are in place to assure the presence of the conditions necessary for all Americans to live longer, healthier lives. To support the creation of an effective intersectoral public health system, the committee identified six areas of action and change. These are reflected in the recommendations made to the potential public health system actors described in this report, but they are equally applicable to other components of the public health system not specifically addressed. Action and change are needed to:

1. Adopt a **population health approach** that builds on evidence of the multiple determinants of health;
2. Strengthen the governmental public health infrastructure—the **backbone** of any public health system;
3. Create a new generation of **partnerships** to build consensus on health priorities and support community and individual health actions;
4. Develop appropriate systems of **accountability** at all levels to ensure that population health goals are met;

5. Assure that action is based on **evidence**; and

6. Acknowledge **communication** as the key to forging partnerships, assuring accountability, and utilizing evidence for decision making and action.

The unique responsibility of government to assure action for health has been discussed and will be discussed further. The essence of the intersectoral public health system described in this report is partnerships linking those who contribute their expertise, resources, and perspectives to the process of assuring population health. Government agencies are subject to more formal systems of accountability through the political process, yet the success of specific activities for health depends on the setting of standards for program and workforce performance and in meeting the needs of the populations served. Emphasizing evidence as the basis for policies and programs acknowledges that information and data should form the basis for effective planning and decision making at all levels and among all partners within the public health system. There is strong and growing evidence that "healthy" public policy must include consideration of domains that are not traditionally associated with health but whose influences have health consequences (e.g., the education, business, housing, and transportation domains). Finally, improving communications is an essential component in the activities of all potential public health system actors. Improving communications capacity will involve, among other things, investment of resources, efficient adoption of cutting-edge technologies, training of workers, and even change in institutional cultures.

The vision of *healthy people in healthy communities* can be achieved only if the governmental backbone of the public health system is strong; intersectoral partnerships create environments and conditions conducive to the best population health; accountability is valued and practiced by all stakeholders; evidence is effectively developed, shared, and translated into practice; and effective communication becomes a priority among all public health partners. In the next section, we describe a number of contextual changes and trends that will influence the kinds of health problems we will face as a society and the strategies we select to address them.

BROAD TRENDS INFLUENCING THE NATION'S HEALTH

This report examines some reasons for the nation's current health status and proposes measures and actors that will help improve and continually assure the nation's health in the future. As noted, there is a need to transform social norms and strengthen the potential for more effective partnerships within a public health system to ensure that they will promote and protect population health. A number of factors create both opportunities and threats as we work to reach this goal. These include (1) population growth and demographic change (a population growing larger, older, and more racially and ethnically diverse, with a higher incidence of chronic disease); (2) unprecedented technological and scientific advances that create new channels for information and communication, as well as novel ways of preventing and treating disease; and (3) the geopolitical and economic challenge of globalization, including international terrorism (Brownson and Kreuter, 1997; Levy, 1998; Koplan and Fleming, 2000; McKinlay and Marceau, 2000). Some of these factors offer unprecedented opportunities for global and national health improvement, whereas others pose threats that make it more difficult to achieve the best conditions necessary for the nation's health.

Population Growth and Demographic Change

The U.S. population will become much grayer in the twenty-first century, and strengthening community and individual capacities and resources to support good health at all ages will be essential. As the Baby Boom generation ages into retirement, the proportion of the U.S. population over age 65 is projected to reach 13.3 percent by 2010 and 18.5 percent by 2025 (Bureau of the Census, 1996; Campbell, 1997). In 21 states, the elderly population is expected to at least double between 1995 and 2025 (Campbell, 1997). The nation has also seen a doubling of the number of centenarians, from 30,000 to 60,000, over the past several years (Portnoi, 1999).

The graying of America doubtlessly will be accompanied by some changes in the population's needs for health care, long-term care, and other services. This trend especially underscores the importance of services and social supports to promote healthy aging. Although care needs for the elderly have declined somewhat in recent years, there are concerns about society's ability to respond effectively to the needs of this demographic group (Wolf, 2001). An aging population will require effective means of chronic disease prevention and management to help older people maintain the best possible levels of health and function. Although some health problems may be inevitable because of biologic and genetic factors, research is pointing to new opportunities for promoting health at older ages (Fried, 2000). For example, community-based interventions to support behavioral changes such as increases in physical activity and good nutrition may partially reverse some health damage and may help prevent the occurrence of additional problems (Andrews, 2001). Furthermore, earlier investments in health promotion and disease prevention could produce benefits at younger ages, before irreparable damage has occurred and before the chances for healthful, functional aging are reduced (Khaw, 1997; Andrews, 2001). Also, public policy could expand the social, economic, and lifestyle options available to aging populations (Jacobzone, 2000). Aging healthfully promises not only psychosocial benefits and the ability to remain functional and independent for as long as possible but may also result in medical cost savings (Reed et al., 1998).

The increasing number of elderly Americans will also draw increased attention to the need (shared by many others, including children and city dwellers) for adequate housing, safe and appropriate urban design, and for easily accessible transportation systems that allow for the continuation of both subsistence activities like grocery shopping and social interactions like participation in senior citizens' groups (NRC, 2001). Moreover, it has already given rise to a well-defined political constituency (e.g., through organizations like the American Association of Retired Persons [AARP]) and can be expected to influence the medical and population-level health research agendas (NRC, 2001).

The United States is also becoming more racially and ethnically diverse through both immigration and natural growth (Day, 1996). The proportion of the population accounted for by Hispanics, African Americans, Asian Americans and Pacific Islanders, and Native Americans is expected to rise from 28 percent in 2000 to 32 percent by 2010 (IFTF, 2000). Although diversity enriches American culture and strengthens America's democracy, it also challenges the systems that traditionally have provided for the health and welfare of American society. For example, minority groups are underrepresented among the population of health care professionals, and many health care workers are not sufficiently skilled in the delivery of culturally competent care. Additionally, the health system itself (as the broader sociocultural environment in which it is embedded) is characterized by complex undercurrents of pervasive inequities and institutional racism, which lead to stereotypes, biases, and uncertainties that result in unequal treatment of racial and ethnic minority patients (IOM, 2002). New immigrant groups also bring their own perceptions about the role of government, the meaning of community, and the definition of health and illness; and these must be considered in creating better ways to achieve a healthy nation.

Continuing disparities in health status and the outcomes of health care demonstrate the need for a greater effort to ensure equitable access to and services from the health care delivery system for people of different backgrounds (IOM, 2002). With an increasingly diverse population, the nation will need a more highly developed knowledge base concerning the social determinants of health and a continuing reassessment and improved understanding of the ways in which social, cultural, and ecological factors shape health behaviors and influence health status (IFTF, 2000).

Technological and Scientific Advances

In this age of technology, the acquisition of new scientific knowledge and capabilities is occurring at unprecedented speed. However, the new knowledge and capabilities in fields like biotechnology also carry ethical, social, and economic ramifications, and raise concerns about the risks of new technologies (Khoury et al., 2000). Some advances, like highly sophisticated medical instruments and better pharmaceuticals, seem most pertinent to the personal health care delivery system, but others are highly relevant for the protection of population health. Developments in genetics, for example, have shed new light on disease causation, thus providing new opportunities for intervention for disease prevention and health promotion (Khoury et al., 2000; Omenn, 2000).

Genomics is expected to transform the practice of medicine from disease screening and diagnostics to treatment. In fact, some health care may come to involve the detection of disease at the gene level, permitting preventive treatment before the disease even begins to unfold (PricewaterhouseCoopers, 1999). However, the promise of genetics is constrained by an incomplete understanding of interactions among genes and between genes and the environment (Austin et al., 2000). This not only poses research challenges but also raises other contentious issues concerning the causes of ill health, personal rights and responsibilities, and the possibility of achieving health equity. For example, can individual choices and behaviors be leveraged against genetic heritage and broader ecological factors in a way that is fair? Additionally, new genetic technologies may compromise efforts to improve overall population health if they lead to the stigmatization and exclusion of certain groups. Furthermore, genetic testing raises a complexity of issues regarding matters such as privacy, cost, employment, and insurability. Ultimately, the benefits of genetic research must be weighed against, and perhaps considered in conjunction with, interventions on behavioral and population-level factors in disease causation (Willett, 2002).

The technological advances in the medical and biological sciences are only rivaled by the recent decade's rapid developments in information and communication technology. The increase in personal computer use and access to the ever-expanding offerings of the Internet present both opportunities and challenges to the goal of improving the health of the population. The Internet is a ready and popular medium for exchanging health information and news and for facilitating political and group mobilization to influence policy. Although the wider availability of health information may empower and inform consumers, erroneous or misleading information may also pose a danger to health.

The partners in the public health system must ensure that emerging communication and information technologies are used effectively to promote the concepts and messages of public health. Public health partners must also become engaged in countering or critiquing media and social messages, products, and patterns that are potentially detrimental to health. Such a responsibility implies that health departments, health care delivery systems, and perhaps others engaged in population-oriented health efforts will be expected to construct and maintain a presence on the World Wide Web and use cyber methodologies to educate and inform consumers and communities. The public health system must gain greater skills to meet the challenge of using the mass media to promote health and to keep pace with the communication revolution. In this Information Age, high-quality web sites, e-newsletters, and Internet Q-and-A columns may become the primary means of delivering health messages, replacing the familiar brochures and posters.

U.S. technological expertise creates an important international dimension. The United States is a magnet for foreign graduate students in science, technology, and health, American specialists are a cornerstone of the international health community, and the nation is a world leader in high-technology exports. The National Research Council report *The Pervasive Role of Science, Technology, and Health in Foreign Policy* considers science, technology, and health developments as "such a pervasive force, they cannot be isolated from the fundamental concept of foreign policy" (NRC, 1999: 2). The report calls on the leadership of the State Department to take a series of steps to increase the department's capability to identify and act on science, technology, and health opportunities in countries of strategic importance and to coordinate these efforts within the department and with other cabinet agencies.

Globalization and Health

The increasing diversity of the average American community is an illustration of what has been occurring on the global scale as people with various backgrounds, nationalities, and ethnicities are migrating or working in places far from their native lands and diverse languages and cultures mix and mingle in cities, towns, and suburbs. Globalization is reflected in both positive and negative developments that include increased trade, travel, migration and demographic changes, food security issues, environmental degradation and unsustainable consumption patterns, the evolution and dissemination of technology and communications, and an increasingly global media (Navarro, 1998; Yach and Bettcher, 1998).

Globalization is a strong influence on population-level health both locally and internationally, and its ultimate impact will depend on society's response (Beaglehole and Bonita, 1998; McMichael and Beaglehole, 2000). Global health issues include, for example, health risks arising from certain infectious diseases, ozone depletion, and lifestyle changes, all of which transcend national borders. There are other factors that are (to various degrees) regulated at national borders, such as food and pharmaceutical quality and safety and the ability of health professionals to practice in countries other than those in which they were trained (Lee, 2001). In addition, socioeconomic determinants of health, such as income and employment status, are often influenced by the global economy. The liberalization of trade may benefit health status and outcomes by facilitating the diffusion of biomedical technologies and international food and agricultural safety standards (Bettcher et al., 2000). However, greater openness to trade may also have negative implications if the global economy engages in practices detrimental to health; examples include the export of tobacco products in developing world markets and the production and dumping of environmental toxins such as methylmercury (Keigher and Lowery, 1998; Sen and Bonita, 2000).

Information and communication technologies, especially those that use the Internet, are increasing at such a scope and rate that they are critical influences on populations through their transmission of knowledge. Their effects on health can range from making the most esoteric specialists available for consultation virtually anywhere in the world, to providing up-to-date scientific literature to isolated researchers and clinicians, to providing information directly to the public about health and illness. Barriers to realizing the health benefits of a global information society were identified in an expert survey reported for project G8-ENABLE, sponsored by the European Institute for Health and Medical Sciences in Surrey, United Kingdom. These barriers include the security of personal information, data standardization, intellectual property and reports, and network and messaging technologies, as well as education, culture, and cost (Rogers and Reardon, 1999). Aside from concerns about exacerbation of the knowledge gap between developed and developing countries, communication, especially popular culture reflected in the entertainment media, can create images and expose a population to behaviors that may introduce unhealthy practices (e.g., in diet and risk behavior) into cultures previously free of them.

With the increasing cross-border flows of people, pharmaceuticals, and food, countries cannot adequately protect their populations through unilateral domestic or foreign policy action; they must collaborate with other countries and within the frameworks of international agreements. The World Health Organization is a forum for setting standards and developing protocols on issues like international travel health standards, tobacco control (the Framework Convention on Tobacco Control), the quality of pharmaceuticals, and food quality and safety. Several issues may benefit from high levels of involvement from countries like the United States, with its wealth and scientific expertise. These issues include a lack of funding for research on diseases and injuries that disproportionately affect the developing world (i.e., the "10/90 gap" [Davey, 2000]), the weakness in the research infrastructure in many developing countries, and the need to address issues of intellectual property involved in making basic drugs available to nations without their own production capacity.

Some have rightly urged that health should be included in America's core foreign policy agenda (Kassalow, 2001) and that our nation must become engaged in matters of global health law (Fidler, 2002). In some instances like bioterrorism and infectious diseases it is a matter of national security, and in others it is a matter of national self-interest and positive identity (IOM, 1997). National-level assessments and policies regarding the health of the population must consider global factors, porous borders, and increasingly mobile people and germs. Historically overshadowed by trade and military issues, the health of the public has in recent years gained preeminence as an issue of national security. This turn of events has been precipitated by the global devastation wrought by HIV/AIDS, the emergence and reemergence of infectious disease, concerns about states that develop and accumulate biological weapons, and fear of bioterrorism (Fidler, 2002). Concern about global health issues led to an unprecedented session of the United Nations Security Council in 1999—the first ever on a health issue—on the global threat of HIV/AIDS. A public–private Global Fund to fight HIV/AIDS, malaria, and TB was established to provide resources to tackle these threats effectively; however, funding commitments to date have fallen far short of the goal. In fact, the current average overseas development aid funds are about 0.2 percent of the gross national product of industrialized countries, well below the 0.7 percent goal agreed upon internationally. U.S. spending is below the average (Kaul and Faust, 2001).

As world economies have become interconnected and interdependent, global health can no longer remain the domain of a few specialists because its repercussions are significant for our economy, our place in the world, and the cultural and human heritage that the populations of the world share. Microbes can weaken national security, impair economies, and destabilize societies. Surveillance efforts, public health research, the training of the workforce, the scope of laboratory activities, and local public health activities should all reflect the global community of which the United States is a part and the global threats and opportunities that the nation and the world confront.

Although this committee was convened to consider the best ways to assure the nation's health in the new century, America is connected to the world through trade, travel, migration, and communication. In a sense, the recommendations put forth in this report have some relevance to considerations of global health. Intersectoral collaboration of the type described in this report is necessary across nations to address common threats and to share information and technologies that will help to protect the health of all.

The future challenges just outlined are complex and far reaching. It is imperative that a strong public health system, with engaged partners, be in place to deal with these challenges if we are to promote and protect the nation's health today and tomorrow.

CONCLUDING OBSERVATIONS

Health is shaped by both innate factors (e.g., genes, age, and sex) and other influences from the social, economic, natural, built, and political environments, ranging from the availability of shelter and food to questions of social connectedness and behavior. These multiple determinants of health, among others, constitute a reality that makes it impossible for one entity or one sector alone to bring about population health improvement. The broader efforts of many sectors and entities are needed within the context of a larger societal commitment to health. This commitment must be reflected in policies and programs at the national, state, and local levels that engage a broad spectrum of society—individual citizens and nongovernmental entities, health care providers, businesses, academic institutions, the media, and others—to work effectively together as a public health system and individually to create the conditions that allow people in the United States to be as healthy as they can be. Such a commitment will require political will that has yet to be mobilized.

Before exploring in more depth the potential role of each partner in the public health system, it is important to review the broad determinants of health that operate at the community and the societal levels to influence the health of individuals and populations.

REFERENCES

Acheson D. 1998. Independent Inquiry into Inequalities in Health. London: The Stationery Office.

Anderson G, Hussey PS. 2001. Comparing health system performance in OECD countries. Health Affairs 20(3):219–232.

Andrews GR. 2001. Promoting health and function in an aging population. British Medical Journal 322(7288):728–729.

ASPH (Association of Schools of Public Health). 1999. Demonstrating excellence in academic public health practice. Washington, DC: ASPH Council of Public Health Practice Coordinators. Available online at www.asph.org/uploads/demon.pdf. Accessed November 3, 2002.

Austin MA, Peyser PA, Khoury MJ. 2000. The interface of genetics and public health: research and educational challenges. Annual Review of Public Health 21:81–99.

Beaglehole R, Bonita R. 1998. Public health at the crossroads: which way forward? Lancet 351(9102):590–592.

Beaglehole R, Bonita R. 2000. Reinvigorating public health. Lancet 356(9232):786.
Beauchamp DE. 1988. The Health of the Republic: Epidemics, Medicine, and Moralism as Challenges to Democracy. Philadelphia: Temple University Press.
Bettcher DW, Yach D, Guidon GE. 2000. Global trade and health: key linkages and future challenges. Bulletin of the World Health Organization 78:521–534.
Brandt AM, Gardner M. 2000. Antagonism and accommodation: interpreting the relationship between public health and medicine in the United States during the 20th century. American Journal of Public Health 90(5):707–715.
Brewin B. 2001. Anthrax threat exposes IT ills. Computerworld, October 22.
Brownson RC, Kreuter MW. 1997. Future trends affecting public health: challenges and opportunities. Journal of Public Health Management 3(2):49–60.
Bureau of the Census. 1996. 65+ in the United States. Current Population Reports, Special Studies, P23–190. Washington, DC: Government Printing Office.
Campbell P. 1997. Population Projections: States, 1995–2025. U.S. Bureau of the Census, Current Population Reports, Population Projections, P25–1131. Washington, DC: U.S. Bureau of the Census.
CDC (Centers for Disease Control and Prevention) and ATSDR (Agency for Toxic Substances Disease Registry). 2001. A Global and National Implementation Plan for Public Health Workforce Development. Draft dated January 5, 2001. Atlanta, GA: CDC and ATSDR.
Daniels N. 1985. Just Health Care. New York: Oxford University Press.
Davey S. 2000. The 10/90 Report on Health Research 2000. Geneva: Global Forum for Health Research.
Day JC. 1996. Population projections of the United States by age, sex, race and Hispanic origin: 1995 to 2050. U.S. Bureau of the Census, Current Population Reports, P25–1130. Washington, DC: Government Printing Office.
Deaton A. 2002. Policy implications of the gradient of health and wealth. Health Affairs 21(2):13–30.
DHHS (Department of Health and Human Services). 2000. Healthy People 2010, Vol. 1, p. 2–4 and p. 2–5. Available online at http://www.health.gov/healthypeople/document/tableofcontents.htm. Accessed October 5, 2001.
DHHS. 2001. Health, United States, 2001 with Urban and Rural Health Chartbook. Atlanta, GA: National Center for Health Statistics, Centers for Disease Control and Prevention, Department of Health and Human Services.
DHHS. 2002. Health, United States, 2002 with Chartbook on Trends in the Health of Americans. Atlanta, GA: National Center for Health Statistics, Centers for Disease Control and Prevention, Department of Health and Human Services.
Duffy J. 1990. The Sanitarians: A History of American Public Health. Urbana: University of Illinois Press.
Fidler D. 2002. A globalized theory of public health law. Journal of Law, Medicine, & Ethics 30:150–161.
Fraser MR. 1999. Information technology and local health departments. Presentation to the NACCHO Board Annual Meeting, Dearborn, Michigan, July 1999. Available online at www.naccho.org/GENERAL156.cfm. Accessed October 25, 2002.
Fried LP. 2000. Epidemiology of aging. Epidemiologic Reviews 22(1):95–106.
Gostin LO. 2000. Public Health Law: Power, Duty, Restraint. Berkeley and New York: University of California Press and Milbank Memorial Fund.
Gostin LO. 2002. Public Health Law and Ethics: A Reader. Berkeley and New York: University of California Press and Milbank Memorial Fund.
The Hastings Center. 2000. Description of the project on civic health. Available online at www.thehastingscenter.org/OldSite/prog4_4.htm. Accessed October 25, 2002.

Hoyert DL, Arias E, Smith BL, Murphy SL, Kochanek KD. 2001 Deaths: Final Data for 1999. National Vital Statistics Reports 49(8).

IFTF (Institute for the Future). 2000. Health & Health Care 2010: The Forecast, the Challenge. Prepared by the Institute for the Future with support from the Robert Wood Johnson Foundation. San Francisco, CA: Jossey-Bass Publishers.

IOM (Institute of Medicine). 1988. The Future of Public Health. Washington, DC: National Academy Press.

IOM. 1997. America's Vital Interest in Global Health: Protecting Our People, Enhancing Our Economy, and Advancing Our International Interests. Washington, DC: National Academy Press.

IOM. 1998. The Future of Public Health. Washington, DC: National Academy Press.

IOM. 1999. The Pervasive Role of Science, Technology, and Health in Foreign Policy: Imperatives for the Department of State. Washington, DC: National Academy Press.

IOM. 2000. Ending Neglect: The Eliminations of Tuberculosis in the United States. Washington, DC: National Academy Press.

IOM. 2001. Health and Behavior. Washington, DC: National Academies Press.

IOM. 2002. Unequal Treatment: Confronting Racial and Ethnic Disparities in Health Care. Washington, DC: National Academies Press.

Jacobzone S. 2000. Coping with aging: international challenges. Health Affairs 19(3):213–224.

Jee M, Or Z. 1999. Health outcomes in OECD countries: a framework of health indicators for outcome oriented policy–making. OECD Labour Market and Social Policy Occasional Paper No. 36 (DEELSA/ELSA/WD(98)7). Available online at www1.oecd.org/els/social/docs.htm. Accessed October 5, 2001.

Kass NE. 2001. An ethics framework for public health. American Journal of Public Health 91(11):1776–1782.

Kassalow JS. 2001. Why Health Is Important to US Foreign Policy. New York: Council on Foreign Relations and the Milbank Memorial Fund. Available online at www.milbank.org/Foreignpolicy.html. Accessed October 25, 2002.

Kaul I, Faust M. 2001. Global public goods: taking the agenda forward. International Journal of Public Health 79(9):869–874.

Keigher SM, Lowery CT. 1998. The sickening implications of globalization. Health and Social Work 23:153–158.

Khaw K. 1997. Healthy aging. British Medical Journal 315(7115):1090–1096.

Khoury MJ, Burke W, Thomson EJ. 2000. Genetic and public health: a framework for the integration of human genetics into public health practice. In Khoury MJ, Burke W, Thomson EJ (Eds.). Genetics and Public Health in the 21st Century: Using Genetic Information to Improve Health and Prevent Disease. New York: Oxford University Press.

Kindig DA. 1997. Purchasing Population Health: Paying for Results. Ann Arbor, MI: University of Michigan Press.

Kinney ED. 2002. Administrative law and the public's health. Journal of Law, Medicine & Ethics 30:212–223.

Koplan JP, Fleming DW. 2000. Current and future public health challenges. Journal of the American Medical Association 284:1696–1698.

Lasker R, the Committee on Medicine and Public Health. 1997. Medicine and Public Health the Power of Collaboration. New York: The New York Academy of Medicine.

Last J. 1995. Dictionary of Epidemiology, 3rd ed. New York: Oxford University Press.

Lee K. 2001. Globalization: a new agenda for health, pp. 13–29. In McKee M, Garner P, Stott R (Eds.). International Cooperation in Health. Oxford: Oxford University Press.

Levit K, Smith C, Cowan C, Lazenby H, Martin A. 2002. Inflation spurs health spending in 2000. Health Affairs 21(1):172–181.

Levy BS. 1998. Creating the future of public health: values, vision, and leadership. American Journal of Public Health 88(2):188–192.

McGinnis GM, Foege WH. 1993. Actual causes of death in the United States. Journal of the American Medical Association 270(18):2207–2212.

McGinnis JM, Williams-Russo P, Knickman JR. 2002. The case for more active policy attention to health promotion. Health Affairs 21:78–93.

McKinlay J, Marceau L. 2000. US public health and the 21st century: diabetes mellitus. Lancet 356:757–761.

McMichael AJ, Beaglehole R. 2000. The changing global context of public health. Lancet 356:495–499.

Mechanic D. 2002. Disadvantage, inequality and social policy. Health Affairs 21(3):48–76.

Mills RJ. 2002. Health insurance coverage: 2001. U.S. Bureau of the Census, Current Population Reports, P60–220. Washington, DC: U.S. Bureau of the Census.

NACCHO (National Association of County and City Health Officials). 2001. Assessment of local bioterrorism and emergency preparedness. NACCHO Research Brief Number 5, October 2001. Available online at http://www.naccho.org/project48.cfm www.naccho.org/project48.cfm. Accessed October 25, 2002.

Navarro V. 1998. Comment: whose globalization? American Journal of Public Health 88:742–743.

Novak WJ. 1996. The People's Welfare: Law and Regulation in Nineteenth-Century America. Chapel Hill: University of North Carolina Press.

NRC (National Research Council). 1999. The Pervasive Role of Science, Technology, and Health in Foreign Policy: Imperatives for the Department of State. Washington, DC: National Academy Press.

NRC. 2001. Preparing for an Aging World: The Case for Cross-National Research. Washington, DC: National Academy Press.

OECD (Organisation for Economic Co-Operation and Development). 2001. Health data 2001, Table 1: life expectancy in years. Available online at www1.oecd.org/els/health/software/fad.htm. Accessed October 25, 2002.

O'Keohane R. Empathy and international regimes. 1990. In Mansbridge JJ (Ed.). Beyond Self-Interest. Chicago: University of Chicago Press.

Omenn GS. 2000. Public health genetics: an emerging interdisciplinary field for the post-genomic era. Annual Review of Public Health 21:1–13.

Parmet WE. 2002. After September 11: rethinking public health federalism. Journal of Law, Medicine & Ethics 30:201–211.

Petersen A, Lupton D. 1996. The New Public Health: Health and Self in the Age of Risk. London: Sage.

Pew Environmental Health Commission. 1999. Healthy from the start: why America needs a better system to track and understand birth defects and the environment. Pew Environmental Commission.

Portnoi VA. 1999. Progressing from disease prevention to health promotion. Journal of the American Medical Association 282(19):1812–1813.

PricewaterhouseCoopers. 1999. HealthCast 2010^{SM}: smaller world, bigger expectations. Available online at www.pwchealth.com/healthcast2010.html. Accessed October 25, 2002.

Public Health Functions Steering Committee. 1994. The Public Health Workforce: An Agenda for the 21st Century. Full Report of the Public Health Functions Project, U.S. Department of Health and Human Services.

Reed DM, Foley DJ, White LR, Heimovitz H, Burchfiel CM, Masaki K. 1998. Predictors of healthy aging in men with high life expectancies. American Journal of Public Health 88(10):1463–1468.

Reinhardt UE, Hussey PS, Anderson GF. 2002. Trends: cross-national comparisons of health systems using OECD data, 1999. Health Affairs 21(3):168–191.

Rogers R, Reardon J. 1999. Recommendations for International Action: Barriers to a Global Information Society for Health. Report from the Project G8-ENABLE. Amsterdam: IOS Press.

Sen K, Bonita R. 2000. Global health status: two steps forward, one step back. Lancet 356:577–581.

Shain BA. 1996. The Myth of American Individualism: The Protestant Origins of American Political Thought. Princeton, NJ: Princeton University Press.

Starfield B. 1998. Primary Care: Balancing Health Needs, Services, and Technology. New York: Oxford University Press.

Starfield B. 2000. Is US health really the best in the world? Journal of the American Medical Association 284(4):483–485.

Turnock BJ. 2001. Public Health: What It Is and How It Works. Gaithersburg, MD: Aspen Publishers.

Walzer M. 1983. Spheres of Justice: A Defense of Pluralism and Equality. New York: Basic Books.

WBGH (Washington Business Group on Health). 2000. The business interest in a community's health. Washington, DC: Washington Business Group on Health.

Weinberg DH. 1996. A brief look at postwar U.S. income inequality. U.S. Census Bureau Current Population Reports, P60–191.

WHO (World Health Organization). 1946. Constitution of the World Health Organization. New York: WHO Interim Commission.

Willett W. 2002. Balancing life-style and genomics research for disease prevention. Science 296:695–698.

Wolf DA. 2001. Population change: friend or foe of the chronic care system. Health Affairs 20(6):28–42.

Yach D, Bettcher, D. 1998. The globalization of public health, I. Threats and opportunities. American Journal of Public Health 88:735–738.

2

Understanding Population Health and Its Determinants

For most people, thinking about health and health care is a very personal issue. Assuring the health of the public, however, goes beyond focusing on the health status of individuals; it requires a population health approach. As noted in Chapter 1, America's health status does not match the nation's substantial health investments. The work of assuring the nation's health also faces dramatic change, systemic problems, and challenging societal norms and influences. Given these issues, the committee believes that it is necessary to transform national health policy, which traditionally has been grounded in a concern for personal health services and biomedical research that benefits the individual. Such repositioning will affirm and expand existing commitments to reflect a broader perspective. Approaching health from a population perspective commits the nation to understanding and acting on the full array of factors that affect health.

To best address the social, economic, and cultural environments at national, state, and local levels, the nation's efforts must involve more than just the traditional sectors—the governmental public health agencies and the health care delivery system. As has been outlined in the preceding pages, what is needed is the creation of an effective intersectoral public health system. Furthermore, the efforts of the public health system must be supported by political will—which comes from elected officials who commit resources and influence based on evidence—and by "healthy" public policy—which comes from governmental agencies that consider health effects in developing agriculture, education, commerce, labor, transportation, and foreign policy.

This chapter describes the rationale behind a transformed approach to addressing population health problems. This approach identifies key determinants of the nation's health and presents evidence for their consideration in developing effective national strategies to assure population health and support the development of a public health system that blends the strengths and resources of diverse sectors and partners (IOM, 1997).

A POPULATION PERSPECTIVE

For nations to improve the health of their populations, some have cogently argued, they need to move beyond clinical interventions with high-risk groups. This concept was best articulated by Rose (1992), who noted that "medical thinking has been largely concerned with the needs of sick individuals." Although this reflects an important mission for medicine and health care, it is a limited one that does little to prevent people from becoming sick in the first place, and it typically has disregarded issues related to disparities in access to and quality of preventive and treatment services. Personal health care is only one, and perhaps the least powerful, of several types of determinants of health, among which are also included genetic, behavioral, social, and environmental factors (IOM, 2000; McGinnis et al., 2002). To modify these, the nation and the intersectoral public health system must identify and exploit the full potential of new options and strategies for health policy and action.

Three realities are central to the development of effective population-based prevention strategies. First, disease risk is currently conceived of as a continuum rather than a dichotomy. There is no clear division between risk for disease and no risk for disease with regard to levels of blood pressure, cholesterol, alcohol consumption, tobacco consumption, physical activity, diet and weight, lead exposure, and other risk factors. In fact, recommended cutoff points for management or treatment of many of these risk factors have changed dramatically and in a downward direction over time (e.g., guidelines for control of "hypertension" and cholesterol), in acknowledgment of the increased risk associated with common moderately elevated levels of a given risk factor. This continuum of risk is also apparent for many social and environmental conditions as well (e.g., socioeconomic status, social isolation, work stress, and environmental exposures). Any population model of prevention should be built on the recognition that there are degrees of risk rather than just two extremes of exposure (i.e., risk and no risk).

The second reality is that most often only a small percentage of any population is at the extremes of high or low risk. The majority of people fall in the middle of the distribution of risk. Rose (1981, 1992) observed that exposure of a large number of people to a small risk can yield a more absolute number of cases of a condition than exposure of a small number of people to a high risk. This relationship argues for the development of strategies that focus on the modification of risk for the entire population rather than for specific high-risk individuals. Rose (1981) termed the preventive approach the "prevention paradox" because it brings large benefits to the community but offers little to each participating individual. In other words, such strategies would move the entire distribution of risk to lower levels to achieve maximal population gains.

The third reality, provided by Rose's (1992) population perspective, is that an individual's risk of illness cannot be considered in isolation from the disease risk for the population to which he or she belongs. Thus, someone in the United States is more likely to die prematurely from a heart attack than someone living in Japan, because the population distribution of high cholesterol in the United States as a whole is higher than the distribution in Japan (i.e., on a graph of the distribution of cholesterol levels in a population, the U.S. mean is shifted to the right of the Japanese mean). Applying the population perspective to a health measure means asking why a population has the existing distribution of a particular risk, in addition to asking why a particular individual got sick (Rose, 1992). This is critical, because the greatest improvements in a population's health are likely to derive from interventions based on the first question. Because the majority of cases of illness arise within the bulk of the population outside the extremes of risk, prevention strategies must be applicable to a broad base of the population. American society experienced this approach to disease prevention and health promotion in the early twentieth century, when measures were taken to promote sanitation and food and water safety (CDC, 1999b), and in more recent policies on seat belt use, unleaded gasoline, vaccination, and water fluoridation, some of which are discussed later in this chapter.

The committee recognizes that achieving the goal of improving population health requires balancing of the strategies aimed at shifting the distribution of risk with other approaches. The committee does, however, endorse a much wider examination, and ultimately the development, of new population-based strategies. Three graphs illustrate different models for risk reduction (see Figure 2–1).

These hypothetical models assume etiological links exist among all exposures and disease outcomes. Figure 2–1a shows the effects of an intervention aimed at reducing the risk of those in the highest-risk category. In this example, people with the highest body mass index (BMI)[1] are at in-

---

[1] *Body mass index* is a measure of body fat based on height and weight (kilograms divided by meters squared, kg/m^2). A person with a BMI of between 18.5 and 24.9 would be considered of normal weight, whereas a person with a BMI of between 25 and 29.9 would be considered overweight, and someone with a BMI of 30 or greater would be classified as obese. BMIs above normal are associated with an increased risk of morbidity and mortality. A person's BMI is influenced by genes, behavior, the environment, and interactions among these factors.

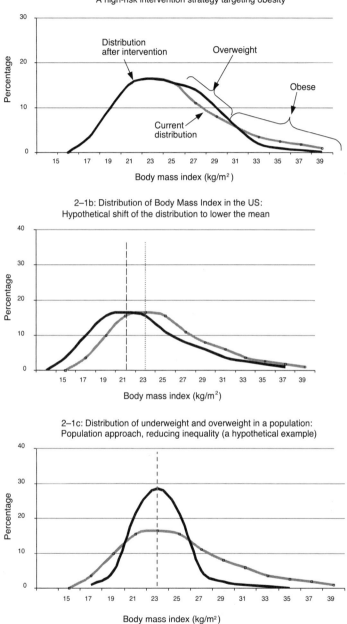

FIGURE 2–1 Models for risk reduction.
SOURCE: Data for current distribution from Schwartz and Woloshin, 1999.

creased risk for cardiovascular heart disease and a plethora of chronic illnesses. Intervening medically, for example, to decrease risk (by lowering levels of obesity, as measured by BMI) ultimately decreases the proportion of the population with the highest BMIs. Such measures among very high-risk individuals may even be endorsed in cases where the "intervention" itself carries a substantial risk of poor outcome or side effects. However, use of such an intervention would be acceptable only in those whose medical risk was very high. Moreover, interventions in high-risk groups may have a limited effect on population outcomes because the greater proportion of those with moderate risk levels may ultimately translate into more chronic disease or other poor health outcomes.

Figure 2–1b illustrates Rose's classic model whereby the greatest benefit is achieved by shifting the entire distribution of risk to a lower level of risk. Because most people are in categories of moderately elevated risk as opposed to very high risk, this strategy offers the greatest benefit in terms of population-attributable risk, assuming that the intervention itself carries little or no risk. The hypothetical example shows what might occur if social policies or other population-wide measures were adopted to promote small decreases in weight in the general population. The committee embraces this kind of model of disease prevention in the case of policies such as seat belt regulation and the reduction of lead levels in gasoline.

The final hypothetical model (Figure 2–1c), although not discussed by Rose explicitly, illustrates a reduction in the distributions of those at highest and lowest risk with no change in the distribution of those with a mean level of risk. This model is appropriate for illustrating phenomena relating to inequality, where redistribution of some good (e.g., income, education, housing, or health care) reduces inequality without necessarily changing the mean of the distribution of that good. One hypothetical example is the association between low income and poor health. In many cases, there is a curvilinear association between these goods and health outcomes, with decreased health gains experienced by those at the upper bounds of the distribution. For example, data on income suggest that there are large differences in the health gains achieved per dollar earned for those at the lower end of the income distribution and fewer differences in the health gains achieved per dollar earned for those at the upper end. Thus, the curvilinear association, if it were a causal one, would suggest that substantial gains in population-level health outcomes may be achieved by a redistribution of some resources without actual changes in the means.

These graphs help to illustrate three different strategies for improving the health of the population. The nation has often endorsed the first strategy without a critical examination of the other two, especially the second one. The American public has grown accustomed to seeing differences in exposures to risk, both environmental and behavioral, and disparities in health outcomes. Acknowledging these gradients fully will help develop true population-based intervention strategies and help the partners who collaborate to assure the public's health move to take effective actions and make effective policies.

Understanding and ultimately improving a population's health rest not only on understanding this population perspective but also on understanding the ecology of health and the interconnectedness of the biological, behavioral, physical, and socioenvironmental domains. In some ways, conventional public health models (e.g., the agent–host–environment triad) have long emphasized an ecological understanding of disease prevention. Enormous gains in the control and eradication of infectious diseases rested upon a deep understanding of the ecology of specific agents and the power of environmental interventions rather than individual or behavioral interventions to control disease. For example, in areas where sanitation and water purification are poor, individual behaviors, such as hand washing and boiling of water, are emphasized to reduce the spread of disease. However, when environmental controls become feasible, it is easy to move to a more "upstream"[2] intervention (like municipal water purification) to improve health. The last several decades of research have resulted in a deeper understanding not only of the physical dimensions of the environment that are toxic but also of a broad range of related conditions in the social environment that are factors in creating poor health. These social determinants challenge the discipline of public health to more fully incorporate them.

Over the past decade, several models have been developed to illustrate the determinants of health and the ecological nature of health (e.g., see Dahlgren and Whitehead [1991], Evans and Stoddart [1990], and Appendix A). Many of these models have been developed in the United Kingdom, Canada, and Scandinavia, where population approaches have started to shape governmental and public health policies. The committee has built on the Dahlgren-Whitehead model—which also guided the Independent Inquiry into Inequalities in Health in the United Kingdom—modifying it to reflect special issues of relevance in the United States (see Figure 2–2). This figure serves as a useful heuristic to help us think about the multiple determinants of population health. It may, for instance, help to illustrate how the health sector, which includes governmental public health agencies and the health care delivery system, must work with other sectors of government such as education, labor, economic development, and agriculture to

---

[2] *Upstream* refers to determinants of health that are somewhat removed from the more "downstream" biological and behavioral bases for disease. Such upstream determinants include "social relations, neighborhoods and communities, institutions, and social and economic policies" (IOM, 2000).

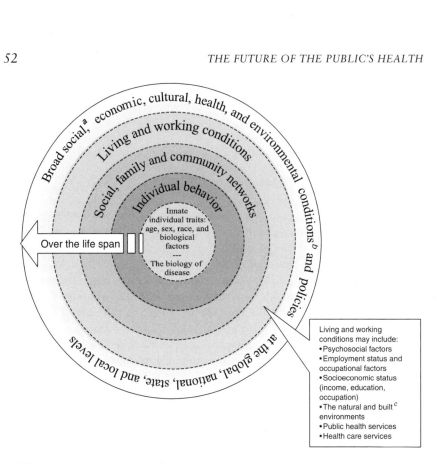

FIGURE 2–2 A guide to thinking about the determinants of population health. NOTES: Adapted from Dahlgren and Whitehead, 1991. The dotted lines between levels of the model denote interaction effects between and among the various levels of health determinants (Worthman, 1999).

[a]Social conditions include, but are not limited to: economic inequality, urbanization, mobility, cultural values, attitudes and policies related to discrimination and intolerance on the basis of race, gender, and other differences.

[b]Other conditions at the national level might include major sociopolitical shifts, such as recession, war, and governmental collapse.

[c]The built environment includes transportation, water and sanitation, housing, and other dimensions of urban planning.

create "healthy" public policy. Furthermore, the governmental sector needs to work in partnership with nongovernmental sectors such as academia, the media, business, community-based organizations and communities themselves to create the intersectoral model of the public health system first alluded to in the 1988 Institute of Medicine (IOM) report and established in this report as critical to effective health action.

Most models of health determinants identify macro-level conditions and policies (social, economic, cultural, and environmental) as potent forces in shaping midlevel (working conditions, housing) and proximate (behavioral, biological) determinants of health. Macro-level or upstream determinants (such as policies and societal norms) and micro-level determinants (such as sex or the virulence of a disease agent) interact along complex and dynamic pathways to produce health at a population level. As mentioned above, exposures at the environmental level may have a greater influence on population health than individual vulnerabilities, although at an individual level, personal characteristics including genetic predispositions interact with the environment to produce disease. For instance, smoking is a complex biobehavioral activity with both significant genetic heritability and nongenetic, environmental influences, and many studies have shown an interaction between smoking and specific genes in determining the risk of developing cardiovascular disease and cancers. It is also important to note that developmental and historical conditions change over time at both a societal level (e.g., demographic changes) and an individual level (e.g., life course issues) and that disease itself evolves as agents change in virulence.

In the pages that follow, the committee provides a concise discussion of the key determinants that constitute the ecology of health, including environmental and social determinants, and elaborates in more detail on the social influences on health. This decision was made in recognition of a longer history in studying the ways in which environment shapes population health.

THE PHYSICAL ENVIRONMENT
AS A DETERMINANT OF HEALTH

At least since the time of Hippocrates' essay "Air, Water and Places," written in 400 B.C.E., humans have been aware of the many connections between health and the environment. Improved water, food, and milk sanitation, reduced physical crowding, improved nutrition, and central heating with cleaner fuels were the developments most responsible for the great advances in public health achieved during the twentieth century. These advantages of a developed nation are taken for granted, but in fact, they could deteriorate without adequate support of the governmental public health infrastructure.

Environmental health problems, historically local in their effects and short in duration, have changed dramatically within the last 25 years. Today's problems are also persistent and global. Together, global warming, population growth, habitat destruction, loss of green space, and resource depletion have produced a widely acknowledged environmental crisis (NRC, 1999). These long-term environmental problems are not amenable to quick technical fixes, and their resolution will require community and societal engagement. At the local and community levels, environmental issues are equally complex and are also related to a range of socioeconomic factors. A brief look at some of the evidence on environmental determinants of health may help shed some light on why health is not equally shared.

The importance of "place" to health status became increasingly clear in the last decades of the twentieth century. The places in which people work and live have an enormous impact on their health. The characteristics of place include the social and economic environments, as well as the natural environment (e.g., air, water) and the built environment, which may include transportation, buildings, green spaces, roads, and other infrastructure (IOM, 2001b). Environmental hazards in workplaces and communities may range from tobacco smoke to pesticides to toxic housing. Rural areas may present increased health risks from pesticides and other environmental exposures, whereas some environmental threats to health can occur because of urban living conditions.

More than three-quarters of Americans live in urban areas (Bureau of the Census, 1993). Although rural Americans experience certain health-related disadvantages (e.g., health care access issues due to transportation and availability) (Slifkin et al., 2000; NCHS, 2001), some of the health effects of the inner city (i.e., decay and crime) are often dramatic and may be related to broader social issues. The "urban health penalty"—the "greater prevalence of a large number of health problems and risk factors in cities than in suburbs and rural areas" (Leviton et al., 2000: 863)—has been frequently discussed and studied (Lawrence, 1999; Freudenberg, 2000; Geronimus, 2000). A variety of political, socioeconomic, and environmental factors shape the health status of cities and their residents by influencing "health behaviors such as exercise, diet, sexual behavior, alcohol and substance use" (Freudenberg, 2000: 837). The negative environmental aspects of urban living—toxic buildings, proximity to industrial parks, and a lack of parks or green spaces, among others—likely affect those who are already at an economic and social disadvantage because of the concentration of such negative aspects in specific pockets of poverty and deprivation (Lawrence, 1999; Maantay, 2001; Williams and Collins, 2001). Urban dwellers may experience higher levels of air pollution, which is associated with higher levels of cardiovascular and respiratory disease (Hoek et al., 2001; Ibald-Mulli et al., 2001; Peters et al., 2001). People who live in aging buildings and in crowded and unsanitary conditions may also experience increased levels of lead in their blood, as well as asthma and allergies (Pertowski, 1994; Pew Environmental Health Commission, 2000; CDC, 2001a). These examples illustrate some of the profound effects of the physical environment on health. The places where people live may expose them to harmful factors.

Methylmercury: A Case Study

The case of methylmercury as an environmental pollutant illustrates the potentially dramatic effects of the physical environment on health. Environmental toxins are a specific form of environmental hazard, caused in most cases by industrial enterprises, and the adverse effects of such toxins on the nervous system have been well documented. High levels of exposure to certain environmental pollutants are known to cause acute effects including convulsions, paralysis, coma, and death. The effects of lead on health and development have been documented for decades, and policy action regarding leaded gasoline and lead-based paints has been taken, with positive effects on child health. However, there is growing concern about emerging evidence that other ubiquitous pollutants such as polychlorinated biphenyls (PCBs) and mercury may cause behavioral problems and affect mood and social adjustment. The adverse impacts of exposure to these pollutants may be most profound during fetal development and early childhood. Amidst growing national concern about developmental disabilities, exposure to mercury in the environment represents an emerging and preventable environmental health threat.

The National Research Council (NRC) report *Toxicological Effects of Methylmercury* (NRC, 2000) examined the evidence of adverse health impacts resulting from exposure to mercury, focusing on consumption of seafood contaminated by releases to the environment. Fossil fuel combustion represents the major source of mercury released to the environment. The deposition of mercury on the land and in surface waters results in conversion to forms that accumulate in the food chain. This bioaccumulation can result in very high concentrations of mercury in some fish, which are the main source of exposure for the population. The developing brain is particularly sensitive to the adverse effects of mercury exposure. Prenatal exposures may interfere with the growth and development of neurons and cause irreversible damage to the nervous system. Infants whose mothers were exposed to high levels in poisoning episodes in Minamata, Japan, and in Iraq were born with severe disabilities, including mental retardation, cerebral palsy, blindness, and deafness (EPA, 1997; NRC, 2000). More recently, epidemiological studies of lower-level exposure from maternal fish consumption have raised concerns about subtle neurodevelopmental deficits.

The NRC report concluded that the evidence of developmental neurotoxic effects from mercury exposure is strong and called for revision of the Environmental Protection Agency (EPA) reference dose that provides public health guidance on acceptable population exposure levels. This conclusion was based on epidemiological studies of low-level chronic exposure from seafood consumption. The population at risk consists of women of childbearing age and their children. Frequent consumers, particularly of fish that tend to accumulate high levels of mercury, may be exposing their unborn children to levels of mercury in the range that has been shown to be associated with developmental deficits. Based upon the available data on fish consumption, the NRC committee estimated that as many as 60,000 newborns may be at risk for adverse neurodevelopmental effects from in utero exposure to mercury. Recently, the Centers for Disease Control and Prevention (CDC) released the first National Exposure Report, which provided dramatic confirmation of the emerging threat of mercury. Ten percent of a national sample of women of childbearing age had mercury levels in their blood within 1/10 of potentially hazardous levels, indicating a narrow margin of safety for many women (CDC, 2001c).

Currently, 40 states have issued fish consumption advisories to reduce exposure to mercury. EPA and the Food and Drug Administration (FDA) have also recently revised their guidance concerning consumption of fish species that have been shown to have high levels of mercury. Ultimately, the threat of mercury can be most effectively reduced through control of the sources of pollution. However, control of sources from the burning of fossil fuels may be decades away. In the meantime, prevention of adverse public health impacts from mercury will require a partnership among health care providers, public health agencies, and others.

The example of methylmercury clearly illustrates the serious impact of just one environmental risk factor. The influences of many other environmental risk factors on health have not been fully documented, and evidence of the influence of environmental factors for some health conditions like asthma is rapidly accumulating (Trust for America's Health, 2001). The association between certain chronic diseases and environmental causes is devastatingly clear, yet knowledge about the scope of environmental health risks and their impact on the public's health is limited. Most states do not track environmental risk factors like pesticides and other hazards or most chronic diseases (such as asthma) and birth defects (Pew Environmental Health Commission, 2001). Certainly, a significant amount of work remains to be done to address the physical environment's powerful influence on health status. A great deal about health determinants in the built and natural environments has been learned in recent decades, but much more is yet to be examined.

THE SOCIAL DETERMINANTS OF HEALTH

Most recently, social epidemiologists and other researchers have focused on identifying the social equivalents of leaded gasoline and environmental tobacco smoke. Among the greatest advances in understanding the factors that shape population health over the last two decades, and clearly since the last Institute of Medicine (IOM, 1988) report on the health of the public, has been the identification of social and behavioral conditions that influence morbidity, mortality, and functioning.

The evidence amassed strongly and consistently points to the importance of these conditions as significant determinants of population health. Because they also feature prominently in the committee's determinants-of-health model, the evidence related to four conditions whose importance is robustly supported is reviewed here: (1) socioeconomic position, (2) race and ethnicity, (3) social networks and social support, and (4) work conditions. Additionally, we discuss the evidence related to a fifth condition that has been and that still is the subject of great interest as well as controversy: ecological-level influences, namely, economic inequality and social capital.[3] The present analysis reviews key evidence related to these five conditions that has been presented more extensively in *Health and Behavior* (IOM, 2001).

Socioeconomic Status and Health

A strong and consistent finding of epidemiological research is that there are health differences among socioeconomic groups. Lower mortality, morbidity, and disability rates among socioeconomically advantaged people have been observed for hundreds of years; and in recent decades, these observations have been replicated using various indicators of socioeconomic status (SES) and multiple disease outcomes (Syme and Berkman, 1976; Kaplan and Keil, 1993). SES is defined in terms of education, income, and occupation. Furthermore, educational differentials in mortality have increased in the United States over the past three decades, leading to a growing inequality, even though mortality rates have dropped for all groups (Feldman et al., 1989; Pappas et al., 1993; Tyroler et al., 1993).

Although it may be measured as level of education or income, SES is a complex phenomenon often based on indicators of relationships to work (occupational position or ranking), social class or status, and access to power. From a policy perspective as well as an etiological perspective, it is important to understand which of the components is critical—for instance, if education is found to be important, the policies that may be implemented would differ from the policies needed if income was found to be the most influential factor. In fact, most research has not tested such competing hypotheses directly, so in the examples that follow, these have not been disaggregated, although the indicators used in each study are explicitly identified.

---

[3] "*Social capital* is defined as the resources available to individuals and to society through social relationships," ranging from material to psychosocial resources (Kawachi et al., 2002).

Several major studies have ascertained that education, income, and occupation, as indicators of SES, are associated with mortality and with mortality due to certain causes. The National Longitudinal Mortality Study found that mortality was strongly associated with all three measures of SES (Rogot et al., 1992; Sorlie et al., 1992, 1995) (see Box 2–1).

The Multiple Risk Factor Intervention Trial followed 320,909 white and African-American men for 16 years (Davey Smith et al., 1996a, 1996b) and found that the median family income in one's zip code of residence was predictive of death from a variety of causes. Heart disease, the leading cause of death in the United States, provides a strong example of the association between SES and mortality. Research has documented the relationship between SES and cardiovascular disease (NCHS, 1992; Kaplan and Keil, 1993), and the British Whitehall longitudinal study of civil servants found that those in the lowest grades of employment were at the highest risk for heart disease (Marmot et al., 1991).

A striking finding that emerges from analyses of occupation- and area-based income measures is the graded and continuous nature of the association between socioeconomic position and mortality, with differences persisting well into the middle socioeconomic ranges (Davey Smith et al., 1990; Blane et al., 1997; Macintyre et al., 1998). For example, in the Whitehall studies (Davey Smith et al., 1990; Marmot et al., 1991), the

---

BOX 2–1
Linking SES to Health:
Findings from the National Longitudinal Mortality Study

- Age-adjusted death rates for white men and women ages 25 to 64 with 0 to 4 total years of education that were 66 and 44 percent higher, respectively, than those for men and women with 5 or more years of college.
- Among African-American men and women ages 25 to 64, the corresponding increases in mortality were 73 and 78 percent, respectively.
- Age-adjusted death rates for white men and women with annual family incomes of less than $5,000 were 80 and 30 percent higher, respectively, than those for their counterparts in households with incomes of $50,000 or more.
- When income was used as an indicator of SES, men in African-American households earning less than $5,000 were twice as likely to die during follow-up than those in families earning $50,000 or more. Poor African-American women were 80 percent more likely to die than their wealthier counterparts.

SOURCES: Rogot et al. (1992) and Sorlie et al. (1992, 1995).

individuals in each employment grade had worse health and a higher rate of mortality than those in the grade above.

Although many of the studies that focused on occupation-, education-, or area-level SES showed a gradient that is virtually linear, studies that focus on income often show somewhat different results. For example, in work by Backlund and colleagues (1996), the association between (increasing) income and (decreasing) mortality is clearly curvilinear, with the decline in the mortality rate with increasing income greatest among those in groups earning less than $25,000 per year but with the decline with increasing income being much less among those earning between $25,000 and $60,000 per year. This curvilinear relationship suggests diminishing returns of income as one approaches the highest income categories, although some association may persist. This curvilinear association between income and health is what lays the framework for findings that more egalitarian societies (i.e., those with a less steep differential between the richest and the poorest) have better average health, because a dollar at the bottom "buys" more health than a dollar at the top. Whether SES has a linear or curvilinear relationship with health has enormous implications for understanding both the etiologic associations and the policy implications of this research. In either case, however, it is important to note that a "threshold" model focused exclusively on the very poorest segments and ignoring others near the bottom and the working poor will not address the relatively poor population health outcomes for the U.S. population as a whole. The major reason for this is because there are groups in the moderate-risk categories of working poor and working class who contribute disproportionately large numbers to death rates and poor health outcomes.

SES is linked to health status through multiple pathways (such as distribution of health care, psychosocial condition, toxic physical environments, and health-related behaviors), but these relationships have not yet been fully elucidated. It is also likely that some degree of reverse causation influences the strength of these associations. Studies in which education rather than income or occupation is used as an indicator of SES are stronger in this regard since most people are not influenced by serious chronic diseases related to cardiovascular disease, stroke, or cancer in ways that inhibit their level of educational attainment in their adolescence and early twenties. Furthermore, although many studies have included a broad range of covariates in their multivariable analyses, it is of course possible that unobserved attributes account for some observed disparities. There is ample evidence that SES is strongly related to access to and the quality of preventive care, ambulatory care, and high-technology procedures (Kaplan and Keil, 1993); but health care appears to account for a small percentage of the variation in health status among different SES groups. It has been argued that differential access to health care programs and services is not entirely responsible for socioeconomic differentials in health (Wilkinson, 1996), because causes of death that apparently are not amenable to medical care show socioeconomic gradients similar to those for potentially treatable causes (Mackenbach et al., 1989; Davey Smith et al., 1996a). Furthermore, similar gradients persist in countries with universal coverage, such as the United Kingdom.

Despite the past century's great advances in sanitation, which have contributed to the sharp increase in life expectancy observed among all socioeconomic groups, the socioeconomic gradient in health status persists. It has been proposed, and to some extent documented, that the gap in health status by SES may still be attributable to the effects of crowded and unsanitary housing, air and water pollution, environmental toxins, an inadequate food supply, poor working conditions, and other such deficits that have historically affected and that still disproportionately affect those in the lower socioeconomic strata (USPHS, 1979; Williams, 1990; Adler et al., 1994; Sargent et al., 1995; McLoyd, 1998). Studies that incorporate assessments of material deprivation and aspects of the physical environment will be important to explicate these important potential pathways.

Considerable evidence links low SES to adverse psychosocial conditions. People in lower socioeconomic positions are not only more materially disadvantaged, but also have higher levels of job and financial insecurity; experience more unemployment, work injuries, lack of control, and other social and environmental stressors; report fewer social supports; and more frequently, have a cynically hostile or fatalistic outlook (Berkman and Syme, 1979; Karasek and Theorell, 1990; Adler et al., 1994; Heaney et al., 1994; Bosma et al., 1997).

There is most often, especially in the United States, a striking and consistent association between SES and risk-related health behaviors such as cigarette smoking, physical inactivity, a less nutritious diet, and heavy alcohol consumption. This patterned behavioral response has led Link and Phelan (1995) to speak of situations that place people "at risk of risks." Understanding why "poor people behave poorly" (Lynch et al., 1997) requires recognition that specific behaviors formerly attributed exclusively to individual choice have been found to be influenced by the social context. The social environment influences behavior by shaping norms: enforcing patterns of social control (which can be health promoting or health damaging); providing or denying opportunities to engage in particular behaviors; and reducing or producing stress, for which engaging in specific behaviors (such as smoking) might be an effective short-term coping strategy (Berkman and Kawachi, 2000). Both physical and social environments place constraints on individual choice. Over time, those with more economic and social resources have tended to adopt health-promoting behaviors and reduce risky behaviors at a faster rate than those with fewer economic resources.

Socioeconomic disparities in health in the United States are large, are persistent, and appear to be increasing over recent decades, despite the general improvements in many health outcomes. The most advantaged American men and women experience levels of longevity that are the highest in the world. However, less advantaged groups experience levels of health comparable to those of average men and women in developing nations of Africa and Asia or to Americans about half a century ago (Berkman and Lochner, 2002). Furthermore, these wide disparities coupled with the large numbers of people in these least-advantaged groups contribute to the low overall health ranking of the United States among developed, industrialized nations. A major opportunity for us to improve the health of the U.S. population rests on our capacity to either reduce the numbers of the most disadvantaged men, women, and children in the highest risk categories or to reduce their risks for poor health.

Racial and Ethnic Disparities in Health

A substantial body of research documents the relationship between racial and ethnic disparities and differences in health status. Numerous studies have shown that minority populations may experience burdens of disease and health risk at disproportionate rates because of complex and poorly understood interactions among socioeconomic, psychosocial, behavioral, and health care-related factors (NCHS, 1998; DHHS, 2000; IOM, 2002). Although Americans in general experienced substantial improvements in life expectancy at all ages throughout the twentieth century, substantial gaps in life expectancy, morbidity, and functional status remain between white and minority populations. Life expectancy at birth for African Americans in 1990 was the same as that for whites in 1950. Even after controlling for income, African-American men and women have lower life expectancies than white men and women at every income level (for example, see Geronimus et al. [1996] and Anderson et al. [1997]). When indicators of SES are considered, these differences, which are often substantial across a diversity of health outcomes, are commonly reduced but remain significant. Few studies have adequately controlled for SES in terms of the inclusion of economic indicators of wealth, homeownership, or other sources of income. Although these indicators should be included, they are unlikely to reduce disparities between African Americans and whites because data suggest that there are even greater disparities in wealth (all assets) than in household income between these two groups (Ostrove et al., 1999). This phenomenon has led researchers to investigate the health effects of discrimination itself. Aspects of discrimination might influence health through any number of mechanisms, including SES. However, conceptualizing discrimination (whether it applies to racial or ethnic minorities, women, homosexuals, or groups of different ages) as a stressful experience that can influence disease processes through a number of potential pathways is a major advance in scientific thinking over the past decade (Krieger and Sidney, 1996). Additionally, although many disparities are measured across broad racial and ethnic classifications, there is significant health status differentiation or "hidden heterogeneity" within, for instance, Asian-American and Pacific Islander populations (NCHS, 1998). The acknowledgment of disparities itself may generalize or aggregate groups that are highly heterogeneous because of variations ranging from the date of immigration and level of acculturation to genetic, social, and cultural differences (Williams and Collins, 1995; Korenbrot and Moss, 2000).

African Americans and other minority populations experience worse health from infancy to old age. Although the national infant mortality rate has decreased over the years to about 7 per 1,000, the rate among African-American infants is nearly twice as high, 14 per 1,000, and that among American Indians is 9.3 per 1,000, whereas it is 5.8 per 1,000 among whites (NCHS, 2002).

Rates of illness such as asthma are much higher among African Americans than among whites, as are levels of obesity, diabetes, and other cardiovascular risk factors that are often established in adolescence and young adulthood. For example, the prevalence of obesity among African Americans is 29.3 percent and that among Hispanics is 21.5 percent, whereas it is 18.5 percent among whites (CDC, 2002). In 2000, the rate of diabetes-related mortality in non-Hispanic African Americans was 49.4 (per 100,000), whereas it was 32.4 in Hispanics and 20.8 in non-Hispanic whites (CDC, 2001b). Rates of death due to HIV/AIDS are 31.9 among African Americans and 3.7 among whites (CDC, 2000).

Some of the racial and ethnic differences in health status may be associated with the fact that minority populations often encounter the health care system in very different ways in terms of both access and quality of care (Fiscella et al., 2000). For a variety of reasons—both structural (having to do with the health care system itself) and financial or cultural—racial and ethnic minorities encounter barriers to health care that often result in less than optimal care and worse outcomes (Carlisle et al., 1997; Epstein and Ayanian, 2001; IOM, 2002). For example, many studies have concluded that African-American patients are significantly less likely than white patients to receive certain revascularization procedures to treat coronary artery disease (Epstein and Ayanian, 2001). Barriers to care may include linguistic differences, a lack of insurance or difficulties with payment, immigration status, social issues such as trust and some pervasive but subtle forms of racism and discrimination, and even logistical problems related to distance and transportation (Thomas, 2001; IOM, 2002). African-American and Hispanic children are more likely to be uninsured than white children and are less likely to have a usual source of health care (Weinick and Krauss, 2000). Recent research indicates that disparities in access persist even after controlling for socioeconomic circumstances and health insurance coverage status (Roetzheim et al., 1999; Weinick and Krauss, 2000). Among other disparities in health care, African Americans have been shown to be less likely to receive certain diagnostic testing; adequate pain medication; early-stage diagnoses of cancer; dialysis as initial treatment for end-stage renal disease, placement on a kidney transplant waiting list, or a kidney transplant; and preventive rather than acute asthma control measures (IOM, 2002). Hispanics are also likely to experience similarly unequal access to health care services (IOM, 2002). With regard to treatment for HIV infection, once tested, HIV-infected African Americans are less likely to receive antiretroviral and related therapies (IOM, 2002). This is in the context of the fact that HIV infection is spreading more rapidly among African Americans and Hispanics than among whites.

Although many studies indicate that certain racial differences in health persist among people of similar SES, it is also true that many minority groups are likely to be poorer and more disadvantaged than whites. This overlap along both racial and economic lines creates a kind of "double jeopardy," which is associated with substantially increasing risks for poor health. In terms of the association between poverty and minority status, in 1998, for instance, 10 percent of non-Hispanic white children lived in poverty, whereas 36.4 percent of African-American children and 33.6 percent of Hispanic children lived in poverty (CDC, 2000). When health outcomes are examined by level of education of the mother, family income, and ethnicity and race, enormous differences emerge between the least-advantaged African-American children and the most advantaged white children. For instance, among African-American children living below the poverty line, 22 percent have elevated blood lead levels, whereas 6 percent of African-American children in high-income families and slightly more than 2 percent of white children in high-income families have elevated blood lead levels. These patterns are persistent and are seen for other outcomes such as low birth weight and hospitalizations for asthma (NCHS, 1998). Such pronounced disparities have led to a presidential initiative targeted at ethnic and racial health disparities in six specific areas (White House, 1998; Office of Minority Health, 2000). Also, the elimination of health disparities is a goal of *Healthy People 2010* (DHHS, 2000).

Social Connectedness and Health

The association between social connectedness and health has received much attention in recent years. Concepts of social connectedness relate to social integration at the broadest level, social networks, social support, and loneliness. Social connectedness may be conceptualized as a societal characteristic related to civic trust and social capital. This area-level experience is discussed in a later section. This section reviews the evidence that the structure of social ties is related to health outcomes and discusses pathways that may link such social experiences to health. People form ties to others the moment they are born. The survival of newborns depends upon their attachment to and nurturance by others over an extended period of time (Baumeister and Leary, 1995). The need to belong does not stop in infancy, but rather, affiliation and nurturing social relationships are essential for physical and psychological well-being throughout life.

Over the past 20 years, 13 large prospective cohort studies in the United States, Scandinavia, and Japan have shown that people who are isolated or disconnected from others are at increased risk of dying prematurely from various causes, including heart disease, cerebrovascular disease, cancer, and respiratory and gastrointestinal conditions (Berkman and Syme, 1979; Blazer, 1982; House et al., 1982, 1988; Welin et al., 1985; Schoenbach et al., 1986; Orth-Gomer and Johnson, 1987; Cohen, 1988; Kaplan et al., 1988; Seeman et al., 1988, 1993; Sugisawa et al., 1994; Seeman, 1996; Pennix et al., 1997). Studies of large cohorts of people enrolled in health maintenance organizations or occupational cohorts also report that social integration is critical to survival, although it may not be as critical an influence on the onset of disease (Vogt et al., 1992; Kawachi et al., 1996).

Powerful epidemiological evidence supports the notion that social support, especially intimate ties and the emotional support provided by them, is associated with increased survival and a better prognosis among people with serious cardiovascular disease (Orth-Gomer et al., 1988; Berkman et al., 1992; Case et al., 1992; Williams et al., 1992) and strokes (Friedland and McColl, 1987; Colantonio et al., 1992, 1993; Glass et al., 1993; Morris et al., 1993). The lack of social support, expressed in terms of conflict or loss of intimate ties, is also associated with health outcomes and risk factors such as neuroendocrine changes in women (Kiecolt-Glaser et al., 1997), high blood pressure (Ewart et al., 1991), elevated plasma catecholamine concentrations (Malarkey et al., 1994), and autonomic activation (Levenson et al., 1993). Caregivers of relatives with progressive dementia are characterized by impaired wound healing (Kiecolt-Glaser et al., 1995, 1998). Social conflicts have been shown to increase susceptibility to infection (Cohen et al., 1998).

Several studies have recently shown that older men and women with high levels of social engagement and networks have slower rates of cognitive decline (Bassuk et al., 1999; Fratiglioni et al., 2000) and better survival independent of physical activity (Glass et al., 2000). The pathways by which social networks might influence health are multiple and include pathways related to health behaviors, health care, access to material resources such as jobs, and direct physiological responses leading to disease development and prognosis. For instance, evidence suggests that, in general, social network size or connectedness is inversely related to risk-related behaviors. People who are socially isolated are more likely to engage in such behaviors as tobacco and alcohol consumption, to be physically inactive, and to be overweight (Berkman and Glass, 2000). Behavioral pathways such as these do not appear to account for a large part of the association between social isolation and poor health, but they are important to consider. It is important to note that networks themselves have generally been shown to exert powerful influences on the behavior of both adolescents and adults, so that networks can either promote health or increase risk depending on the norms of the networks themselves.

Experimental work with animals and humans indicates that social isolation can have a direct effect on physiologic function and subsequent diseases. Animals that are isolated in adulthood, that experience maternal separation, or that are not nurtured in infancy develop more atherosclerosis; have poor, inefficient, or exaggerated neuroendocrine responses; and may have higher levels of immunosuppression (Nerem, 1980; Shively et al., 1989; Suomi, 1991; Meaney et al., 1996). Among humans and primates, those who lack affiliation and strong social networks have been shown to be more likely to develop colds, have stronger stress responses in terms of neuroendocrine reactions and higher levels of cardiovascular reactivity, and have altered immune responses (Glaser et al., 1992, 1999; Kirschbaum et al., 1995; Cohen et al., 1997; Sapolsky et al., 1997; Roy et al., 1998; Cacioppo et al., 2000). There is limited research on whether access to material goods and resources is a mechanism through which social networks might influence health, and this is an important area for investigation. We do know, however, that networks have the capacity to provide informational and instrumental support effectively. Although much of the research in this area examines the effects of close relationships and social support, there is also evidence that weak social ties may also have indirect positive effects on health and well-being. For instance, a classic investigation of how people find jobs suggests that weak ties to others may be more helpful in enabling people to find jobs, providing access to one of the most critical life opportunities. Whereas one's close friends and relatives (who are likely to belong to the same social circles) may often provide redundant information, weak social ties (e.g., a friend of a friend) may allow individuals to tap into new sets of information (Granovetter, 1995). Instrumental and informational support, two critical components of the support paradigm, relate to help with practical matters such as grocery shopping; rides to the doctor; and information about health care, behavior, and risk. Finally, many of the observational data linking social connectedness to health outcomes do not permit us to rule out issues of reverse causation or the possibility that some unobserved condition explains these associations. More experimental work is needed to answer these questions completely. Much of the experimental work cited here supports the concept that social isolation increases the risk for poor health. However, a recent clinical trial, Enhancing Recovery in Coronary Heart Disease, aimed at improving social support to reduce mortality and reinfarction among subjects after myocardial infarction, found no effect (NIH, 2001). Developing both clinical and population-based experimental studies is the next step in this work.

A large body of evidence accumulated over the last two decades consistently points to the importance of social connectedness, and incorporation of this evidence would involve the inclusion of nurturing community and social networks. As we think of broad social determinants of health that could be influenced to improve health, social connections may be one example that has the support of a number of sectors. Because social relationships influence health through such a myriad of pathways, broad health improvements may be facilitated by considering and enacting policies that support social connections.

Work-Related Conditions and Health

Two decades of research show that the workplace not only generates adverse health effects due to economic circumstances such as downsizing and unemployment or to work conditions such as job demands, control, latitude, and threatened job loss (Karasek and Theorell, 1990), but also generates protective health effects such as social ties that may help counteract the physical and mental adverse effects of work stressors (Buunk and Verhoeven, 1991). The "demand–control" model was developed to describe the psychosocial work environment (Karasek and Theorell, 1990), and other empirical studies have tested the predictive validity of the model with respect to physical health, for instance, by examining the effects of reward relative to effort (Sigerist, 1996).

It has been hypothesized that job strain (the combination of a psychologically demanding workplace and a low level of job control) leads to adverse health outcomes, and findings show that job control is an important component of health-promoting work environments (Johnson et al., 1996; North et al., 1996; Bosma et al., 1997, 1998; Theorell et al., 1998). Schnall and colleagues (1994) found that lower levels of job control (the opportunity to use and develop skills and to exert authority over workplace decisions) were predictive of adverse cardiovascular disease outcomes in 17 of 25 studies, whereas high psychological demands of work had similarly negative effects in only 8 of 23 studies.

The links between unemployment and health have been investigated by

European researchers and, to a somewhat more limited extent, U.S. researchers. Although longitudinal studies of European populations have demonstrated a significant relationship between unemployment and higher standardized mortality ratios (SMRs), even after adjusting for age and social status (Moser et al., 1984, 1986, 1987; Costa and Segnan, 1987; Iversen et al., 1987; Martikainen, 1990; Kasl and Jones, 2000; Stefansson, 1991), U.S. data based on the U.S. National Longitudinal Mortality Study (Sorlie and Rogot, 1990) have shown no significant association between age, education, and income-adjusted SMRs and unemployment for either men or women. However, other U.S. epidemiological findings associate unemployment or risk of job loss with health conditions such as depression and engagement in negative health behaviors such as substance abuse, poor diet, and inactivity (Dooley et al., 1996). Analysis of panel data from the U.S. Epidemiologic Catchment Area study suggested that the 1-year incidence of clinically significant alcohol abuse was greater among those who had been laid off than among those who had not (Catalano et al., 1993). Examination of cases of job loss due to factory closures is important because worker characteristics in such cases have no effect on the loss of jobs. Morris and Cook (1991) reviewed longitudinal studies of factory closures and found that the job loss experience exerts a negative effect on physical health.

The impact of threatened job loss has received increased attention recently. European studies found negative effects on health because of threatened job loss or organizational change, although there were no significant differential trends in weight, blood pressure, or blood glucose over time.

The Whitehall II cohort of British civil servants (Ferrie et al., 1995, 1998) found that white-collar workers under threat of major organizational change (elimination or transfer to the private sector) may experience adverse changes in self-rated health, long-standing illness, sleep patterns, and number of physical symptoms and may experience minor psychiatric morbidity. Longitudinal data on male Swedish shipyard workers threatened with job loss and on stably employed controls (Mattiasson et al., 1990) showed that serum cholesterol concentrations increased significantly among the former group. In a study of Finnish government workers (Vahtera et al., 1997), downsizing was associated with increased medically certified sick leave. Among American automobile workers (Heaney et al., 1994), extended periods of job insecurity were associated with increased physical symptoms. However, workers who remain in an organization after a downsizing do not experience a decline in well-being, despite an increase in work demands (Parker et al., 1997). Contrary to work conditions related to involuntary job loss, retirement does not appear to have negative health consequences (Moen, 1996; Kasl and Jones, 2000).

Ecological-Level Influences:
The Importance of Place in Population Health

Social characteristics of individuals are closely related to health. Among the most important findings to emerge from public health research over recent years is the extent to which characteristics of areas exert independent effects on health. This ecological[4] approach has been rediscovered and is now embedded in a multilevel framework. The major idea is that characteristics of places—neighborhoods, schools, work sites, and even nations— carry with them health risks for the individuals who live in those environments. The health risk conferred by these places is above and beyond the risk that individuals carry with them. Thus, we might view characteristics of physical environments (e.g., parks and buildings) as well as social environments (e.g., levels of inequality and civic trust) as truly properties of places, not individuals. In this section, the committee reviews evidence related to two aspects of places—economic inequality and social capital— that are assessed at an ecological level to examine their effects on health. These findings are relatively new and undoubtedly will be refined with further research. Economic inequality may exert an effect on health in addition to the effect of individual income on health. Such an effect may be particularly robust for people in the United States who are at the lower ends of the distribution.

The United States is among the richest countries in the world, yet it is also one of the most (and increasingly) unequal in terms of the distribution of its wealth as measured by a wide and growing gap between the best-off and the worst-off quintiles (Weinberg, 1996; Jencks, 2002) (see Box 2–2). At a national level, the hypothesis linking income inequalities and health would predict that two countries with the same average income but different income distributions would experience different patterns of mortality, with the country with the more even distribution having a longer life expectancy overall. Cross-national studies initially supported an association between income equality and population longevity, but more recent research, which includes newer and more accurate data for more countries, suggests that the area-level effects of inequality across nations may not hold over time (Lynch et al., 2001; Gravelle et al., 2002; Rodgers, 2002). Recent studies have shown the cross-national correlation between economic inequality and mortality to be very weak or virtually nonexistent (Kunst et al., 1998). Furthermore, in several countries (Canada, for example), inequalities at the level of provinces or neighborhoods within cities often have been found to be not significant in terms of health status. In the United

---

[4] "Ecological" refers to the ecology or the combined characteristics (e.g., the social and economic characteristics) of places.

BOX 2–2
Income Inequality in the United States

- In 1968, the wealthiest 20 percent of U.S. households earned an average of $73,754, whereas the poorest 20 percent of households earned $7,202 (Atkinson et al., 1995).
- In 1994, the inflation-adjusted average income of the top 20 percent of households had jumped to $105,945, whereas the average income of the bottom 20 percent of households had grown to only $7,762 (Brown et al., 1997).
- The "best-off" 1 percent of the American population owns 40 to 50 percent of the nation's wealth (Hacker, 1997; Wolff, 2000).
- In 2001, the poverty rate was 11.7 percent; that is, 32.9 million people lived below the poverty thresholds (Proctor and Dalaker, 2002).

States, however, data are more consistent in supporting the area-level effect of inequality net of individual effect. For example, Kaplan and colleagues (1996) and Kennedy and colleagues (1996) independently found that the degree of household income inequality in the 50 states was associated with the state-level variation in total mortality, as well as with the state-level variations in infant mortality and rates of death from coronary heart disease, cancer, and homicide. The findings persisted after controlling for urban–rural proportion and for health behavior variables such as cigarette smoking rates.

Lynch and colleagues (1998) observed a relationship between income inequality and mortality at the level of U.S. metropolitan areas. Although income inequality is strongly correlated with poverty ($R = 0.73$), the adverse effect of income inequality on health outcomes does not appear to be explained entirely by the fact that places that exhibit income inequality have greater concentrations of poor people, who in turn have a higher risk of mortality (compositional effects). There is also evidence of a contextual effect of income inequality directly on individual health (Wilkinson, 1992; Kennedy et al., 1998; Soobader and LeClere, 1999). Kennedy and colleagues (1998) reported that people residing in states with the greatest income inequality were 1.25 times more likely to report being in fair or poor health than were those living in the most egalitarian states. The effect of income inequality was statistically significant and independent of absolute income levels.

These findings pose the challenge of explaining why the effects of inequality are more significant and conclusive in the United States than in other developed nations. Some (Kawachi and Kennedy, 1997) have argued that inequality is associated with a lack of investment in education, development, and social services and is also related to weak civic and social bonds—or a lack of trust—between people (Wilkinson, 1996; Kawachi et al., 1997; Kawachi and Berkman, 2000). Some countries buffer the effects of inequality with stronger social service programs. Investigators have argued that U.S. analyses have not adequately considered other state-level or country-level social and demographic factors (e.g., racial composition) that may not be "downstream" in the causal chain linking inequality to health (Deaton and Lubotsky, 2001). These questions remain challenges to a new field. However, it is important to note that these studies are all examining the contextual or area-level effects of inequality, net of individual or "compositional" effects. No one has disputed the strong and consistent effects of SES on individual health. New research on area-level efforts related to neighborhoods, work sites, and states and even across countries poses considerable methodological challenges (Deaton, 2002). Nonetheless, such research holds great potential to help us understand the ways in which both the social and the physical (built and natural) environments may affect health and behavior.

Social participation and integration can also be conceived of as both individual and societal characteristics (Kawachi and Kennedy, 1997). Some investigators have started to conceptualize these dimensions at an ecological or group level. At the group level, a socially cohesive society, or one in which most citizens are socially integrated, is one that is endowed with stocks of "social capital," which consists partly of moral resources such as trust between citizens and norms of reciprocity. This has led investigators to examine the area-level effects of these domains. Particular interest has been focused on the relationship between social capital and health. At a group level, more socially integrated societies seem to have lower rates of crime, suicide, and mortality from all causes and a better overall quality of life (Wilkinson, 1996; Kawachi and Kennedy, 1997; Kawachi and Berkman, 2000).

Kawachi and colleagues (1997) analyzed social capital indicators across the United States in relation to state-level death rates. The per capita density of membership in voluntary groups was inversely correlated with age-adjusted mortality from all causes. Density of civic association, group membership, and levels of interpersonal trust (i.e., percentage of citizens endorsing the expectation that altruistic behaviors will be returned in kind at some future time) were also associated with lower mortality. Kawachi and colleagues (1999) also carried out a multilevel study of the relationship between the above indicators of state-level social capital and individual self-rated health. A strength of this study was the availability of information on individual medical and behavioral confounding variables, including health insurance coverage, cigarette smoking, and being overweight, and on sociodemographic characteristics, such as household income, education, and whether one lived alone. Even after adjustment for these variables, people residing in states with low levels of social capital were more likely to report fair or poor health. The odds ratio for fair or poor health in association with living in areas with the lowest levels of interpersonal trust as opposed to the highest levels of interpersonal trust was 1.41.

There are several plausible mechanisms by which social cohesion might influence health through contextual effects. At the neighborhood level, social capital might influence health behaviors by promoting the more rapid diffusion of health information. Sampson and colleagues (1997) provide evidence that "collective efficacy," or the extent to which neighbors are willing to exert social control over deviant behavior, plays an important role in preventing crime and delinquency. Neighborhood social capital also could affect health by increasing access to local services and amenities (Sampson et al., 1997). Finally, neighborhood social capital could influence health through direct psychosocial pathways by providing social support and acting as the source of self-esteem and mutual respect.

Although there has been a great deal of interest in these area-level studies of social capital, there has also been a fair amount of skepticism regarding their validity. Several social scientists (Portes and Landolt, 1996; Sandefur and Laumann, 1998; Durlauf, 1999) have voiced concerns about the ambiguity of the concept, the potential for social capital to lead to undesirable outcomes related to the exclusion of certain groups, and insufficient attention to the determinants of social capital itself or the causal patterning between it and other social conditions. Future studies will be strengthened with the addition of items tapping the conceptual richness of the domain of social capital and the capacity to distinguish it from other closely related constructs of social networks and SES.

POPULATION-LEVEL PREVENTIVE INTERVENTIONS

The evidence presented and discussed in this chapter aims to demonstrate that taking into account the environmental and social determinants of health is essential to creating effective population-level interventions for health improvement. Health risk is related to a complex of social, economic, and political factors that both surpass and powerfully interact with "downstream" elements such as individual behaviors, biological traits, and access to health care services. There have been few empirical tests of population-based approaches to health promotion that focused on risk-related social conditions, but in an effort to understand how such approaches might work, several examples are presented to illustrate the effectiveness and efficiency (e.g., cost) of population-based interventions to prevent disease and promote health.

Preventive interventions at the population level may be classified as universal, selective, and indicated, borrowing the classification developed by Gordon (IOM, 1994b). A *universal* measure is one that would be desirable for everyone in an eligible population. It would focus on shifting the entire population distribution rather than on targeting only relatively high-risk individuals, as illustrated earlier in this chapter. It would likely involve an agreed-on public policy requiring broad-based public understanding and political support. A *selective* preventive measure is one that is desirable only when an individual is a member of a subgroup of the population whose risk of becoming ill is above average. These are the more traditional population-oriented public health education interventions targeted toward the high-risk segments of the population. Finally, an *indicated* preventive measure is one that is applicable to persons who, on examination, manifest a risk factor, condition, or abnormality that identifies them individually as being at high risk for the future development of a disease. This type of intervention, usually provided in the context of clinical practice, deals only with individuals diagnosed with a disease, not with the nameless statistical subset of a population as in selective preventive measures. For example, a universal preventive measure for heart disease could include the provision of general advice to consume a diet low in fat accompanied by a regulatory policy requiring food labeling. A selective intervention could include a program focusing on diet and behavioral changes for overweight individuals who do not exercise regularly, and an indicated preventive measure might include antihypertensive medication for those diagnosed as hypertensive.

Although many studies have looked at the effectiveness of preventive measures, few have studied universal, population-level strategies. In some cases, however, such as tobacco use prevention and automobile-related injury prevention population-based strategies (e.g., laws) have been used successfully, largely because of recognition of the broad determinants of health. Results of these interventions indicate that, at least in some cases, a population-level strategy or, to use Gordon's classification, a universal measure may be more optimal and cost-effective than interventions targeted further downstream (i.e., at the individual level). Acting on the most upstream level of determinants of health typically means the level of national policy. This may help shift national norms and values that lead to the passage, adoption, and ultimately, success of the respective legislation, as in the case of seat belt legislation, which has steadily and gradually normalized this behavior across America, or tobacco policy, which has curbed the use of tobacco (e.g., through changes in the social landscape of outdoor advertising and sanctions on smoking in the workplace and public places such as restaurants). Alternately, upstream policy interventions may also refer to modifying the broader, social determinants of health such as income (e.g., through the provision of earned income tax credits and minimum wage increases), education, and social connectedness.

Policy making at the national, state, and local levels has the potential to positively shape population health by addressing specific elements of the determinants of health, such as inadequate housing, unavailability of family-friendly social and work policies, lack of public transportation, lack of safe public spaces, and so forth. The health consequences of contaminated water and leaded gasoline have been well elaborated. It is now time to determine their social equivalents—elements of the social environment that influence health status—and take action to shape them in support of population health. Such action may focus not only on education, decent housing, and a living wage but also on the political choices that move the broad (social and other) determinants of health in a positive direction. For example, certain health care disparities (e.g., disparities in access and quality) are created in part by political choices and by allowing public and private insurance programs to limit coverage for preventive health care and for conditions related to mental health, substance abuse, and oral health.

Seat Belt Laws

Federal legislation has been an important strategy in reducing motor vehicle injuries (IOM, 1998). Between 1966 and 1970, highway safety acts authorized the federal government to set safety standards for new vehicles and equipment (e.g., standard safety belts for all automobile occupants) and to develop a coordinated national highway safety program, established in 1970 as the National Highway and Traffic Safety Administration.

A number of early studies found seat belts to be cost-effective (Warner, 1982). A more recent report outlines the benefits of safety belts based on medical and financial information from the Crash Outcome Data Evaluation System. A 1996 report to Congress revealed that safety belts are highly effective in reducing morbidity and mortality and in decreasing the severity of injuries (e.g., the inpatient charge for unbelted accident victims was 55 percent greater than the charge for those who wore seat belts) (NHTSA, 1996). Other evidence suggests smaller, although still significant, differences between injuries experienced by belted and unbelted accident victims. National averages indicate that for each occupant involved in a crash, medical costs average $2,930 for restrained riders and $5,630 for unrestrained riders (in 1995 dollars) (Miller et al., 1998).

Although there are ethnic differences in seat belt use, rates of seat belt use are higher in states that implement and enforce restraint laws (Davis et al., 2001; Schiff and Becker, 2002). Seat belt laws have had a significant impact on modifying behavior and thus decreasing risk and improving health outcomes across the population. Such strong effects for any single piece of legislation illustrate that this orientation can be effective. A meta-analysis of research regarding the effectiveness of interventions to increase the use of seat belts found that both primary seat belt laws (a motorist can be stopped for not wearing a seat belt) and secondary seat belt laws (a motorist stopped for other reasons can also be cited for not wearing a seat belt), as well as enhanced enforcement policies (e.g., more officers and checkpoints for seat belts), are effective (Dinh-Zarr, 2001). An economic analysis found that the benefit–cost ratio for passage of a seat belt law was $260 per new user. The benefit–cost ratio per quality-adjusted life year showed that all three interventions offered net cost savings (Miller, 2001). The case of seat belt legislation demonstrates that such upstream or population-level measures aiming to prevent disease and disability may be effective in transforming social norms and ultimately changing behavior.

The Case of Tobacco

Tobacco prevention and cessation efforts have offered many lessons about the links between behavior and disease and how to intervene effectively to improve population health. CDC described the "antismoking campaign" dating from the first Surgeon General's report as one of the major public health successes of the second half of the twentieth century (Warner, 2000). Effective antismoking campaigns are generally comprehensive, multidimensional interventions involving several aspects of prevention and control. One of the most important lessons learned from the tobacco experience is that the social context or social environment serves as a potent force in shaping smoking behavior. Therefore, measures such as creating educational and information-filled environments (from counteradvertising to truthful labeling and Surgeon General's warnings) and enacting regulations to restrict smoking in buildings or public spaces and to control tobacco marketing and sales (to minors) have been effective in changing smoking behavior.

School-based antismoking interventions constitute an effective prevention strategy, although one that is resource intensive (and thus not sufficiently accessible), given the state-of-the-art programs needed to assure success (DHHS, 1994; Warner, 2000). The *Growing Up Tobacco Free* report (IOM, 1994a) has detailed three categories of tobacco prevention strategies: information dissemination approaches, effective education approaches, and social influence approaches. According to that report, the former two strategies fail to address the relationship between the acquisition of knowledge and behavior and the addictive nature of tobacco, nor do they address the social context in which smoking occurs, which often involves peer pressure and norms about use. The third strategy (the social influence approach) was developed to address the deficiencies of earlier strategies, and in a meta-analysis of 143 adolescent drug use prevention programs, it was found that peer programs based on this strategy had the greatest effects on all outcome measures for the average school-based population (Tobler, 1986). Multiple levels of influence and multiple determinants affect the uptake of smoking, from individual characteristics and behaviors to population-level advertising and availability. Also, as noted earlier in the context of generic population health improvement, upstream approaches, including action at the community or population level, may be more cost-effective than downstream approaches directed at specific individuals (Corbett, 2001). Such measures, it seems, make use of the characteristics of social networks and relationships that may be used as elements to further protect health. Although recognizing the importance of approaches that go beyond individuals and their behavior, use of a social influences strategy may not work well if it is used alone, as in the case of the Hutchinson Smoking Prevention Project, a long-term randomized trial that used a school-based social influences approach and concluded that it lacked long-term effectiveness to deter smoking (Peterson et al., 2000). According to Warner (2000), success is more likely when a broad array of multisectoral, multilevel, upstream interventions is used.

Such upstream measures include taxation of cigarettes, which appears to affect tobacco consumption among youth and adults and both the initiation and the cessation of tobacco-smoking (Chaloupka et al., 2002). It also appears to have a more powerful impact among lower-income groups than higher-income groups, an important concept because most of the educational interventions are believed to be more effective among more highly educated groups (Evans and Farelly, 1998; Warner, 2000). Overall, on average it appears that an approximately 10 percent increase in the price of cigarettes will produce a 4 percent reduction in demand. Policies based on taxation have the potential to have a significant impact on smoking rates nationwide (Warner, 2000), although the effectiveness of taxation on teenagers becomes somewhat attenuated in adulthood, underscoring the need for interventions on several fronts (Glied, 2002). An added benefit of tax increases is the production of revenue while the level of consumption declines. Cigarette taxation is an excellent example of a cost-effective preventive strategy aimed at the entire population. It is serving to broaden the face of policy interventions in public health, leading to consideration of taxation in relation to alcohol consumption, unhealthy diets, and even gun control. It is feasible that such economic disincentives could affect a broad range of other social and behavioral conditions as well.

In a recent effort to develop a model for evaluating the outcomes of youth-targeted tobacco prevention and control programs, the Social Science Research Center at Mississippi State University developed a Social Climate Survey. Baseline data were obtained in 1999, and national data were added to the model in 2000 for comparison purposes. The Social

Climate Survey measures beliefs, norms, and practices related to tobacco use, sale, taxation, and regulation in seven social institutional areas: family and friendship groups, education, government and political order, work, health and medical care, recreation/leisure/sports, and mass communication or culture. Data from the surveys have indicated that implementation of a comprehensive, multidimensional approach to tobacco prevention and cessation will affect the social climate in which decisions regarding tobacco use are made (McMillen et al., 2001).

Some of the most striking examples of the environmental embeddedness and social implications of health risk come from the study of alcohol and tobacco product advertising. For example, a study of billboards in Chicago was compared to census data and demonstrated that the density of advertising for alcohol was five times higher in poor and minority urban wards than in other geographic areas and that the density of advertising for tobacco products was three times higher (Hackbarth et al., 1995). An observational study of tobacco billboard advertising in St. Louis used geographic information systems and found that advertisements were concentrated in low-income and minority neighborhoods, as well as in close proximity to public school property (Luke et al., 2000). Such data support recent efforts to control tobacco advertising, adding this to the arsenal of taxation and limits on smoking in public places.

THE PUBLIC HEALTH SYSTEM IN ACTION: A SCENARIO

In this section, the committee uses the specific scenario of a risk to population health—namely, obesity—to present and discuss the contributions that communities, the health care delivery system, employers and business, the media, academia, and the governmental public health infrastructure can make to improve health. Food and eating are integral to the life of individuals and communities. Families, friends, and neighbors gather around meals; and both the process of eating and the food itself are heavily imbued with cultural, social, and even emotional meaning. This helps explain why eating and nutrition perfectly exemplify the influence of multiple determinants on health. The development of obesity itself is influenced by multiple determinants of health, from the genetic to the social and environmental, and the public health partners must consider these many dimensions in formulating their responses.

Obesity: Magnitude and Future Trends

The problems of overweight and obesity in America have reached epidemic proportions and threaten the health and quality of life of millions of adults and children. According to CDC's 1999 *National Health and Nutri-*

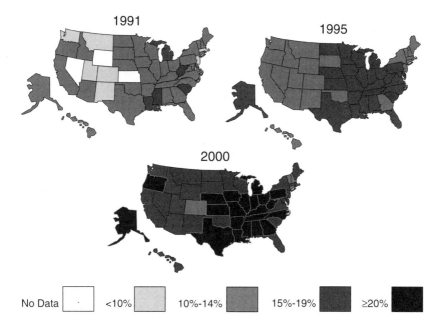

FIGURE 2–3 Obesity trends among U.S. adults: Behavioral Risk Factor Surveillance System (BRFSS), 1991, 1995, 2000.
NOTE: Obesity is BMI 30, or –30 lbs overweight for 5 '4" woman.
SOURCE: CDC (www.cdc.gov/nccdphp/dnpa/obesity/trend/maps/slide/003.htm), citing Mokdad et al. (1999).

tion Examination Survey, more than 61 percent of adults are either overweight or obese and at least 13 percent of children ages 6 to 11 and 14 percent of adolescents ages 12 to 19 are overweight. The prevalence of obesity among adults has grown by nearly 20 percent over the past 30 years, and the number of children who are overweight has tripled in the same period (see Figure 2–3) (CDC, 2001a).

Obesity is a growing concern because it poses a higher risk and results in a higher incidence of health conditions such as diabetes, cardiovascular disease, stroke hypertension, osteoarthritis, and certain cancers than other risk factors (NIH, 1998; Allison et al., 1999; Must et al., 1999; Williamson, 1999; Tataranni and Bogardus, 2001; Tuomilehto et al., 2001).

The human and economic costs are impossible to ignore. Every year an estimated 300,000 U.S. adults die of causes that may be attributed to obesity; in addition, others suffer from chronic disease and an impaired quality of life (Allison et al., 1999; Mokdad et al., 2000). According to another estimate, as many as 309,000 to 582,000 deaths in 1990 were

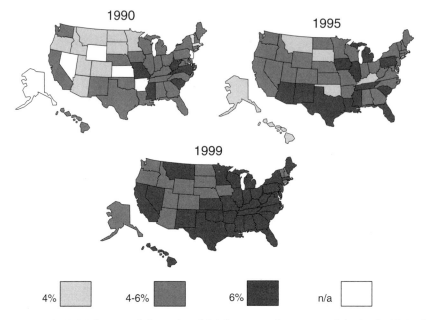

FIGURE 2–4 Diabetes and Gestational Diabetes trends among adults in the United States: BRFSS 1990, 1995, and 1999.
SOURCES: CDC (www.cdc.gov/diabetes/pubs/glance.htm) and Mokdad et al. (2000).

associated with poor diet and inadequate physical activity (McGinnis and Foege, 1993). Should the number of overweight and obese Americans continue to grow at its current rate, obesity will surpass tobacco as the most preventable cause of death and illness in the United States. Additionally, the estimated direct and indirect costs associated with obesity are $100 billion annually (Wolf and Colditz, 1998), and this figure does not take into consideration the cost of treating the uninsured or the personal impact of obesity on quality of life.

The fact that the prevalence and incidence of type II diabetes mellitus (see Figure 2–4) have increased exemplifies the association between weight and health. The rise in the rate of obesity during the past decade has been paralleled by a 25 percent increase in the rate of type II diabetes (Harris et al., 1998). The rapid and large rate of increase in obesity among children is especially alarming, given that childhood obesity is clearly associated with obesity in adulthood and subsequent health problems. For instance, until recently, type I diabetes was the most prevalent type of diabetes among children. However, new studies have shown that the rate of type II diabetes is increasing dramatically and that 85 percent of children with type II diabetes are either overweight or obese (ADA, 2000). Approximately 63 percent of the total direct costs associated with obesity are related to type II diabetes (Wolf and Colditz, 1998).

Although the prevalence and growth of obesity affect all segments of the population, there are notable trends among certain segments. Men are more likely to be overweight, whereas women are more likely to be obese. Obesity also increases with age until the mid-60s; this may be partly because Americans over the age of 65 are more likely to be malnourished. The prevalence of obesity among African Americans and Hispanics, especially women, is significantly higher than that among other populations. People with lower education and income levels also have increased rates of obesity, as do people living in the southeastern region of the United States (CDC, 2000).

The causes of obesity are both complex and multifaceted. Although genetic factors do play a role in determining whether a person has a propensity for obesity, nutritional, behavioral, and environmental factors are more significant (Hill and Peters, 1998). Americans are consuming more calories, eating higher-calorie foods, and exercising less than ever before. Work is more likely to be sedentary than in the past; and more time is spent watching television, playing video games, or using computers. High-calorie food choices are widely available and easily affordable as more Americans turn to fast food and prepared meals on a daily basis. Furthermore, food portions have become "supersized," surpassing the Department of Agriculture and Department of Health and Human Services (DHHS) recommended dietary guidelines for how much food Americans should consume each day. At the same time, the number of physical education programs in schools is declining, and people in some communities lack access to affordable and nutritional food options and safe areas in which to exercise (Hill and Peters, 1998; CDC, 1999a; Crespo et al., 2001; Dietz, 2001; French et al., 2001).

The association between obesity and socioeconomic factors illustrates the value of a population perspective and the need to consider the multiple determinants of health in addressing population health improvement.

Engaging Partners

Changing patterns in infectious diseases typically attract attention and significant mobilization of funding and action. Chronic disease has often been less of a priority for public health and health care organizations, but the evidence of escalating obesity in the United States is alarming and should motivate widespread action to contain and reverse the effects of this silent epidemic. Such concerted action cannot be undertaken successfully by governmental public health agencies alone; it requires the resources and efforts of other partners within the public health system. Taking action to address the problem of obesity also requires that all entities in the public health system engage in partnerships; demonstrate accountability to their patients, communities, clients, employers, and each other; make program and policy decisions based on the evidence (e.g., community assessments and effectiveness data); and communicate effectively with other partners and the public. For example, communities and community-based organizations can assess the extent of overweight and obesity in the community and engage in a range of activities, from traditional, modestly successful methods that involve the provision of education and information to more innovative and powerful efforts to change the community conditions that make sedentary living and unhealthy eating "the path of least resistance." They can encourage the adoption of active lifestyles by working with community development and planning agencies to make parks and playing fields safe and accessible. As discussed in Chapter 4, communities can also make changes in their physical surroundings, by engaging in a variety of activities to improve neighborhood safety and livability, and by increasing the amount of green space and the recreational options available to children. Schools can become sites for community recreation centers that are affordable and easy to access. Communities could also facilitate the formation of community walk groups that meet on a regular basis to exercise together and share knowledge and success stories. The recently launched Hearts N'Parks program sponsored by the National Heart, Lung, and Blood Institute and the National Recreation and Park Association is getting communities interested and mobilized to become physically active by planning a variety of community and educational activities (NIH, 2002).

In the area of nutrition, school cafeterias can also modify their offerings to support better food choices by students. Through partnerships with schools, communities can work to change children's eating and physical activity habits by providing support and information to help teachers and school staff modify curricula and change cafeteria menus, and by not permitting vending machines with sugar- and fat-laden products in the school setting. For example, the Los Angeles Unified School District discontinued soda vending on all school premises in the district, thus removing an element that has been linked to childhood obesity (Wood, 2002). Communities could also develop relationships with farmers to make fresh fruits and vegetables more readily available and affordable through weekly markets. Neighborhood restaurants and grocery stores could offer and advertise healthier foods. In partnership with local media, health officials, large and small businesses, and others, community groups can spearhead public awareness campaigns and emphasize the importance of physical activity and the opportunities available, as well as the need to make healthy food choices, within a context of enhanced access, affordability, and cultural appropriateness.

The health care delivery system can provide training and resources to all health care providers and professionals to recognize and monitor individuals who are overweight or obese and to inform and educate patients about the risks and the changes that they can make and the benefits that they will receive. Health care plans should base administrative policy decisions on the evidence (e.g., the association between eating, exercise, and chronic disease and the three times greater likelihood that patients who are counseled about weight loss by their health care providers will actually try to lose weight). The health care sector should also work to adopt the National Institutes of Health's (NIH's) 1998 *Clinical Guidelines on the Identification, Evaluation, and Treatment of Overweight and Obesity in Adults* and partner with researchers to establish treatment protocols (e.g., pharmacotherapy and surgery) that are safe, effective, and tailored to individual needs and circumstances. Health care systems and providers should also communicate and work collaboratively with health departments and community-based and national associations and advocacy groups focused on educating the public about the link between obesity and chronic disease.

Businesses and employers can play a major role in carrying out some essential public health services. The contributions of employers may range from providing health insurance plans that offer comprehensive preventive services to supporting research about and implementation of workplace promotion of weight management (e.g., by providing healthy cafeteria and vending machine alternatives and the space, equipment, and time for physical activity). Food industry businesses may also provide point-of-sale nutritional information and healthier menu options.

The news and entertainment media can play a unique part in addressing the problem of obesity. The media can serve primarily as a source of information about the associations between physical activity and nutrition, weight, and chronic disease. Through reporting and entertainment, the media creates a forum for discussing Americans' increasing girth, its implications for overall health, the social and cultural correlates, and related issues that may increase awareness. Local media may collaborate with local health officials to communicate locally relevant information and to highlight opportunities for community-based physical activity. By taking part in tackling this major population health concern, the media can better fulfill its accountability to the public to provide accurate and timely information.

The academic setting can make many contributions to addressing obesity and its impact on overall population health, especially to the evidence base. For example, research has demonstrated that educational approaches aimed at improving individual knowledge and action about food choices and exercise have been largely ineffective at preventing weight gain (Nestle and Jacobson, 2000; Jeffery, 2001). Academic research is necessary to enhance current monitoring and surveillance tools to more accurately track obesity, eating habits, and physical activity among all adults, children, specific populations, and states. Also needed is the development of more precise and consistent assessment tools for measuring obesity and overweight among children. It is also important for academia to continue to support, evaluate, and implement projects related to environmental conditions and policies for their impact on decreasing obesity and increasing healthy eating habits and physical activity. Academia can also disseminate data more broadly to interested parties on initiatives, programs, and policies that are effective and document and analyze how obesity affects mental health, development, and socialization; continue to research the relationship between obesity and various medical conditions; and develop prevention and treatment protocols to address them. Academic researchers can continue to evaluate treatment strategies made available by advances in technology, pharmacokinetics, and genetic research.

The role of the governmental public health infrastructure in responding to the obesity epidemic is multifaceted. Such efforts may include supporting the activities of other partners, funding NIH and academic research on obesity, helping to develop the Dietary Guide for Americans (a collaboration between DHHS and the Department of Agriculture), and spearheading a variety of initiatives such as food labeling. The role of the federal government in addressing obesity is essential, as it sets the pace for the nation and underscores this as a critical issue in assuring population health. In June 2002, in the wake of the 2001 Surgeon General's report on obesity, President George W. Bush launched a new initiative, HealthierUS, that encourages Americans to pursue physical activity, healthy eating, and other healthy choices and to get preventive screenings (White House, 2002). In July 2002, CDC launched a multicultural Youth Media Campaign (entitled "VERB: It's what you do.") targeting youth across the nation (DHHS, 2002). The campaign encourages children between ages 9 and 13 to choose a "verb" (e.g., swim, run, or bowl) that fits their personality and interests and to start applying that verb in their daily lives. The campaign aims to engage children in a type of physical activity that they enjoy and, ultimately, to help them reap the related benefits of enhanced self-esteem, social connectedness, confidence, and discipline. At the local level of governmental public health agencies, health departments may administer or collaborate with the Department of Agriculture's Women, Infants and Children (WIC) food supplementation program that provides nutritious foods and education to mothers and children up to age 5. They may also collaborate with local school programs and engage in many other community-based efforts that target overweight and obesity through a wide range of activities.

CONCLUDING OBSERVATIONS

In the previous sections, the committee has outlined what population health means in terms of understanding not only the risks of various exposures to individuals but also the importance of incorporating concepts related to the distribution of risk in populations. This chapter has outlined a way to understand how social, environmental, and biological conditions shape population health. Population-based interventions, such as tobacco control policies, show that it is possible to implement cost-effective strategies that benefit society as a whole and improve the health of many segments of the population. Population health improvements will have to focus attention on both overall improvement in the nation's health and reduction of the disparities in health, as recommended by *Healthy People 2010*. To achieve this goal, the nation will have to develop innovative strategies for interventions for a broad set of health determinants. Many of the determinants of health are part of the broad economic and social context and, thus, beyond the direct control of administrators in public- and private-sector health care organizations. Action on these strategies at the national level will require an alignment of public policy in the agriculture, commerce, education, and treasury sectors of government, among others, to promote health. This includes providing resources to support the population-based research necessary to further our understanding of the social etiology of disease and disability. Efforts to curb tobacco use have a 50-year history from the appearance of the first surgeon general's report. There is now a high level of consensus and political will to act. Effective public health systems must be vehicles to accelerate such efforts to save thousands of lives that will otherwise be lost. The special role of the governmental public health infrastructure is to advocate for and educate others about the evidence to support such policy actions and to assure that the public health system—the diverse array of individuals and organizations that must act together for health at the community level—is both committed to and equipped for implementation of a coordinated set of strategies to attain the highest levels of health for the nation. The next chapters of this report explore the potential role of each component of the public health system in achieving this goal.

Assurance is one of the three core public health functions put forth by the 1988 IOM report *The Future of Public Health*. The special role of the governmental public health infrastructure in this mission will be that of steward, facilitator, and supporter rather than actor in every situation, because assuring a healthy nation cannot be accomplished through a single plan of action or through the efforts of a single governmental agency or sector of the economy. Instead, it will require a coordinated set of strategies that must be implemented by all Americans—as individuals, families and community members, businesses and workers, and citizens. With each sector of society assuming a portion of the responsibility for improving the health of the nation, it becomes increasingly possible to achieve the nation's true potential for a population with excellent health and the fewest possible disparities.

The chapters that follow discuss several partners within a redefined public health system that has as its backbone the governmental public health infrastructure but that includes the resources, perspectives, and actions of other stakeholders who are partners in the public health system. Each of these partners can increase the relevance of its contributions to population health by considering the multiple determinants of health, especially those that contribute to unequal opportunities for good health.

REFERENCES

Adler NE, Boyce T, Chesney MA, Cohen S, Folkman S, Kahn RL, Syme SL. 1994. Socioeconomic status and health: the challenge of the gradient. American Psychologist 49(1):15–24.

Allison DB, Fontaine KR, Manson JE, Stevens J, VanItallie TB. 1999. Annual deaths attributable to obesity in the United States. Journal of the American Medical Association 282(16):1530–1538.

American Diabetes Association (ADA). 2000. Type 2 diabetes in children and adolescents. Pediatrics 105(3, Pt. 1):671–680.

Anderson RT, Sorlie P, Backlund E, Johnson N, Kaplan GA. 1997. Mortality effects of community socioeconomic status. Epidemiology 8:42–47.

Atkinson AB, Rainwater L, Smeeding TM. 1995. Income Distribution in OECD Countries: Evidence from the Luxembourg Income Study. Paris: Organization for Economic Cooperation and Development.

Backlund E, Sorlie PD, Johnson NJ. 1996. The shape of the relationship between income and mortality in the United States: evidence from the National Longitudinal Mortality Study. Annals of Epidemiology 6(1):12–20.

Bassuk SS, TA Glass, LF Berkman. 1999. Social disengagement and incident cognitive decline in community-dwelling elderly persons. Annals of Internal Medicine 131(3):165–173.

Baumeister RF, Leary MR. 1995. The need to belong: desire for interpersonal attachments as a fundamental human motivation. Psychological Bulletin 117:497–529.

Berkman L, Syme S. 1979. Social networks host resistance and mortality: a nine-year follow-up of Alameda County residents. American Journal of Epidemiology 109:186–204.

Berkman L, Glass T. 2000. Social integration social networks social support and health. In Berkman L, Kawachi I (Eds.). Social Epidemiology. New York: Oxford University Press.

Berkman L, Kawachi I (Eds.). 2000. Social Epidemiology. New York: Oxford University Press.

Berkman LF, Lochner KA. 2002. Social determinants of health: meeting at the crossroads. Health Affairs 21(2):291–293.

Berkman LF, Leo-Summers L, and Horwitz RI. 1992. Emotional support and survival after myocardial infarction: a prospective population-based study of the elderly. Annals of Internal Medicine 117:1003–1009.

Blane D, Bartley M, Davey Smith G. 1997. Disease aetiology and materialistic explanations of socioeconomic mortality differentials. European Journal of Public Health 7:385–391.

Blazer D. 1982. Social support and mortality in an elderly community population. American Journal of Epidemiology 115:684–694.

Bosma H, Marmot MG, Hemingway H, Nicholson AC, Brunner E, Stansfeld SA. 1997. Low job control and risk of coronary heart disease in Whitehall II (prospective cohort) study. British Medical Journal 314:558–565.

Bosma H, Peter R, Siegrist J, Marmot M. 1998. Two alternative job stress models and the risk of coronary heart disease. American Journal of Public Health 88:68–74.

Brown LR, Renner M, Flavin C. 1997. Vital Signs 1997. New York: W. W. Norton and Company.

Bureau of the Census. 1993. United States 1790–1990. Table 4. Available online at www.census.gov/population/censusdata/table-4.pdf. Accessed October 10, 2002.

Buunk BP, Verhoeven K. 1991. Companionship and support at work: a microanalysis of the stress-reducing features of social interactions. Basic and Applied Social Psychology 12:243–258.

Cacioppo JT, Ernst JM, Burleson MH, McClintock MK, Malarkey WB, Hawkley LC, Kowalewski RB, Paulsen A, Hobson JA, Hugdahl K, Spiegel D, Bernston GG. 2000. Lonely traits and concomitant physiological processes: the MacArthur social neuroscience studies. International Journal of Psychophysiology 35:143–154.

Carlisle DM, Leake BD, Shapiro MF. 1997. Racial and ethnic disparities in the use of cardiovascular procedures: associations with type of health insurance. American Journal of Public Health 87(2):263–267.

Case RB, Moss AJ, Case N, McDermott M, Eberly S. 1992. Living alone after myocardial infarction. Journal of the American Medical Association 267:515–519.

Catalano R, Dooley D, Wilson G, Hough R. 1993. Job loss and alcohol abuse: a test using data from the Epidemiologic Catchment Area Project. Journal of Health and Social Behavior 34:215–225.

CDC (Centers for Disease Control and Prevention). 1999a. Neighborhood safety and the prevalence of physical inactivity—selected states, 1996. Morbidity and Mortality Weekly Report 48:143–146.

CDC. 1999b. Ten great public health achievements—United States, 1900–1999. Morbidity and Mortality Weekly Report 48(12):241–243.

CDC. 2000. The Fact Book 2000/2001. Available online at http://www.cdc.gov/maso/factbook/main.htm. Accessed August 12, 2002.

CDC. 2001a. CDC FactBook 2000/2001: Profile of the Nation's Health. Atlanta, GA: CDC.

CDC. 2001b. State trends in health and mortality. Prepared by the National Center for Health Statistics, CDC. Available online at http://www.cdc.gov/nchs/datawh/statab/morttables.htm. Accessed October 14, 2002.

CDC. 2001c. Blood and hair mercury levels in young children and women of childbearing age—United States, 1999. Morbidity and Mortality Weekly Report 50(8):140–143.

CDC. 2002. Prevalence of obesity among U.S. adults, by characteristics. Data from the Behavioral Risk Factor Surveillance System (1991–2000). Available online at http://www.cdc.gov/nccdphp/dnpa/obesity/trend/prev_char.htm. Accessed October 13, 2002.

Chaloupka FJ, Cummings KM, Morley CP, Horan JK. 2002. Tax, price and cigarette smoking: evidence from the tobacco documents and implications for tobacco company marketing strategies. Tobacco Control 11(Suppl. 1):I62–I72.

Cohen S. 1988. Psychosocial models of the role of social support in the etiology of physical disease. Health Psychology 7:269–297.

Cohen S, Doyle WJ, Skoner DP, Rabin BS, Gwaltney JM Jr. 1997. Social ties and susceptibility to the common cold. Journal of the American Medical Association 277:1940–1944.

Cohen S, Frank E, Doyle WJ, Skoner DP, Rabin BS, Gwaltney JM. 1998. Types of stressors that increase susceptibility to the common cold in healthy adults. Health Psychology 17:214–223.

Colantonio A, Kasl S, Ostfeld A. 1992. Depressive symptoms and other psychosocial factors as predictors of stroke in the elderly. American Journal of Epidemiology 136:884–894.

Colantonio A, Kasl SV, Ostfeld AM, and Berkman LF. 1993. Psychosocial predictors of stroke outcomes in an elderly population. Journal of Gerontology 48:S261–S268.

Corbett KC. 2001. Susceptibility of youth to tobacco: a social ecological framework for prevention. Respiration Physiology 128:103–118.

Costa G, Segnan N. 1987. Unemployment and mortality. British Medical Journal (Clinical Research Edition) 294:1550–1551.

Crespo CJ, Smit E, Troiano RP, Bartlett SJ, Macera CA, Andersen RE. 2001. Television watching, energy intake, and obesity in US children: results from the third National Health and Nutrition Examination Survey, 1988–1994. Archives of Pediatrics and Adolescent Medicine 155(3):360–365.

Dahlgren G, Whitehead M. 1991. Policies and Strategies to Promote Social Equity in Health. Stockholm: Institute for the Futures Studies.

Davey Smith G, Shipley MJ, Rose G. 1990. Magnitude and causes of socioeconomic differentials in mortality: further evidence from the Whitehall Study. Journal of Epidemiology and Community Health 44:265–270.

Davey Smith G, Neaton JD, Wentworth D, Stamler R, Stamler J. 1996a. Socioeconomic differentials in mortality risk among men screened for the Multiple Risk Factor Intervention Trial II. Black men. American Journal of Public Health 86:497–504.

Davey Smith G, Wentworth D, Neaton JD, Stamler R, Stamler J. 1996b. Socioeconomic differentials in mortality risk among men screened for the Multiple Risk Factor Intervention Trial. I. White men. American Journal of Public Health 86:486–496.

Davis JW, Bennink L, Kaups KL, Parks SN. 2002. Motor vehicle restraints: primary versus secondary enforcement and ethnicity. Journal of Trauma 52(2):225–228.

Deaton A. 2002. Policy implications of the gradient of health and wealth. Health Affairs 21(2):13–30.

Deaton A, Lubotsky D. 2001. Mortality, inequality and race in American cities and states. Working Paper No. 8370. Cambridge, MA: National Bureau of Economic Research, Inc.

DHHS (Department of Health and Human Services). 2000. Healthy People 2010, Vol. I. A Systematic Approach to Health Improvement. Available online at www.health.gov/healthypeople/Document/html/uih/uih_2.htm. Accessed November 16, 2001.

DHHS. 2002. HHS launches new campaign to encourage physical activity and healthy behaviors for kids: "VERB: It's what you do." aims to spark "activity movement" among kids. DHHS press release. Available online at www.hhs.gov/news/press/2002press/20020717b.html. Accessed August 9, 2002.

Dietz WH. 2001. The obesity epidemic in young children. Reduce television viewing and promote playing. British Medical Journal 322(7282):313–314.

Dinh-Zarr TB, Sleet DA, Shults RA, Zaza S, Elder RW, Nichols JL, Thompson RS, Sosin DM. 2001. Reviews of evidence regarding interventions to increase the use of safety belts. American Journal of Preventive Medicine 21(4 Suppl.):48–65.

Dooley D, Fielding J, Lennart L. 1996. Health and unemployment. Annual Review of Public Health 17:449–465.

Durlauf S. 1999. The case "against" social capital. Research Paper No. 9929. Social Systems Research Institute, University of Wisconsin, Madison. Available online at http://www.ssc.wisc.edu/econ/Durlauf/research.html. Accessed October 14, 2002.

EPA (Environmental Protection Agency). 1997. Mercury study report to Congress. Volume I, Executive Summary. Washington, DC: EPA.

Epstein AM, Ayanian JZ. 2001. Racial disparities in medical care. New England Journal of Medicine 344(19):1471–1473.

Evans RG, Stoddart GL. 1990. Producing health, consuming healthcare. Social Science and Medicine 31(12):1347–1363.

Ewart CK, Taylor CB, Kraemer HC, Agras WS. 1991. High blood pressure and marital discord: not being nasty matters more than being nice. Health Psychology 10:155–163.

Feldman J, Makuc D, Kleinman J, Cornoni-Huntley J. 1989. National trends in educational differentials in mortality. American Journal of Epidemiology 129:919–933.

Ferrie J, Shipley M, Marmot M, Stansfeld S, Davey Smith G. 1995. Health effects of anticipation of job change and non-employment: longitudinal data from the Whitehall II study. British Medical Journal 311:1264–1269.

Ferrie J, Shipley M, Marmot M, Stansfeld S, Davey Smith G. 1998. The health effects of major organisational change and job insecurity. Social Science and Medicine 46:243–254.

Fiscella K, Franks P, Gold MR, Clancy CM. 2000. Inequality in quality: addressing socioeconomic, racial, and ethnic disparities in health care. Journal of the American Medical Association 283(19):2579–2584.

Fratiglioni L, Wang HX, Ericsson K, Maytan M, Winblad B. 2000. Influence of social network on occurrence of dementia: a community-based longitudinal study. Lancet 355:1315–1319.

French SA, Story M, Jeffery RW. 2001. Environmental influences on eating and physical activity. Annual Review of Public Health 22:309–335.

Freudenberg N. 2000. Time for a national agenda to improve the health of urban populations. American Journal of Public Health 90(6):837–840.

Friedland J, McColl M. 1987. Social support and psychosocial dysfunction after stroke: buffering effects in a community sample. Archives of Physical Medicine and Rehabilitation 68(8):475–480.

Geronimus AT. 2000. To mitigate, resist or undo: addressing structural influences on the health of urban populations. American Journal of Public Health 90(6):867–872.

Geronimus AT, Bound J, Waidmann TA, Hillemeier MM, Burns PB. 1996. Excess mortality among blacks and whites in the United States. New England Journal of Medicine 335:1552–1558.

Glaser R, Kiecolt-Glaser JK, Bonneau RH, Malarkey W, Kennedy S, Hughes J. 1992. Stress-induced modulation of the immune response to recombinant hepatitis B vaccine. Psychosomatic Medicine 54:22–29.

Glaser R, Rabin B, Chesney M, Cohen S, Natelson B. 1999. Stress-induced immunomodulation: implications for infectious diseases? Journal of the American Medical Association 281:2268–2270.

Glass TA, Matchar DB, Belyea M, Feussner JR. 1993. Impact of social support on outcome in first stroke. Stroke 24(1):64–70.

Glass TA, Dym B, Greenberg S, Rintell D, Roesch C, Berkman LF. 2000. Psychosocial intervention in stroke: Families in Recovery from Stroke Trial (FIRST). American Journal of Orthopsychiatry 70(2):169–181.

Glied S. 2002. Youth tobacco control: reconciling theory and empirical evidence. Journal of Health Economics 21(1):117–135.

Granovetter M. 1995. Getting a Job: A Study of Contacts and Careers. Cambridge, MA: Harvard University Press.

Gravelle H, Wildman J, Sutton M. 2002. Income, income inequality and health: what can we learn from aggregate data? Social Science and Medicine 54(4):577–589.

Hackbarth DP, Silvestri B, Cosper W. 1995. Tobacco and alcohol billboards in 50 Chicago neighborhoods: market segmentation to sell dangerous products to the poor. Journal of Public Health Policy 16(2):213–230.

Hacker A. 1997. Money: Who Has How Much and Why. New York: Scribner.

Harris MI. 1998. Diabetes in America: epidemiology and scope of the problem. Diabetes Care 21(Suppl. 3):C11–C14.

Heaney C, Israel B, House J. 1994. Chronic job insecurity among automobile workers: effects on job satisfaction and health. Social Science and Medicine 38:1431–1437.

Hill JO, Peters JC. 1998. Environmental contributions to the obesity epidemic. Science 280(5368):1371–1374.

Hoek G, Brunekreef B, Fischer P, van Wijnen J. 2001. The association between air pollution and heart failure, arrhythmia, embolism, thrombosis, and other cardiovascular causes of death in a time series study. Epidemiology 12(3):355–357.

House J, Robbins C, Metzner H. 1982. The association of social relationships and activities with mortality: prospective evidence from the Tecumseh Community Health Study American. Journal of Epidemiology 116:123–140.

House JS, Landis KR, Umberson D. 1988. Social relationships and health. Science 241(4865):540–545.

Ibald-Mulli A, Stieber J, Wichmann HE, Koenig W, Peters A. 2001. Effects of air pollution on blood pressure: a population-based approach. American Journal of Public Health 91(4):571–577.

IOM (Institute of Medicine). 1988. The Future of Public Health. Washington, DC: National Academy Press.

IOM. 1994a. Growing up Tobacco Free: Preventing Nicotine Addition in Children and Youths. Washington, DC: National Academy Press.

IOM. 1994b. Reducing Risks for Mental Disorders: Frontiers for Preventive Intervention Research. Washington, DC: National Academy Press.

IOM. 1997. Improving Health in the Community. Washington, DC: National Academy Press.

IOM. 1998. Reducing the Burden of Injury: Advancing Prevention and Treatment. Washington, DC: National Academy Press.

IOM. 2000. Promoting Health: Intervention Strategies from Social and Behavioral Research. Washington, DC: National Academy Press.

IOM. 2001. Health and Behavior. Washington, DC: National Academy Press.

IOM. 2002. Unequal Treatment: Confronting Racial and Ethnic Disparities in Health Care. Washington, DC: The National Academies Press.

Iversen L, Andersen O, Andersen P, Christoffersen K, Keiding N. 1987. Unemployment and mortality in Denmark 1970–80. British Medical Journal 295:879–884.

Jeffery RW. 2001. Public health strategies for obesity treatment and prevention. American Journal of Health Behavior 25:252–259.

Jencks C. 2002. Does inequality matter? Daedalus Summer:49–65. Available online at www.daedalus.amacad.org/issues/winter2002/Jencks.pdf. Accessed October 2, 2002.

Johnson JV, Stewart W, Hall EM, Fredlund P, Theorell T. 1996. Long-term psychosocial work environmental and cardiovascular mortality among Swedish men. American Journal of Public Health 86:324–331.

Kaplan G, Salonen J, Cohen R, Brand R, Syme S, Puska P. 1988. Social connections and mortality from all causes and cardiovascular disease: prospective evidence from eastern Finland. American Journal of Epidemiology 128:370–380.

Kaplan GA, Keil JE. 1993. Socioeconomic factors and cardiovascular disease: a review of the literature. Circulation 88:1973–1998.

Kaplan GA, Pamuk E, Lynch JW, Cohen RD, Balfour JL. 1996. Inequality in income and mortality in the United States: analysis of mortality and potential pathways. British Medical Journal 312:999–1003.

Karasek R, Theorell T. 1990. Healthy Work. New York: Basic Books.

Kasl S, Jones B. 2000. The impact of job loss and retirement on health. In Berkman L, Kawachi I (Eds.). Social Epidemiology. New York: Oxford University Press.

Kawachi I, Berkman L. 2000. Social cohesion, social capital and health. In Berkman L, Kawachi I (Eds.). Social Epidemiology. New York: Oxford University Press.

Kawachi I, Kennedy BP. 1997. Socioeconomic determinants of health: health and social cohesion: why care about income inequality? British Medical Journal 314:1037–1040.

Kawachi I, Colditz GA, Ascherio A, Rimm EB, Giovannucci E, Stampfer MJ, Willett WC. 1996. A prospective study of social networks in relation to total mortality and cardiovascular disease in men in the USA. Journal of Epidemiology and Community Health 50:245–251.

Kawachi I, Kennedy B, Lochner K, Prothrow-Stith D. 1997. Social capital, income inequality and mortality. American Journal of Public Health 87:1491–1498.

Kawachi I, Kennedy BP, Glass R. 1999. Social capital and self-rated health: a contextual analysis. American Journal of Public Health 89:1187–1193.

Kawachi I, Subramanian SV, Almeida-Filho N. 2002. A glossary for health inequalities. Journal of Epidemiology and Community Health 56:647–652.

Kennedy BP, Kawachi I, Prothrow-Stith D. 1996. Income distribution and mortality: cross-sectional ecologic study of the Robin Hood Index in the United States. British Medical Journal 312:1004–1007.

Kennedy BP, Kawachi I, Glass R, Prothrow-Stith D. 1998. Income distribution, socioeconomic status and self rated health in the United States: multilevel analysis. British Medical Journal 317:917–921.

Kiecolt-Glaser JK, Marucha PT, Malarkey WB, Mercado AM, Glaser R. 1995. Slowing of wound healing by psychological stress. Lancet 346:1194–1196.

Kiecolt-Glaser JK, Glaser R, Cacioppo JT. 1997. Marital conflict in older adults: endocrinological and immunological correlates. Psychosomatic Medicine 59:339–349.

Kiecolt-Glaser JK, Page GG, Marucha PT, MacCallum RC, Glaser R. 1998. Psychological influences on surgical recovery: perspectives from psychoneuroimmunology. American Psychologist 53:1209–1218.

Kirschbaum C, Klauer T, Filipp SH, Hellhammer DH. 1995. Sex-specific effects of social support on cortisol and subjective responses to acute psychological stress. Psychosomatic Medicine 57(1):23–31.

Korenbrot CC, Moss NE. 2000. Preconception, prenatal, perinatal and postnatal influences on health, pp. 125–169. In Promoting Health: Intervention Strategies from Social and Behavioral Research. Washington, DC: National Academy Press.

Krieger N, Sidney S. 1996. Racial discrimination and blood pressure: the CARDIA study of young black and white adults. American Journal of Public Health 86(10):1370–1378.

Kunst AE, Groenhof F, Mackenbach J, European Union Working Group on Socioeconomic Inequalities in Health. 1998. Occupational class and cause specific mortality in middle aged men in 11 European countries: comparison of population based studies. British Medical Journal 316:1636–1642.

Lawrence J. 1999. Urban health: an ecological perspective. Review of Environmental Health 14(1):1–10.

Levenson RW, Carstensensen LL, Gottman JM. 1993. Long-term marriage: age gender and satisfaction. Psychology and Aging 8:301–313.

Leviton LC, Snell E, McGinnis M. 2000. Urban issues in health promotion strategies. American Journal of Public Health 90(6):863–866.

Link B, Phelan J. 1995. Social conditions as fundamental causes of disease. Journal of Health and Social Behavior (Special Issue):80–94.

Luke D, Esmundo E, Bloom Y. 2000. Smoke signs: patterns of tobacco billboard advertising in a metropolitan region. Tobacco Control 9:16–23.

Lynch J, Kaplan GA, Pamuk ER, Cohen RD, Heck KE, Balfour JL, Yen IH. 1998. Income inequality and mortality in metropolitan areas of the United States. American Journal of Public Health 88:1074–1080.

Lynch J, Davey Smith G, Hillemeiera M, Shawe M, Raghunathanb T, Kaplan G. 2001. Income inequality, the psychosocial environment, and health: comparisons of wealthy nations. Lancet 358(9277):194–200.

Lynch JW, Kaplan GA, Salonen JT. 1997. Why do poor people behave poorly? Variation in adult health behaviors and psychological characteristics by stages of the socioeconomic life course. Social Science and Medicine 44:809–819.

Maantay J. 2001. Zoning, equity, and public health. American Journal of Public Health 91(7):1033–1041.

Macintyre S, Ellaway A, Der G, Ford G, Hunt K. 1998. Do housing tenure and car access predict health because they are simply markers of income or self-esteem? A Scottish study. Journal of Epidemiology and Community Health 52:657–664.

Mackenbach JP, Stronks K, Kunst AE. 1989. The contribution of medical care to inequalities in health: differences between socioeconomic groups in decline of mortality from conditions amenable to medical intervention. Social Science and Medicine 29:369–376.

Malarkey WB, Kiecolt-Glaser JK, Pearl D, Glaser R. 1994. Hostile behavior during marital conflict alters pituitary and adrenal hormones. Psychosomatic Medicine 56:41–51.

Marmot MG, Davey Smith G, Stansfield S, Patel C, North F, Head J, White I, Brunner E, Feeney A. 1991. Health inequalities among British civil servants: the Whitehall II Study. Lancet 337:1387–1393.

Martikainen P. 1990. Unemployment and mortality among Finnish men 1981–5. British Medical Journal 301:407–411.

Mattiasson I, Lindegarde F, Nilsson J, Theorell T. 1990. Threat of unemployment and cardiovascular risk factors: longitudinal study of quality of sleep and serum cholesterol concentrations in men threatened with redundancy. British Medical Journal 301:461–465.

McGinnis JM, Foege WH. 1993. Actual causes of death in the United States. Journal of the American Medical Association 270(18):2207–2212.

McGinnis JM, Williams-Russo P, Knickman JR. 2002. The case for more active policy attention to health promotion. To succeed, we need leadership that informs and motivates, economic incentives that encourage change, and science that moves the frontiers. Health Affairs 21(2):78–93.

McLoyd VC. 1998. Socioeconomic disadvantage and child development. American Psychologist 53(2):185–204.

McMillen RC, Frese W, Cosby AG. 2001. The National Social Climate of Tobacco Control, 2000–2001. Starkville, MS: Social Science Research Center, Mississippi State University.

Meaney MJ, Diorio J, Francis D, Widdowson J, LaPlante P, Caldji C, Sharma S, Seckl JR, Plotsky PM. 1996. Early environmental regulation of forebrain glucocorticoid receptor gene expression: implications for adrenocortical responses to stress. Developmental Neuroscience 18(1–2):49–72.

Miller T, Lestina D, Spicer R. 1998. Highway crash costs in the United States by driver age, blood alcohol level, victim age, and restraint use. Accident Analysis and Prevention 30(2):137–150.

Miller TR. 2001. The effectiveness review trials of Hercules and some economic estimates for the stables. American Journal of Preventive Medicine 21(4 Suppl.):9–12.

Moen P. 1996. A life course perspective on retirement gender and well being. Journal of Occupational Health Psychology 1:131–144.

Mokdad AH, Serdula MK, Dietz WH, Bowman BA, Marks JS, Koplan JP. 1999. The spread of the obesity epidemic in the United States, 1991–1998. Journal of the American Medical Association 282(16):1519–1522.

Mokdad AH, Ford ES, Bowman BA, Nelson DE, Engelgau MM, Vinicor F, Marks JS. 2000. Diabetes trends in the U.S.: 1990–1998. Diabetes Care 23(9):1278–1283.

Morris J, Cook D. 1991. A critical review of the effect of factory closures on health. British Journal of Industrial Medicine 48:1–8.

Morris PL, Robinson RG, Andrzejewski P, Samuels J, Price TR. 1993. Association of depression with 10-year poststroke mortality. American Journal of Psychiatry 150(1):124–129.

Moser K, Fox A, Jones D. 1984. Unemployment and mortality in the OCPS Longitudinal Study. Lancet 2(8415):1324–1329.

Moser K, Fox A, Jones D, Goldblatt P. 1986. Unemployment and mortality: further evidence from the OCPS Longitudinal Study 1971–1981. Lancet 1(8477):365–367.

Moser K, Goldblatt P, Fox A, Jones D. 1987. Unemployment and mortality: comparison of the 1971 and 1981 longitudinal study census samples. British Medical Journal 294:86–90.

Must A, Spadano J, Coakley EH, Field AE, Colditz G, Dietz WH. 1999. The disease burden associated with overweight and obesity. Journal of the American Medical Association 282(16):1523–1529.

NCHS (National Center for Health Statistics). 1992. Vital Statistics of the United States 1992. Washington DC: Government Printing Office.

NCHS. 1998. Health, United States, 1998. With Socioeconomic Status and Health Chartbook. Atlanta, GA: National Center for Health Statistics, Centers for Disease Control and Prevention, Department of Health and Human Services.

NCHS. 2001. Health, United States, 2001. With Urban and Rural Health Chartbook. Atlanta, GA: National Center for Health Statistics, Centers for Disease Control and Prevention, Department of Health and Human Services.

NCHS. 2002. Health, United States, 2002. With Chartbook on Trends in the Health of Americans. DHHS Publication No. 1232. Atlanta, GA: National Center for Health Statistics, Centers for Disease Control and Prevention, Department of Health and Human Services.

Nerem RM, Levesque MJ, Cornhill JF. 1980. Social environment as a factor in diet-induced atherosclerosis. Science 208(4451):1475–1476.

Nestle M, Jacobson MF. 2000. Halting the obesity epidemic: a public health policy approach. Public Health Reports 115(1):12–24.

NHTSA (National Highway Traffic Safety Administration). 1996. Report to Congress on benefits of safety belts and motorcycle helmets, based on data from the Crash Outcome Data Evaluation System (CODES). DOT HS 808–347. Washington, DC: Department of Transportation.

NIH (National Institutes of Health). 1998. Clinical Guidelines on the Identification, Evaluation, and Treatment of Overweight and Obesity in Adults. The Evidence Report. Rockville, MD: National Heart, Lung, and Blood Institute, National Institutes of Health.

NIH. 2001. Study finds no reduction in deaths or heart attacks in heart disease patients treated for depression and low social support. News Release, November 12, 2001, National Heart, Lung and Blood Institute, National Institutes of Health, Rockville, MD.

NIH. 2002. About Hearts N' Parks. Available online at http://www.nhlbi.nih.gov/health/prof/ heart/obesity/hrt_n_pk/. Accessed October 14, 2002.

North FM, Syme SL, Feeney A, Shipley M, Marmot M. 1996. Psychosocial work environment and sickness absence among British civil servants: the Whitehall II study. American Journal of Public Health 86:332–340.

NRC (National Research Council). 1999. Our Common Journey: A Transition Toward Sustainability. Washington, DC: National Academy Press.

NRC. 2000. Toxicological Effects of Methylmercury. Washington, DC: National Academy Press.

Office of Minority Health. 2000. Assessment of State Minority Health Infrastructure and Capacity to Address Issues of Health Disparity. Developed by COSMOS Corporation for the Office of Minority Health, Office of Public Health and Science, Department of Health and Human Services. Available online at http://www.omhrc.gov/omh/sidebar/cossmo/cover. htm. Accessed October 14, 2002.

Orth-Gomer K, Johnson J. 1987. Social network interaction and mortality: a six-year follow-up study of a random sample of the Swedish population. Journal of Chronic Diseases 40:949–957.

Orth-Gomer K, Unden AL, Edwards ME. 1988. Social isolation and mortality in ischemic heart disease. A 10-year follow-up study of 150 middle-aged men. Acta Medica Scandinavica 224(3):205–215.

Ostrove JM, Feldman P, Adler NE. 1999. Relations among socioeconomic status indicators and health for African-Americans and whites. Journal of Health Psychology 4(4):451–463.

Pappas G, Queen S, Hadden W, Fisher G. 1993. The increasing disparity in mortality between socioeconomic groups in the US, 1960–1986. New England Journal of Medicine 329:103–109.

Parker S, Chmiel N, Wall T. 1997. Work characteristics and employee well-being within a context of strategic downsizing. Journal of Occupational Health Psychology 2:289–303.

Pennix BW, van Tilburg T, Kriegsman DM, Deeg DJ Boeke AJ, van Eijk JT. 1997. Effects of social support and personal coping resources on mortality in older age: the Longitudinal Aging Study, Amsterdam. American Journal of Epidemiology 146:510–519.

Pertowski C. 1994. Lead poisoning, pp. 311–320. In From Data to Action: CDC's Public Health Surveillance for Women, Infants, and Children. Centers for Disease Control and Prevention Maternal & Child Health Monograph. Available online at http://www.cdc.gov/nccdphp/drh/datoact/. Accessed October 14, 2002.

Peters A, Dockery DW, Muller JE, Mittleman MA. 2001. Increased particulate air pollution and the triggering of myocardial infarction. Circulation 103(23):2810–2815.

Peterson AV, Kealey KA, Mann SL, Marek PM, Sarason IG. 2000. Hutchinson Smoking Prevention Project: long-term randomized trial in school-based tobacco use prevention—results on smoking. Journal of the National Cancer Institute 92(24):1979–1991.

Pew Environmental Health Commission. 2000. America's environmental health gap: why the country needs a nationwide health tracking network. Pew Environmental Health Commission, Johns Hopkins University School of Public Health. Available online at http://healthyamericans.org/resources/ files/healthgap.pdf. Accessed October 2, 2002.

Pew Environmental Health Commission. 2001. Transition report to the new administration: strengthening our public health defense against environmental threats. Pew Environmental Health Commission, Johns Hopkins University School of Public Health. Available online at http://healthyamericans.org/ resources/files/transition.pdf. Accessed October 2, 2002.

Portes A, Landolt P. 1996. The downside of social capital. The American Prospect 26:18–21.

Proctor BD, Dalakar J. 2002. Poverty in the United States: 2001. Current Population Reports, P60–219. Washington, DC: Bureau of the Census, Department of Commerce.

Rodgers GB. 2002. Income and inequality as determinants of mortality: an international cross-section analysis. International Journal of Epidemiology 31(3):533–538.

Roetzheim RG, Pal N, Tennant C, Voti L, Ayanian JZ, Schwabe A, Krischer JP. 1999. Effects of health insurance and race on early detection of cancer. Journal of the National Cancer Institute 91(16):1409–1415.

Rogot E, Sorlie P, Johnson N. 1992. Life expectancy by employment status income and education in the National Longitudinal Mortality Study. Public Health Reports 107:457–461.

Rose G. 1981. Strategy of prevention: lessons from cardiovascular disease. British Medical Journal 282:1847–1851.

Rose G. 1992. The Strategy of Preventive Medicine. Oxford: Oxford University Press.

Roy MP, Steptoe A, Kirschbaum C. 1998. Life events and social support as moderators of individual differences in cardiovascular and cortisol reactivity. Journal of Personality and Social Psychology 75(5):1273–1281.

Sampson RJ, Raudenbush SW, Earls F. 1997. Neighborhoods and violent crime: a multilevel study of collective efficacy. Science 277:918–924.

Sandefur RF, Laumann OE. 1998. A paradigm for social capital. Rationality and Society 10(4):481–501.

Sapolsky RM, Alberts SC, Altmann J, 1997. Hypercortisolism associated with social subordinance or social isolation among wild baboons. Archives of General Psychiatry 54(12):1137–1143.

Sargent JD, Brown MJ, Freeman JL, Bailey A, Goodman D, Freeman D. 1995. Childhood lead poisoning in Massachusetts communities: its association with sociodemographic and housing characteristics. American Journal of Public Health 85(4):528–534.

Schiff M, Becker T. 1996. Trends in motor vehicle traffic fatalities among Hispanics, non-Hispanic whites and American Indians in New Mexico, 1958–1990. Ethnicity & Health 1(3):283–291.

Schnall P, Landsbergis P, Baker D. 1994. Job strain and cardiovascular disease. Annual Review of Public Health 15:381–411.

Schoenbach V, Kaplan B, Freedman L, Kleinbaum D. 1986. Social ties and mortality in Evans County Georgia. American Journal of Epidemiology 123:577–591.

Schwartz LM, Woloshin S. 1999. Changing disease definitions: implications for disease prevalence. Analysis of the Third National Health and Nutrition Examination Survey, 1988–1994. Effective Clinical Practice 2(2):76–85.

Seeman T. 1996. Social ties and health: the benefits of social integration. Annals of Epidemiology 6:442–451.

Seeman T, Kaplan G, Knudsen L, Cohen R, Guralnik J. 1988. Social network ties and mortality among the elderly in the Alameda County Study. American Journal of Epidemiology 126:714–723.

Seeman T, Berkman L, Kohout F, LaCroix A, Glynn R, Blazer D. 1993. Intercommunity variation in the association between social ties and mortality in the elderly: a comparative analysis of three communities. Annals of Epidemiology 3:325–335.

Shively CA, Clarkson TB, Kaplan JR. 1989. Social deprivation and coronary artery atherosclerosis in female cynomolgus monkeys. Atherosclerosis 77(1):69–76.

Sigerist J. 1996. Adverse health effects of high-effort/low-reward conditions. Journal of Occupational Health Psychology 1:27–41.

Slifkin R, Goldsmith L, Ricketts T. 2000. Race and place: urban-rural differences in health for racial and ethnic minorities. North Carolina Rural Health Research Program, University of North Carolina at Chapel Hill, Cecil G. Sheps Center for Health Services Research, Working Paper No. 66. Available online at www.shepscenter.unc.edu/research_programs/Rural _Program/wp.html. Accessed October 10, 2002.

Soobader MJ, LeClere FB. 1999. Aggregation and the measurement of income inequality: effects on morbidity. Social Science and Medicine 48:733–744.

Sorlie P, Rogot E. 1990. Mortality by employment status in the National Longitudinal Mortality Study. American Journal of Epidemiology 132:983–992.

Sorlie P, Rogot E, Anderson R, Johnson N, Backlund E. 1992. Black-white mortality differences by family income. Lancet 340:346–350.

Sorlie P, Backlund E, Keller JB. 1995. US mortality by economic, demographic, and social characteristics: the National Longitudinal Mortality Study. American Journal of Public Health 585:949–956.

Stefansson C. 1991. Long-term unemployment and mortality in Sweden 1980–1986. Social Science and Medicine 32:419–423.

Sugisawa H, Liang J, Liu X. 1994. Social networks social support and mortality among older people in Japan. Journal of Gerontology 49:S313.

Suomi SJ. 1991. Early stress and adult emotional reactivity in rhesus monkeys. Ciba Foundation Symposium 156:171–183.

Syme S, Berkman L. 1976. Social class susceptibility and sickness. American Journal of Epidemiology 104:1–8.

Tataranni PA, Bogardus C. 2001. Changing habits to delay diabetes. New England Journal of Medicine 344(18):1390–1392.

Theorell T, Tsutsumi A, Hallquist J, Reuterwall C, Hogstedt C, Fredlund P, Emlund N, Johnson JV. 1998. Decision latitude job strain and myocardial infarction: a study of working men in Stockholm. The SHEEP Study Group Stockholm Heart Epidemiology Program. American Journal of Public Health 88:382–388.

Thomas SB. 2001. The color line: race matters in the elimination of health disparities. American Journal of Public Health 91(7):1046–1048.

Tobler NS. 1986. Meta-analysis of 143 adolescent drug prevention programs: quantitative outcome results of program participants compared to a control or comparison group. Journal of Drug Issues 16(4):537–567.

Trust for America's Health. 2001. Short of breath: our lack of response to the growing asthma epidemic and the need for nationwide tracking. Available online at http://healthyamericans.org/resources/files/shortofbreath.pdf. Accessed October 10, 2002.

Tuomilehto J, Lindstrom J, Eriksson JG, Valle TT, Hamalainen H, Ilanne-Parikka P, Keinanen-Kiukaanniemi S, Laakso M, Louheranta A, Rastas M, Salminen V, Uusitupa M. 2001. Prevention of type 2 diabetes mellitus by changes in lifestyle among subjects with impaired glucose tolerance. New England Journal of Medicine 344(18):1343–1350.

Tyroler HA, Wing S, Knowles MG. 1993. Increasing inequality in coronary heart disease mortality in relation to educational achievement profiles of places of residence United States 1962 to 1987. Annals of Epidemiology 3:S51–S54.

USPHS (U.S. Public Health Service). 1979. Healthy People: the Surgeon General's report on health promotion and disease prevention. DHEW (PHS) Publication No. 79–55071. Washington, DC: U.S. Public Health Service.

Vahtera J, Kivimaki M, Pentti J. 1997. Effect of organizational downsizing on health of employees. Lancet 350:1124–1128.

Vogt TM, Mullooly JP, Ernst D, Pope CR, Hollis JF. 1992. Social networks as predictors of ischemic heart disease, cancer, stroke, and hypertension: incidence survival and mortality. Journal of Clinical Epidemiology 45:659–666.

Warner KE. 1982. Mandatory passive restraint systems in automobiles: issues and evidence. Technology and handicapped people. Background Paper No. 1. Office of Technology Assessment, U.S. Congress. Washington, DC: Government Printing Office

Warner KE. 2000. The need for, and value of, a multi-level approach to disease prevention: the case of tobacco control, pp. 417–449. In Promoting Health: Intervention Strategies from Social and Behavioral Research. Institute of Medicine. Washington, DC: National Academy Press.

Weinberg DH. 1996. A Brief Look at Postwar US Income Inequality. Census Bureau Current Population Reports, P60–191. Washington, DC: U.S. Bureau of the Census, Department of Commerce.

Weinick RM, Krauss NA. 2000. Racial/ethnic differences in children's access to care. American Journal of Public Health 90(11):1771–1774.

Welin L, Tibblin G, Svardsudd K, Tibblin B, Ander-Peciva S, Larsson B, Wilhelmsen L. 1985. Prospective study of social influences on mortality. The study of men born in 1913 and 1923. Lancet 1(8434):915–918.

The White House. 1998. President Clinton announces new racial and ethnic health disparities initiative. White House fact sheet, February 21, 1998. Available online at http://raceandhealth.hhs.gov/sidebars/sbwhats.htm. Accessed August 19, 2002.

The White House. 2002. President Bush launches HealthierUS initiative. Press release. Available online at www.whitehouse.gov/news/releases/2002/ 06/20020620-6.html. Accessed August 9, 2002.

Wilkinson RG. 1992. Income distribution and life expectancy. British Medical Journal 304:165–168.

Wilkinson RG. 1996. Unhealthy Societies: The Afflictions of Inequality. London: Routledge.

Williams DR. 1990. Socioeconomic differentials in health: a review and redirection. Social Psychology Quarterly 53:81–99.

Williams DR, Collins C. 1995. U.S. socioeconomic and social differences in health: patterns and explanations. Annual Review of Sociology 21:349–386.

Williams DR, Collins C. 2001. Racial residential segregation: a fundamental cause of racial disparities in health. Public Health Reports 116(5):404–416.

Williams RB, Barefoot JC, Califf RM, Haney TL, Saunders WB, Pryor DB, Hlatky MA, Siegler IC, Mark DB. 1992. Prognostic importance of social and economic resources among medically treated patients with angiographically documented coronary artery disease. Journal of the American Medical Association 267(4):520–524.

Williamson DF. 1999. The prevention of obesity. New England Journal of Medicine 341(15):1140–1141.

Wolf AM, Colditz GA. 1998. Current estimates of the economic cost of obesity in the United States. Obesity Research 6(2):97–106.

Wolff E. 2000. Reconciling Alternative Estimates of Wealth Inequality from the Survey of Consumer Finances. American Enterprise Institute Seminar on Economic Inequality, February 9, 2000.

Wood D. 2002. A farewell to fizz from LA lunchrooms. The Christian Science Monitor, August 30, 2002, p. 1.

Worthman CM. 1999. Epidemiology of human development, pp. 47–104. In Panter-Brick C, Worthman CM (Eds.). Hormones, Health, and Behavior: A Socio-Ecological and Lifespan Perspective. Cambridge: Cambridge University Press.

3

The Governmental Public Health Infrastructure

The success or failure of any government in the final analysis must be measured by the well-being of its citizens. Nothing can be more important to a state than its public health; the state's paramount concern should be the health of its people.

Franklin Delano Roosevelt
(quoted in Gostin, 2000)

An effective public health system that can assure the nation's health requires the collaborative efforts of a complex network of people and organizations in the public and private sectors, as well as an alignment of policy and practice of governmental public health agencies at the national, state, and local levels. In the United States, governments at all levels (federal, state, and local) have a specific responsibility to strive to create the conditions in which people can be as healthy as possible. For governments to play their role within the public health system, policy makers must provide the political and financial support needed for strong and effective governmental public health agencies.

Weaknesses in the nation's governmental public health infrastructure were clearly demonstrated in the fall of 2001, when the once-hypothetical threat of bioterrorism became all too real with the discovery that many people had been exposed to anthrax from letters sent through the mail. Communication among federal, state, and local health officials and with political leaders, public safety personnel, and the public was often cumbersome, uncoordinated, incomplete, and sometimes inaccurate. Laboratories were overwhelmed with testing of samples, both real and false. Many of these systemic weaknesses were well known to public health professionals, but resources to address them had been insufficient. A strong and effective governmental public health infrastructure is essential not only to respond to crises such as these but also to address ongoing challenges such as preventing or managing chronic illnesses, controlling infectious diseases, and monitoring the safety of food and water.

The fragmentation of the governmental public health infrastructure is in part a direct result of the way in which governmental roles and responsibilities at the federal, state, and local levels have evolved over U.S. history. This history also explains why the nation lacks a comprehensive national health policy that could be used to align health-sector investment, governmental public health agency structure and function, and incentives for the private sector to work more effectively as part of a broader public health system. In this chapter, the committee reviews the organization of governmental public health agencies in the United States. The chapter then examines some of the most critical shortcomings in the public health infrastructure at the federal, state, and local levels: the preparation of the public health workforce, inadequate information systems and public health laboratories, and organizational impediments to effective management of public health activities. The committee recommends steps that must be taken to respond to these challenges so that governmental public health agencies can meet their obligations within the public health system to protect and improve the population's health.

The committee believes that the federal and state governments share a responsibility for assuring the public's health. From a historical and constitutional perspective, public health is largely a local and state function. The role of the states and localities is a primary and important one. The federal government, however, has the resources, expertise, and the obligation to assess the health of the nation and to make recommendations for its improvement. Ensuring a sound public health infrastructure is an urgent matter, and the committee urges the federal government to engage in planning for national and regional funding to accomplish this.

PRIOR ASSESSMENTS OF THE PUBLIC HEALTH INFRASTRUCTURE

In 1988, *The Future of Public Health* (IOM, 1988) reported that the American public health system, particularly its governmental components, was in disarray. In that report, the responsible committee sought to clarify the nature and scope of public health activities and to focus specifically on the roles and responsibilities of governmental agencies. Aiming to provide a set of directions for public health that could attract the support of the broader society, the committee produced findings and made recommendations dealing with three basic issues:

1. The mission of public health
2. The government's role in fulfilling this mission and
3. The responsibilities unique to each level of government

The mission of public health was specified as "fulfilling society's inter-est in assuring conditions in which people can be healthy" (IOM, 1988: 7). The government's role in fulfilling this mission was described in terms of three core functions of public health practice: assessment of health status and health needs, policy development, and assurance that necessary services are provided. States were considered to have primary public responsibility for health, but it was considered essential that residents of every community have access to public health protections through a local component of the public health system. The public health obligations of the federal govern-ment included informing the nation about public health policy issues, aid-ing states and localities in carrying out their public health functions in a coordinated manner, and setting national health goals and standards. The report also contained recommendations for a review of the statutory basis for public health, the establishment of the governmental public health infra-structure as the clear organizational hub for public health activities, better linkages to other government agencies with health-related responsibilities, and strategies to strengthen the capacities of public health agencies to per-form the core functions. A complete listing of the recommendations from that report can be found in Appendix C.

Responding to Disarray

The Future of Public Health provided the public health community with a common language and a focus for reform, and progress has been made. In Washington, Illinois, and Michigan, for example, revisions of the state public health codes resulted in the inclusion of mandatory provisions for funding and the distribution of services to all communities "no matter how small or remote," as recommended by the Institute of Medicine (IOM) (1988). In 1994, the Public Health Functions Working Group, a committee convened by the Department of Health and Human Services (DHHS) with representa-tives from all major public health constituencies, agreed on a list of the essential services of public health. This list of services translates the three core functions into a more concrete set of activities, called the 10 Essential Public Health Services (see Box 3–1). These essential services provide the foundation for the nation's public health strategy, including the *Healthy People 2010* objectives concerning the public health infrastructure (DHHS, 2000) (see Appendix D) and the development of National Public Health Performance Standards (CDC, 1998) for state and local public health systems.

At least four subsequent National Academies reports have made a strong case for sustained federal action both domestically and internation-ally to strengthen the public health infrastructure (IOM, 1992, 1997a, 1997b; NRC, 2002). The federal government has yet to take the initiative to develop a comprehensive, long-term plan to build and sustain the financ-

---

BOX 3–1
The 10 Essential Public Health Services

Assessment
1. Monitor health status to identify community health problems
2. Diagnose and investigate health problems and health hazards in the community

Policy Development
3. Inform, educate, and empower people about health issues
4. Mobilize community partnerships to identify and solve health problems
5. Develop policies and plans that support individual and community health efforts

Assurance
6. Enforce laws and regulations that protect health and ensure safety
7. Link people to needed personal health services and assure the provision of health care when otherwise unavailable
8. Assure a competent public health and personal health care workforce
9. Evaluate effectiveness, accessibility, and quality of personal and population-based health services

Serving All Functions
10. Research for new insights and innovative solutions to health problems

SOURCE: Public Health Functions Steering Committee (1994).

---

ing for this infrastructure at the state and local levels to ensure the availability of the essential health services to all people, and this is a critical concern. The federal government has, however, developed and funded various new programs and organizational units, which, if effectively coordinated, could serve as important components of a more systematic program. The Centers for Disease Control and Prevention (CDC) established (in 1989) the Public Health Practice Program Office and strengthened university-based Centers for Prevention Research (initiated in 1983). CDC also developed Public Health Leadership Institutes (initiated in 1992) at the national and regional levels and the National Public Health Training Network (initiated in 1993). Both programs respond to recommendations to improve the overall leadership competencies of public health practitioners. In 1993, CDC began discussions of a modern and uniform approach to public health surveillance, and it has moved forward with the development of a National Electronic Disease Surveillance Network. More recently, CDC has worked with states to establish the Health Alert Network (initiated in 1999) to improve information and communication systems for both routine and emergency use and the Centers for Public Health Preparedness (launched in 2000) to improve linkages between local health agencies and academic centers. These programs provided important services in the aftermath of September 11, 2001.

Many units within CDC have contributed to strengthening the public health infrastructure. The National Center for Chronic Disease Prevention and Health Promotion, for example, has led the effort to develop statewide population-based cancer registries, a tracking system for cardiovascular disease, and a program for the early detection of breast and cervical cancer (CDC, 2002). The National Center for Environmental Health also contributed to the improvement of public health monitoring and assessment functions when it developed a biomonitoring program to measure people's exposures to 27 different chemicals by analyzing human blood and urine samples. This program offers the first national assessment of people's exposure to 24 chemicals for which exposures were not previously assessed and 3 for which exposures were previously assessed. In 2002, the center began developing a nationwide environmental public health tracking network in response to a Pew Environmental Health Commission report entitled *America's Environmental Health Gap: Why the Country Needs A National Health Tracking Network* (Pew Environmental Health Commission, 2000; www.cdc.gov/nceh/tracking/background.htm). Among CDC initiatives are the development of immunization registries and a guide to community preventive services (www.cdc.gov).

Limited Progress

Despite this progress, the committee found that in many important ways, the public health system that was in disarray in 1988 remains in disarray today. Many of the recommendations from *The Future of Public Health* have not been put into action. There has been no fundamental reform of the statutory framework for public health in most of the nation. Funding for the public health infrastructure has recently increased to support the infrastructure that relates to bioterrorism and emergency preparedness but may still be insufficient. Furthermore, governmental and nongovernmental support (both political and financial) and advocacy for the report's recommendations have been limited. Progress is mixed in strengthening public health agencies' capacities to address environmental health problems, in building linkages with the mental health field, and in meeting the health care needs of the medically indigent. In addition, new information and technological challenges face the system today. In a recent review of the nation's public health infrastructure for the U.S. Senate Appropriations Committee, CDC (2001d) pointed to the need for further efforts to address gaps in workforce capacity and competency, information and data systems, and the organizational capacities of state and local health departments and laboratories.

Finding continued disarray in the public health system is especially disturbing because the nation faces increasingly diverse threats and challenges. The early detection of and the response to these threats will depend on capacity and expertise within the public health system at every level. The gaps in the system warrant urgent remediation. Many of these basic reforms also require actions from agencies that are outside the direct control of governmental public health agencies but whose policies and programs can have important health consequences, such as the Environmental Protection Agency (EPA) (environment) and the Departments of Agriculture (nutrition and food safety), Labor (working conditions), and Treasury (economic development). This support has not been forthcoming from elected or appointed government officials (including those in control of budgets), and stakeholders in the broader public health system—who should have been partners in the vision of creating a healthier nation—have yet to be effectively mobilized in this effort.

In the next section, the committee provides an overview of the special role of governmental public health agencies (at the federal, tribal, state, and local levels). The section addresses the legal framework for governmental responsibility and its authorities for protecting the health of the people as well as the organization of the governmental public health infrastructure.

THE ROLE OF GOVERNMENTS IN PUBLIC HEALTH: AN OVERVIEW AND LEGAL FRAMEWORK

Governments at every level—federal, tribal, state, and local—play important roles in protecting, preserving, and promoting the public's health and safety (Gostin, 2000, 2002). In the United States, the government's responsibility for the health of its citizens stems, in part, from the nature of democracy itself. Health officials are either directly elected or appointed by democratically elected officials. To the extent, therefore, that citizens place a high priority on health, these elected officials are held accountable to ensure that the government is able to monitor the population's health and intervene when necessary through laws, policies, regulations, and expenditure of the resources necessary for the health and safety of the public.

The U.S. Constitution provides for a national government, with power divided among the legislative, executive, and judicial branches, each with distinct authority. The states have adopted similar schemes of governance. In health matters, the legislative branch creates health policy and allocates the resources to implement it. In the executive branch, health departments and other agencies must act within the scope of legislative authority by implementing legislation and establishing health regulations to enforce health policy. The judiciary's task is to interpret laws and resolve legal disputes. Increasingly, the courts have exerted substantial control over public health policy by determining the boundaries of government power (Gostin, 2000). The separation of powers provides a system of checks and balances to ensure that no single branch of government can act without some degree of oversight and control by another.

Modern public health agencies wield considerable power to make rules to control private behavior, interpret statutes and regulations, and adjudicate disputes about whether an individual or a company has conformed to health and safety standards. In the area of health and safety (which is highly complex and technical), public health agencies are expected to have the expertise and long-range perspective necessary to assemble the facts about health risks and to devise solutions.

Role of State and Local Governments in Assuring Population Health

States and their local subdivisions retain the primary responsibility for health under the U.S. Constitution.[1] To fulfill this responsibility, state and local public health authorities engage in a variety of activities, including monitoring the burden of injury and disease in the population through surveillance systems; identifying individuals and groups that have conditions of public health importance with testing, reporting, and partner notification; providing a broad array of prevention services such as counseling and education; and helping assure access to high-quality health care services for poor and vulnerable populations. State and local governments also engage in a broad array of regulatory activities. They seek to ensure that businesses conduct themselves in ways that are safe and sanitary (through the institution of measures such as inspections, licenses, and nuisance abatements) and that individuals do not engage in unduly risky behavior or pose a danger to others (through the provision of services such as vaccinations, directly observed therapy, and isolation), and they oversee the quality of health care provided in the public and private sectors.

Role of Tribal Governments in Assuring Population Health

Although their legal status varies, tribal governments have a unique sovereignty and right to self-determination that is often based on treaties with the federal government. Under these treaties, the federal government

---

[1] The 10th Amendment enunciates the plenary power retained by the states: "The powers not delegated to the United States by the Constitution, nor prohibited by it to the States, are reserved to the States respectively, or to the people."

has an obligation to provide tribes with certain services, including health-related services. In addition, American Indians and Alaska Natives are eligible as individual citizens to participate in state health programs. However, in some instances, tribal–state relations are strained, and there are often misunderstandings about the relative responsibilities of states and tribes for the financing of health care and population-based public health services. Until the mid-1970s, the federal government directly provided health care services to American Indians living on reservations and to Alaska Natives living in villages through the Indian Health Service (IHS), an agency within DHHS. In 1975, the Indian Self-Determination and Education Assistance Act (P.L. 93–638) established two other options for obtaining these services: (1) tribal governments can contract with IHS to provide the services or (2) administrative control, operation, and funding for the services can be transferred to a tribal government (IHS, 2001c). In the mid-1970s, legislation also authorized funding health services for American Indians living in urban areas.[2] The operation of IHS programs depends on annual discretionary appropriations, which are generally considered inadequate (Noren et al., 1998; IHS, 2001a). Some tribes are able to supplement IHS funding, but many cannot. Many tribes have health directors and operate extensive public health programs that include environmental safety and community health education, as well as direct curative and preventive services.

Role of the Federal Government in Assuring Population Health

The federal government acts in six main areas related to population health: (1) policy making, (2) financing, (3) public health protection, (4) collecting and disseminating information about U.S. health and health care delivery systems, (5) capacity building for population health, and (6) direct management of services (Boufford and Lee, 2001). For most of its history, the U.S. Supreme Court has granted the federal government broad powers under the Constitution to protect the public's health and safety. Under the power to "regulate Commerce . . . among several states" and other constitutional powers, the federal government acts in areas such as environmental protection, occupational health and safety, and food and drug purity (Gostin, 2000). The federal government may set conditions on the expenditure of federal funds (e.g., require adoption of a minimum age of 21 for legal consumption of alcoholic beverages to receive Federal-Aid Highway

---

[2] According to 1990 Census Bureau data, about 56 percent of the American Indian and Alaska Native population lived in urban areas (IHS, 2001b). Census data for 2000 show a similar pattern, with 57 percent of individuals who identify themselves solely as Native American or Alaska Native living in metropolitan areas (Forquera, 2001).

Funds), tax commodities whose use results in risky behavior (e.g., cigarettes), reduce taxes for socially desirable behaviors (e.g., for voluntary employer provision of health care), and regulate persons and businesses whose activities may affect interstate commerce (e.g., manufacturers of pharmaceuticals and vaccines so that they are safe and effective).

The judicial branch also can shape federal health policy in many ways. It can interpret public health statutes and determine whether agencies are acting within the scope of their legislative authority. The courts can also decide whether public health statutes and regulations are constitutionally permissible. The Supreme Court has made many decisions of fundamental importance to the public's health. The court has upheld the government's power to protect the public's health (e.g., require vaccinations), set conditions on the receipt of public funds (e.g., set a minimum drinking age), and affirmed a woman's right to reproductive privacy (e.g., a right to contraception and abortion). Gostin (2000) notes that although the courts generally have been permissive on matters of public health, stricter scrutiny has come when there is any appearance of discrimination against a suspect class or invasion of a fundamental right, such as bodily integrity.

Public Health Law: The Need for State Reforms

Because primary responsibility for protection of the public's health rests with the states, their laws and regulations concerning public health matters are critical in determining the appropriateness and effectiveness of the governmental public health infrastructure. At present, however, the law relating to public health is scattered across countless statutes and regulations at the state and local levels and is highly fragmented among the states and territories. Furthermore, public health law is beset by problems of antiquity, inconsistency, redundancy, and ambiguity that make it ineffective, or even counterproductive, in advancing the population's health.

The most striking characteristic of state public health law, and the one that underlies many of its defects, is its overall antiquity. Much of public health law contains elements that are 40 to 100 years old, and old public health statutes are often outmoded in ways that directly reduce their effectiveness and their conformity with modern legal norms in matters such as protection of individual rights.[3] These laws often do not reflect contemporary scientific understandings of health risks or the prevention and treat-

---

[3] For example, a South Dakota statute passed in the late 1800s and last amended in 1977 makes it a misdemeanor for a person infected with a "contagious disease" to "intentionally [expose] himself . . . in any public place or thoroughfare" (S.D. Codified Laws § 34–22–5). Similarly, an 1895 New Jersey statute forbids common carriers to "accept for transportation

ment of health problems. For example, laws aimed at preventing casual transmission of airborne diseases such as influenza and measles have little relevance for control of the sexually transmitted and blood-borne pathogens that are major concerns of health authorities today (Gostin et al., 1999). When many of these statutes were written, the science of public health, in fields such as epidemiology and biostatistics, and of behavior and behavioral interventions, such as client-centered counseling, was in its infancy.

Related to the problem of antiquity is the problem of multiple layers of law. The law in most states consists of successive layers of statutes and amendments, built up over more than 100 years in some cases, in response to changing perceptions of health threats. This is particularly troublesome in the area of infectious diseases, which forms a substantial part of state health codes. Colorado's disease control statute, for example, has separate sections for venereal diseases, tuberculosis, and HIV. All three sections authorize compulsory control measures, but they vary significantly in the procedures required and the public health philosophy expressed. Whereas the venereal disease statute simply empowers compulsory examination whenever health officials deem it necessary, the HIV section sets out a list of increasingly intrusive options (requiring use of the least restrictive) and places the burden of proof on the health department to show a danger to public health (Gostin et al., 1999).

Because health codes in each state and territory have evolved independently, they show profound variations in their structures, substance, and procedures for detecting, controlling, and preventing injury and disease. In fact, statutes and regulations among American jurisdictions vary so significantly in definitions, methods, age, and scope that they defy orderly categorization. There is, however, good reason for greater uniformity among the states in matters of public health. Health threats are rarely confined to single jurisdictions, instead posing risks across regions or the entire nation.

State laws do not have to be identical. There is often a justification for the differences in approaches among the states if there are divergent needs or circumstances. There is also a case for states' acting as laboratories to determine the best approach. Nevertheless, a certain amount of consistency

---

within this state any person affected with a communicable disease or any article of clothing, bedding, or other property so infected" without a license from the local board of health (N.J. Stat. Ann. § 26:4–11 9). This might have made some sense in a time when diseases such as influenza, diphtheria, and measles were significant sources of serious illness and death, but it serves little purpose today. Although it may be impolite for people with the flu to walk around in public, it is not a major health threat. Furthermore, efforts to isolate people who do not pose a significant health risk would often violate modern disability discrimination law (it was held that the threat of disease did not justify excessively stringent quarantine of a blind plaintiff's guide dog) (see *Crowder v. Kitagawa*, 81 F.3d 1480, 1481, 9th Circuit, 1996).

is vital in public health. Infectious diseases and other health threats do not confine themselves to state boundaries but pose regional or even national challenges. States must be able to engage in surveillance and respond to health threats in a predictable and consistent fashion, using similar legal structures. Consistent public health statutes would help facilitate surveillance and data sharing, communication, and coordinated responses to health threats among the states. Consider the coordination that would be necessary if a biological attack were to occur in the tristate area of New York, New Jersey, and Connecticut. Laws that complicate or hinder data communication among states and responsible agencies would impede a thorough investigation and response to such a public health emergency.

To remedy the problems of antiquity, inconsistency, redundancy, and ambiguity, the Robert Wood Johnson and W. K. Kellogg Foundations' Turning Point initiative launched a Public Health Statute Modernization Collaborative in 2000 "to transform and strengthen the legal framework for the public health system through a collaborative process to develop a model public health law" (Gostin, 2002). The model public health law focuses on the organization, delivery, and funding of essential public health services, as well as the mission and powers of public health agencies. It is scheduled for completion by October 2003, and current drafts are available on the Turning Point website, at http://www.turningpointprogram.org.

The process of law reform took on new urgency after the events of September 11, 2001, and the subsequent intentional dispersal of anthrax through the postal system. In response, the Center for Law and the Public's Health at Georgetown University and Johns Hopkins University drafted the Model State Emergency Health Powers Act (MSEHPA) at the request of CDC (www.publichealthlaw.net). DHHS recommends that each state review its legislative and regulatory needs and requirements for public health preparedness. MSEHPA offers a guide or checklist for governors and legislatures to review their current laws. As of September 2002, three-quarters of the states had introduced a version of MSEHPA, and 19 states had adopted all or part of the act (Gostin et al., 2002). The model act, under review by federal and state officials, defines the purpose of the legislation as giving the governor and other state and local authorities the powers and ability to prevent, detect, manage, and contain emergency health threats without unduly interfering with civil rights and liberties. The legislation would address matters including reporting requirements, information sharing, access to contaminated facilities, medical examination and testing, and procedures for isolation and quarantine (Center for Law and the Public's Health, 2001).

CDC is facilitating the law reform process through its internal Public Health Law Collaborative. Efforts are in place to improve scientific understanding of the interaction between law and public health and to strengthen the legal foundation for public health practice. Through the Public Health Law Collaborative, CDC is joined in its work in public health law by a growing number of partners. These include public health practice associations, academic institutions and researchers, and public policy organizations (www.phppo.cdc.gov/PhLawNet).

The committee finds that the problems of antiquity, inconsistency, redundancy, and ambiguity render many public health laws ineffective or even counterproductive in improving population health. A set of standards and procedures would add needed clarity and coherence to legal regulation. Therefore, **the committee recommends that the Secretary of the Department of Health and Human Services, in consultation with states, appoint a national commission to develop a framework and recommendations for state public health law reform. In particular, the national commission would review all existing public health law as well as the Turning Point[4] Model State Public Health Act and the Model State Emergency Health Powers Act[5]; provide guidance and technical assistance to help states reform their laws to meet modern scientific and legal standards; and help foster greater consistency within and among states, especially in their approach to different health threats.** It is essential that any reform of public health legislation address the powers needed to deal effectively with bioterrorism and other public health emergencies that pose significant threats across state boundaries. Each state could adapt the commission's recommendations to its unique legal structures and particular needs for public health preparedness. Public health is traditionally a state function, so the commission would provide guidance to the states rather than impose standards.

The following section provides a description of the federal, state, and local governmental agencies that are responsible for protecting the health of the public. Later in the chapter, the committee examines certain aspects of the state and local public health infrastructures that are of special concern.

The State and Local Governmental Public Health Infrastructure

Although the states carry the primary constitutional responsibility and authority for public health activities in the United States, public health

---

[4] Turning Point, a program funded by the Robert Wood Johnson and W. K. Kellogg Foundations, works to strengthen the public health infrastructure at the state and local levels across the United States and spearheads the Turning Point National Collaborative on Public Health Statute Modernization.

[5] The Model State Emergency Health Powers Act (MSEHPA) provides states with the powers needed "to detect and contain bioterrorism or a naturally occurring disease outbreak. Legislative bills based on MSEHPA have been introduced in 34 states" (Gostin et al., 2002).

administration first began in cities in the late eighteenth century (Rosen, 1993). The burgeoning social problems of industrial cities convinced legislatures to form more elaborate and professional public health administrations within municipal governments (Duffy, 1990). City boards of health were established to obtain effective agency supervision and control of health threats facing the population. Only after the Civil War did states form boards of health. County and rural health departments emerged in the early twentieth century (Ferrell and Mead, 1936). Today, there are more than 3,000 local public health agencies, 3,000 local boards of health, and 60 state, territorial, and tribal health departments (CDC, 2001b).

Structure and Governance of State and Local Public Health Agencies

The organization and authority granted to state and local public health agencies vary substantially across the country. Every state has an agency with responsibility for public health activities. That agency may be an independent department or a component of a department with broader responsibilities, such as human services programs. In 31 states, the state health officer is also the head of the larger health and human services agency (Turnock, 2000). Physicians and nurses often lead state public health agencies. At the local level, however, general managers with business training rather than formal training in public health or medicine may lead public health agencies.

States differ in terms of the relationship between the state agency and the agencies serving localities within the state. In some states (e.g., Arkansas, Florida, Georgia, and Missouri), the state public health infrastructure is centralized, meaning that the state agency has direct control and authority for supervision of local public health agencies. In other states (e.g., California, Illinois, and Ohio), local public health agencies developed independently from the state agency, in that they are run by counties or townships (rather than the state) and report directly to local boards of health or health commissioners or are governed by cooperative agreements. Still other states (e.g., Iowa and North Dakota) have no local public health agencies and the state public health agency is preeminent (Fraser, 1998).

In a recent report on the local public health agency infrastructure, the National Association of County and City Health Officials (NACCHO) (2001d) identified five types of local public health agencies (see Figure 3–1).

The most common arrangement is a local public health agency (LPHA) serving a single county, ranging from small rural counties (e.g., Issaquena County, Mississippi, with a population less than 1,000) to large metropolitan counties (e.g., Los Angeles County, with a population approaching 10 million). LPHAs may also serve single cities of various sizes (e.g., Kansas City, Missouri, and New York City). A combined city–county local public

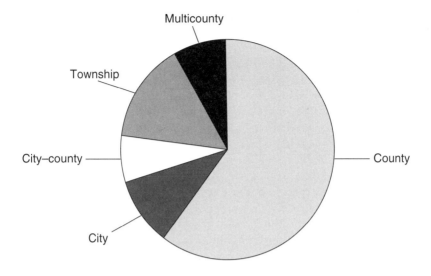

FIGURE 3–1   Types of local public health agencies (LPHAs) across the United States.

health agency is also found (e.g., Seattle-King County, Washington). Township local public health agencies are common in states with strong "home-rule" political systems[6] (e.g., Connecticut, Massachusetts, and New Jersey). City or township health agencies may operate within counties that are also served by county health agencies.

Multicounty local public health agencies often span large geographic areas in the western United States. For example, the Northeast Colorado Health District serves six counties, an area roughly equivalent in size to that of the state of Vermont. In these local public health agencies, health directors may be accountable to multiple county boards of health or to a combined board of health whose membership represents the counties or other units covered by the local public health agency. The multicounty local public health agency category also includes state health department regional offices that act as local public health agencies, an arrangement found in several states (e.g., Alabama, New Mexico, Tennessee, and Vermont).

The governance of state and local public health agencies generally fits

---

[6] Home-rule statutes (in constitutions or by statute) give localities (e.g., cities or counties) powers of self-government. In such cases, localities can exercise police powers independently from the state.

one of three models. In a cabinet model, the head of the agency is appointed by and answers to the governor, mayor, or other executive authority. Under a board-of-health model, the state or local health director reports to an appointed board representing constituencies served by the department. In many cases, however, a board of health functions in a strictly advisory capacity, with no oversight authority. Under an "umbrella" model, the public health agency is part of a larger agency, and the health director either heads the agency or reports to its head. There are considerable variations within these three models.

Even with this great variability in governance at both the state and local levels, there are no data to suggest what an "ideal" state and local agency governance structure might be. Thus, it would be important for state agencies to examine their present governance structures and evaluate mechanisms to make these structures more effective. Doing so should serve to build and strengthen relationships with local public health agencies, coordinate efforts for the delivery of the essential public health services and crisis response services, integrate essential health information, and respond to the changing health needs of the population.

Scope of Agency Responsibilities and Activities

At both the state and local levels, there are differences among public health agencies in terms of the scope of their authority, responsibilities, and activities. At the state level, activities such as immunization, infectious disease control and reporting, health education, and health statistics are common to most public health agencies. States are also responsible for licensing and regulating the institutional and individual providers that deliver health care services. However, states differ in whether the public health agency has responsibility for programs such as mental health and substance abuse, environmental health, and Medicaid. These organizational differences make it more complicated to frame and pursue a coherent national agenda concerning changes and improvements in the governmental public health infrastructure.

A recent NACCHO (2001e) survey of local public health agency infrastructures has helped document the variation in services provided at the local level. Among county health departments, for example, 98 percent provided childhood immunizations (directly or through contract services), 76 percent were responsible for restaurant inspections and licensing, and 31 percent provided dental services. City and township local public health agencies were often less likely to offer services that other types of local public health agencies provided. The most common services provided by local public health agencies include those most associated with traditional public health practice: adult and childhood immunizations, communicable disease control, community assessment, community outreach and education, environmental health services, epidemiology and surveillance, food safety, health education, restaurant inspections, and tuberculosis testing. Services provided by a smaller percentage of local public health agencies included treatment for chronic disease, behavioral and mental health services, programs for the homeless, substance abuse services, and veterinary public health (NACCHO, 2001d).

One widespread change in the scope of local public health agency activities is a reduction in the direct delivery of health care services, especially to Medicaid participants. This is consistent with a national effort to have governmental public health agencies return their attention to the more population-based public health services that had been weakened by the pressing need to provide safety-net services to uninsured individuals. Although some have been unable to do so, many state and local public health agencies now have contracts with managed care organizations and other private providers to serve those populations. A substantial transfer of service delivery from health departments to private providers has also occurred for childhood immunizations under federal and state programs for the purchase and distribution of vaccines (IOM, 2000a). Some researchers have found the partnership between managed care and local public health agencies to be positively associated with the overall scope and perceived effectiveness of local public health activities in terms of their ability to meet population-based community needs (Mays et al., 2001). (See Chapter 5 for additional discussion of the role of health care services providers in the public health system.) However, some local public health agencies have found it difficult to compensate for the loss of revenue that had previously come from the delivery of health care services that have now been transferred to managed care organizations (Wall, 1998; Keane et al., 2001).

THE FEDERAL PUBLIC HEALTH INFRASTRUCTURE

In contrast to state and local public health agencies, the federal government has a limited role in the direct delivery of essential public health services. Nevertheless, it plays a crucial role in protecting and improving the health of the population by providing leadership in setting health goals, policies, and standards, especially through its regulatory powers. It also contributes operational and financial resources: to assure financing of health care for vulnerable populations through Medicare, Medicaid, Community and Migrant Health Centers, and IHS programs; to finance research and higher education; and to support development of the scientific and technological tools needed to improve the effectiveness of the public health infrastructure at all levels.

Organization of the Federal Public Health Infrastructure

At the federal level, the lead entity responsible for public health activities is DHHS. Several key agencies in DHHS comprise the U.S. Public Health Service (PHS): the Agency for Healthcare Research and Quality, CDC, the Agency for Toxic Substances and Disease Registry (ATSDR), the Food and Drug Administration (FDA), the Health Resources and Services Administration (HRSA), IHS, the National Institutes of Health (NIH), and the Substance Abuse and Mental Health Services Administration (SAMHSA). In addition, various White House agencies such as the Office of Science and Technology Policy and the Office of National Drug Control Policy, 14 cabinet-level departments and agencies (e.g., Department of Agriculture, Department of Transportation, EPA, Department of Veterans Affairs [VA], and Department of Defense [DOD]), and more than 10 public corporations and commissions and subcabinet agencies are responsible for certain health programs.

The U.S. Congress oversees the activities of federal agencies through committees that review the authorization of programs and the appropriation of funds. Multiple committees in both the House of Representatives and the Senate have jurisdiction over DHHS programs and health-related activities in other departments. These multiple authorities and congressional jurisdictions are an important reason for the "disarray" noted in previous IOM reports.

Scope of DHHS Responsibilities and Activities

Although activities and responsibilities related to public health are spread throughout the federal government, the committee focused its attention on DHHS and its agencies as the principal federal component of the nation's governmental public health infrastructure and as the principal point of contact for other federal agencies with health or health-related programs and for state and local public health agencies. Reviewed briefly here are DHHS activities related to the previously noted functions of policy making, financing of public health activities, public health protection, collection and dissemination of information about U.S. health and health care delivery systems, capacity building for population health, and direct management of services. Some of these activities are considered in more detail later in this chapter, in conjunction with the discussion of specific concerns regarding weaknesses in the nation's governmental public health infrastructure.

Policy Making

Policy making is a critical function for DHHS and involves the initiation, shaping, and ultimately, implementation of congressional and presidential decisions. It involves the creation and use of an evidence base, informed by social values, so that public decision makers can shape legislation, regulations, and programs. The annual budget cycle is routinely the time when lawmakers present new legislation and renew legislation for existing programs and when DHHS defends proposed program budgets to Congress. Policy making also occurs through program initiatives that do not require legislative action. One of the leading examples in public health is the Healthy People initiative, which establishes national goals and objectives for health promotion and disease prevention. The Healthy People initiative is led by the DHHS Office of Disease Prevention and Health Promotion and now involves all DHHS operating divisions, other federal departments, and partnerships with state and local public health officials, as well as more than 350 national membership organizations, nongovernmental organizations, and corporate sponsors. Although the effort is voluntary, the activity and regular widespread public consultation involved in the initiative have perhaps proved to be the department's most effective nonlegislative policy vehicle for promoting action on population health at the national, state, and local levels (Boufford and Lee, 2001).

Financing of Public Health Activities

Through a variety of mechanisms—grants, contracts, and reimbursements through publicly funded health insurance programs—DHHS is an important financial contributor to the activities of state and local governmental public health agencies, primarily by financing personal health care services through mandatory spending for the entitlement programs of Medicaid. The fiscal year (FY) 2002 budget for Medicaid amounted to $142 billion (OMB, 2001b); in sharp contrast, the DHHS discretionary budget for PHS agencies in FY 2002 was about $41 billion, of which $23.2 billion was designated for NIH. Very little of this discretionary money goes directly to states for governmental public health agency infrastructure.

Public Health Protection

Public health protection is perhaps the most classic public health function of the federal government. In this regard, the federal government uses its surveillance capacity to assess health risks and its standard-setting and regulatory powers to protect the public from health risks: unfair treatment; low-quality services; and unsafe foods, medicines, biologics such as blood and medical devices, as well as environmental and occupational health hazards. In addition to certain regulatory responsibilities, DHHS also develops and maintains a research base that produces the scientific evidence needed to support the regulations in health-related areas that other federal agencies use. The principal regulatory agencies of DHHS are FDA for drugs and biologics, medical devices, and certain foods and the Centers for Medicare and Medicaid Services (CMS) for health care providers. Both CMS and FDA are responsible for regulatory oversight of laboratories (Boufford and Lee, 2001). Other departments and agencies outside DHHS are also responsible for regulations that protect health.[7]

Collection and Dissemination of Information

Timely and reliable data are an essential component of public health assessment, policy development, and assurance at all levels of government. DHHS, particularly the PHS agencies, sponsors a variety of public health and health care data systems and activities. These include national vital and health statistics, household surveys on health and nutrition, health care delivery cost and utilization information, and reporting requirements for programs funded by federal grants or assistance. The National Center for Health Statistics within CDC is the primary agency collecting and reporting health information for the federal government. CMS collects administrative data on the Medicare and Medicaid programs and conducts beneficiary surveys. The Administration for Children and Families and the Administration on Aging also collect data on human services. Other agencies (e.g., the Census Bureau, the Department of Agriculture, and the Department of Labor) also collect data that are important for public health purposes. In addition, the collection and dissemination of research findings can be considered part of this activity.

---

[7] Federal agencies have developed numerous regulatory techniques and decision-making processes to identify and respond to health and safety risks (Gostin, 2000). Agencies can control entry into a field by requiring a license or permit to undertake specified activities; set health and safety standards, conduct inspections to ensure compliance, adjudicate violations, and impose penalties; abate nuisances that threaten the public; dispense grants, subsidies, or other incentives; and influence conduct through a wide variety of informal methods (Gostin, 2000). For example, the Department of Agriculture regulates the safety of meat, poultry, and eggs. EPA regulates air and water pollution, pesticides, and toxic wastes. The Department of Energy oversees radiation-related environmental management, environmental safety and health, and civilian radioactive waste management. The Department of Labor regulates occupational health and safety and self-insured employee benefit plans. The Department of Transportation sets and monitors standards for highway safety. The Bureau of Alcohol, Tobacco, and Firearms in the Department of the Treasury, the Consumer Product Safety Commission, the Federal Trade Commission, and the Occupational Safety and Health Administration also issue regulations that protect the public against health risks (Boufford and Lee, 2001).

Capacity Building for Population Health

The capacity-building function of the federal government centers on ensuring the ability of its own agencies to effectively discharge their responsibilities. It also centers on ensuring that state and local levels of government have the resources—human, financial, and organizational—they need to carry out the responsibilities delegated to them by the federal government or for which they are responsible by law as they work to assure and promote the health of the communities that they serve. In terms of the public health infrastructure, this includes striving for effective collaboration within DHHS, between DHHS and other cabinet departments for domestic and international health policy, and between DHHS and state and local public health departments. With more than 200 categorical public health programs in DHHS and a variety of health-related programs in other federal agencies, the alignment of policies and strategies is challenging. This also makes it difficult to devise an approach to the systematic and accountable long-term investment of federal funding in governmental public health agencies at the state and local levels.

Direct Management of Services

Federal funding supports the delivery of medical care through a variety of categorical grant programs (e.g., for community health centers and maternal and child health services) and insurance programs (e.g., Medicaid and Medicare). However, the direct management of clinical or other services delivered to individuals is a small part of DHHS's role. Under DHHS, direct medical care and public health services are provided primarily by IHS, which serves members of federally recognized American Indian tribes. As tribal governments assume greater responsibility for managing these services, the role of IHS could evolve into that of a payer or purchaser rather than a provider of services. In addition, DOD and VA play larger direct management roles in the provision of health care services for their particular constituencies.

The next section highlights the current status of certain critical components of the public health infrastructure that support the public health system in carrying out essential public health functions. These components include the public health workforce, information and data systems, and public health laboratories. The section also reviews how these components of the infrastructure are critical to emergency preparedness and response activities.

CRITICAL COMPONENTS OF
THE PUBLIC HEALTH INFRASTRUCTURE

The Public Health Workforce

The governmental public health infrastructure at the federal, state, and local levels consists of physical resources (e.g., laboratories), information networks, and human resources (the public health workforce). An adequately sized and appropriately trained workforce performing competently is an essential element of the public health infrastructure. The public health workforce at the federal, state, and local levels must be prepared to respond to an array of needs, such as the assurance of health-related environmental safety, the interpretation of scientific data that can influence health outcomes, or the clarification of vast amounts of highly technical information after a community emergency. In addition to meeting the scientific and technical requirements of public health practice, state and local public health officials are often expected to provide community leadership, manage community reactions, and communicate about risk, protection, and prevention.

Current estimates indicate that approximately 450,000 individuals are working in salaried public health positions, with many more contributing to this mission through nongovernmental organizations or on a voluntary basis (HRSA, 2000). Public health practitioners have training in a variety of disciplines, including the biological and health sciences, psychology, education, nutrition, ethics, sociology, epidemiology, biostatistics, business, computer science, political science, law, public affairs, and urban planning.

Recent studies have shown, however, that the current public health workforce is unevenly prepared to meet the challenges that accompany the practice of public health today. An estimated 80 percent of the current workforce lacks formal training in public health (CDC-ATSDR, 2001). Moreover, the major changes in technology, biomedical knowledge, informatics, and community expectations will continue to challenge and redefine the practice of public health, requiring that current public health practitioners receive the additional, ongoing training and support they need to update their existing skills (Pew Health Professions Commission, 1998).

Training and Education for the Public Health Workforce

Competency-Based Training

Given that early public health efforts in the United States were aimed at improving sanitation, controlling infectious diseases, assuring the safety of food and water supplies, and immunizing children, it is hardly surprising that public health workers at that time were predominantly graduates of schools of medicine, nursing, and the biological sciences. Today, however, the public health workforce has broader responsibilities and must be much more diverse. For example, as part of the performance of essential services, members of the public health workforce must be prepared to engage the community in effective actions to promote mental, physical, environmental, and social health. Advances in biomedical and genomics research and technologies have the potential to change the way public health practitioners think about population-level disease risk and how disease prevention and health promotion activities might be practiced. Moreover, rapidly evolving computer and information technologies and the use of mass media and social marketing have the potential to revolutionize health departments' access to up-to-date surveillance information, disease databases, and communications networks as well as to enhance worker productivity.

The need to strengthen the public health workforce was recognized by IOM in 1988 and has been the focus of a variety of efforts since then. Some of these activities will be discussed in the chapter on the role of academia in the public health system (Chapter 8). A few key efforts focusing on the current workforce (rather than training new workers) are also covered here. In particular, the report *The Public Health Workforce: An Agenda for the 21st Century* (USPHS, 1997) called for greater leadership on workforce issues from national, state, and local public health agencies; use of a standard taxonomy to better assess and monitor workforce composition; competency-based curriculum development; and greater use of new technologies for distance learning. The Taskforce for Public Health Workforce Development, established in 1999 by CDC and ATSDR, recommended six broad strategies for a national public health workforce development agenda (CDC, 2000e):

1. Monitor current workforce composition and project future needs.
2. Identify competencies and develop curricula.
3. Design integrated learning systems.
4. Use incentives to promote public health practice competencies.
5. Conduct and support evaluation and research.
6. Assure financial support for a lifelong learning system in public health.

An almost universal priority for workforce development is ensuring that all public health practitioners have mastery over a basic set of competencies involving generalizable knowledge, skills, and abilities that allow them to effectively and efficiently function as part of their public health organizations or systems (CDC-ATSDR, 2000; DHHS, 2000; CDC, 2001d) (see Appendix E for an extended list of competencies for public health workers). Many experienced public health professionals require a variety of cross-cutting competencies to help them meet the routine and emergent

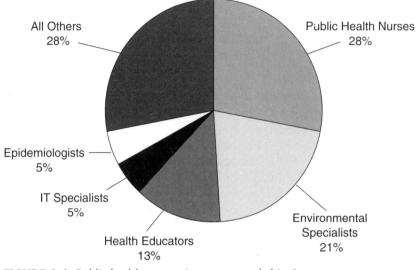

FIGURE 3–2 Public health occupations most needed in 5 years.

challenges of public health, as well as specialized skills and abilities in areas such as maternal and child health, community health, and genomics. In addition, a recent survey of the local public health infrastructure found that several specific public health occupations are projected to be the most needed in the coming 5 years (NACCHO, 2001e). These occupations included public health nurses, epidemiologists, and environmental specialists (NACCHO, 2001e) (see Figure 3–2).

The Council on Linkages between Academia and Public Health Practice[8] has developed a list of 68 core public health competencies in eight domains (see Box 3–2), with different levels of competency expectations for frontline public health workers, senior professional staff, program specialists, and leaders (Council on Linkages between Academia and Public Health Practice, 2001). An expert panel convened by CDC, ATSDR, and HRSA has recommended adoption of this list as the basis for competency-based training of the public health workforce (CDC, 2000e). Use of this list as the basis for training and continuing education for the public health workforce

---

[8] The Council on Linkages between Academia and Public Health Practice is composed of leaders from national organizations representing the public health practice and academic communities. The council grew out of the Public Health Faculty/Agency Forum, which developed recommendations for improving the relevance of public health education to the demands of public health in the practice sector. The council and its partners have focused attention on the need for a public health practice research agenda.

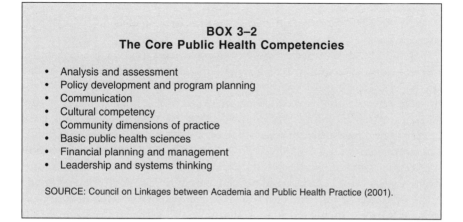

BOX 3–2
The Core Public Health Competencies

- Analysis and assessment
- Policy development and program planning
- Communication
- Cultural competency
- Community dimensions of practice
- Basic public health sciences
- Financial planning and management
- Leadership and systems thinking

SOURCE: Council on Linkages between Academia and Public Health Practice (2001).

was recommended, regardless of the programmatic or categorical focus of the training (CDC, 2000e). Efforts are under way in the various public health training networks to establish models that will contribute to a systematic approach to competency-based training that is linked to the essential services framework and grounded in prior competency validation efforts (CDC, 2000e).

Meeting the Needs for Workforce Development

The issue of workforce training and competency is central to the success of any public health system. Governmental public health agencies have a responsibility to identify the public health workforce needs within their jurisdictions and to implement policies and programs to fill those needs. In addition, an assessment of current competency levels and needs is essential to develop and deliver the appropriate competency-based training, as well as to evaluate the impact of that training in practice settings. Workforce training and education efforts may be conducted in partnership with academia and other relevant and appropriate community partners, and ideally, a percentage of public health employees should be targeted annually for continuing education (DHHS, 2000). These and other issues are discussed in the 2003 IOM report *Who Will Keep the Public Healthy: Educating Public Health Professionals for the 21st Century.*

Training resources for the public health workforce are expanding, spurred by modest funding by HRSA for Public Health Training Centers and by CDC for Public Health Preparedness Centers. By mid-2002, there were 14 Training Centers and 15 Preparedness Centers, which form the backbone of a national public health training network. Both types of centers promote a variety of general workforce development strategies, although the CDC-funded centers place a heavier emphasis on bioterrorism preparedness.

Given the importance of the workforce in carrying out the mission of public health, the committee finds that education and development of the current workforce must continue to be a fundamental priority within the broader efforts to improve the state and local public health infrastructure. Therefore, **the committee recommends that all federal, state, and local governmental public health agencies develop strategies to ensure that public health workers who are involved in the provision of essential public health services demonstrate mastery of the core public health competencies appropriate to their jobs. The Council on Linkages between Academia and Public Health Practice should also encourage the competency development of public health professionals working in public health system roles in for-profit and nongovernmental entities.**

To facilitate ongoing workforce development, the committee encourages public health agencies to engage in training partnerships with academia to ensure the availability of coordinated, continuous, and accessible systems of education. These systems should be capable of addressing a variety of workforce training needs, ranging from education on the basic competencies to continuing education for individuals in the specialized professional disciplines of public health science.

Furthermore, **the committee recommends that Congress designate funds for CDC and HRSA to periodically assess the preparedness of the public health workforce, to document the training necessary to meet basic competency expectations, and to advise on the funding necessary to provide such training.**

Preparing Public Health Leaders

Senior public health officials must have the preparation not only to manage a government agency but also to provide guidance to the workforce with regard to health goals or priorities, interact with stakeholders and constituency groups, provide policy direction to a governing board, and interact with other agencies at all levels of government whose actions and decisions affect the population whose health they are trying to assure (Turnock, 2000). These tasks require a unique and demanding set of talents: professional expertise in the specific subject area; substantive expertise in the content and values of public health; and competencies in the core skills of leadership. Those who have mastery of the skills to mobilize, coordinate, and direct broad collaborative actions within the complex public health system must lead in implementing the actions outlined in this report. They require the skills for vision, communication, and implementation. Although many of these skills are innate for most professionals and other leaders, they need constant refinement and honing.

CDC has pioneered the development and funding of a national Public Health Leadership Institute, and in the intervening dozen years, more than 500 leaders in public health have been exposed to leadership training and skill building (described in more detail in the Academia chapter). Furthermore, a similar network of State and Regional Public Health Leadership Institutes has been funded and, over time, has developed the capacity to work collaboratively through a national network, which permits institutes to benchmark and share best practices and continue the process of learning needed to help with state-of-the art curriculum and educational training efforts. Equally notable has been the development of the Management Academy for Public Health, a joint effort of the major public health philanthropies. Although effort is still at an early stage, this academy has already generated graduates who work hand in glove with senior leadership in public health organizations. Furthermore, the Turning Point Initiative devotes efforts to increasing collaborative leadership across all sectors and at all levels (Larson et al., 2002)

Another key to leadership is continuity in office long enough to exert the leadership and to provide the institutional memory to defend public health agencies and the public health sector from the political winds of the moment. Yet, the committee finds there has been great difficulty in recruiting, developing, and retaining the leaders so vital to the job.

A state health official's term, if that official is a political appointee, is tied to the governor's term. Health officials must work with legislators who operate on 2-year terms. Given that the average tenure of a state health officer is relatively short (an average of 3.9 years and a median of 2.9 years) (ASTHO, 2002), many state health officials find it difficult to create longer-term plans for achieving health goals on shorter-term time frames (Meit, 2001). Additionally, because state health officers report to many governing bodies, they generally have less direct access to policy makers, and state health officials must prioritize the issues that they think deserve the most attention (Meit, 2001). Political factors at the state level can also have a significant impact on the abilities of public health leadership to influence policy. To address the specific issues of discontinuity occasioned by the rapid turnover, particularly of state health officials, the Robert Wood Johnson Foundation has funded a unique State Health Leadership Initiative administered by the National Governors Association to immerse newly appointed officials in a curriculum for political leadership and provide a network of resources and mentors.

Governmental public health leadership is a critical component of the infrastructure that must be strengthened, supported, and held accountable by all of the partners of the public health system and the community at large. For this reason, **the committee recommends that leadership training, support, and development be a high priority for governmental public health agencies and other organizations in the public health system and for schools of public health that supply the public health infrastructure with its professionals and leaders.**

Considering Credentialing as a Tool for Workforce Development

Credentialing is a mechanism that is used to certify specific levels of professional preparation. There are many different forms of credentials, including academic degrees, professional certifications, and licenses. For example, medical credentials include medical degrees to certify successful completion of course work, professional testing (e.g., through medical board exams) to provide evidence of qualification to practice medicine, and medical licensing to establish compliance with state standards for medical practice. An individual credentialed as a Certified Health Education Specialist (CHES) has successfully completed a course of study and passed a competency-based test.

Although some public health workers are credentialed as physicians, nurses, health educators, or environmental health practitioners, few are credentialed within those professions specifically for public health practice. Most physicians working in public health lack board certification in preventive medicine or public health; most nurses working in public health lack credentials in community public health nursing; and most individuals working as health educators lack the CHES credential. Furthermore, no single credentialing or certification process has been established to test the various competencies required for the interdisciplinary field of public health; thus, the majority of the public health workforce (80 percent) lacks credentials (HRSA, 2000).

Given the importance of establishing and maintaining a competent public health workforce, CDC and other public health agencies and organizations, including NACCHO, the Association of State and Territorial Health Officials (ASTHO), the Association of Schools of Public Health, and the American Public Health Association (APHA), are examining the feasibility of creating a credentialing system for public health workers based on competencies linked to the essential public health services framework. CDC (2001d) has recommended the use of credentialing. Such a process would complement efforts to establish national public health performance standards for state and local public health systems based on the essential public health services framework and the related objectives of *Healthy People 2010* (Objective 23–11) (DHHS, 2000). Although this national effort focuses on experienced public health leaders, support is growing for the concept of credentialing at a basic level all public health workers and at an intermediate level the experienced professionals from many disciplines who share the need for higher-level, cross-cutting competencies in the areas of public health practice, community health assessment, policy development, communication, and program development and evaluation.

Certification or credentialing would help establish that public health practitioners have a demonstrated level of accomplishment in and mastery of the principles of public health practice. In terms of building the capacity of the public health workforce, the credentialing process could help document the knowledge, skills, and performance of experienced workers who may not have formal academic training and could encourage other workers to seek additional training to meeting credentialing requirements. An especially important component of this process is that it could play a key role in shaping the training and preparation of future public health practitioners and leaders.

The key challenge is whether and how public health organizations can begin to integrate competency-based credentialing in their hiring, promotion, performance appraisal, and salary structures. Although the idea of credentialing has considerable support at the federal level, states and particularly localities have voiced concerns that workforce credentialing mandates may become too closely tied to federal funding mechanisms. In these situations, the fiscal impact could be grave for public health departments that do not or cannot meet credentialing requirements (community informants, personal communications to the committee, 2001).

The committee finds that in the ongoing debate about public health workforce credentialing, what is most needed is a national dialogue that can address the full range of issues and concerns. Therefore, **the committee recommends that a formal national dialogue be initiated to address the issue of public health workforce credentialing. The Secretary of DHHS should appoint a national commission on public health workforce credentialing to lead this dialogue. The commission should be charged with determining if a credentialing system would further the goal of creating a competent workforce and, if applicable, the manner and time frame for implementation by governmental public health agencies at all levels. The dialogue should include representatives from federal, state, and local public health agencies, academia, and public health professional organizations who can represent and discuss the various perspectives on the workforce credentialing debate.**

Special Need for Communication Skills

The role of communication in public health practice cannot be underestimated. It is crucial for the successful performance of public health's core functions and essential services. Governmental public health agencies must communicate effectively internally as well as externally with other governmental agencies and nongovernmental stakeholders and partners. Informing and advising the public about health promotion and disease prevention are standard duties of both state and local public health agencies, and listening to community voices is also critical for programs to be effective. In emergency situations, public health professionals must have the ability to communicate clearly and effectively—being aggressive and credible enough to command attention—with both the public and other officials about the nature of the health hazards and the steps necessary to minimize health risks.

The response to the discovery of anthrax exposures in the fall of 2001 brought into sharp focus the importance of effective communication in the face of serious health risks. According to *New York Times* medical reporter Dr. Lawrence Altman, lapses and delays in communication with the public and with public health and health care professionals could have made the situation worse had the anthrax exposures been more widespread (Altman, 2001). Altman found that the delay was attributed in part to Federal Emergency Response Act restrictions about disclosing information and to the Federal Bureau of Investigation's (FBI's) criminal investigation. Altman suggested, however, that CDC could have issued information as a part of the parallel public health investigation that was already under way. The initial paucity of information on anthrax and the investigations in the *Morbidity and Mortality Weekly Report* (*MMWR*), one of CDC's most valuable means of quickly informing public health and health care professionals about communicable diseases, was also noted (Altman, 2001). *MMWR*'s editor reported being "out of the [information] loop" for some time (Altman, 2001). It should be noted that CDC used the Health Alert Network many times after September 11, 2001, to alert public health officials and to disseminate information.

The federal government's handling of the anthrax attacks also prompted criticism of DHHS for uncoordinated communication as well as a convoluted and inadequate public communication strategy (Connolly, 2001). For example, as reported by the press, the department's initial decisions to direct all media requests through the Secretary's press office effectively silenced CDC, FDA, and NIH, the agencies with the most relevant expertise (Connolly, 2001). The lack of information from DHHS was also frustrating to other federal, state, and local leaders and governmental public health officials, some of whom learned about new cases and contamination in their states though network and cable television newscasts (Connolly, 2001). The lesson from these and other communication breakdowns is evident: clear and effective communication, both internal and external, is a critical service of the governmental public health infrastructure.

Under more normal circumstances, public health communication is important for gathering information from the community about their health concerns as well as delivering and even "marketing" health information to the public. Because the responsibilities of public health agencies cover all aspects of health, public health officials are in a unique position to provide timely, accurate health-related information to the public on a wide variety of topics, ranging from depression and other mental health issues to obesity and physical activity, environmental health and safety, emergency preparedness, and policies that affect health or health outcomes.

However, few public health agencies have staff members who are trained to interact effectively with the public and to work effectively with the news media. In fact, the most recent examination of the public health workforce indicated that 575 individuals in the public health workforce have the expertise to be classified in the category of "Public Relations/ Media Specialist" (HRSA, 2000). Of these 575 people, most are working in DHHS and other federal health agencies. Of the others, 115 are working in state and territorial public health agencies and 12 are working in voluntary agencies (HRSA, 2000).

Given the tremendous potential of the mass media and evolving information technologies, such as the Internet, to influence the knowledge, normative beliefs, and behavior patterns of individuals and groups, governmental public health agencies must be prepared to use these communication tools. The public health workforce must have sufficient expertise in communications to be able to engage diverse audiences with public health information and messages and to work with the media to ensure the accuracy of the health-related information they convey to the public. For example, public health officials can develop relationships with journalists and assist them in accurately representing health risks and interpreting the significance of new research findings so that reporting on public health issues is accurate and members of the public can make informed decisions about protecting their health.

For these reasons, the committee finds that communication skills and competencies are crucial to the effective performance of the 10 essential public health services and the practice of public health at the federal, state, and local levels. Therefore, **the committee recommends that all partners within the public health system place special emphasis on communication as a critical core competency of public health practice. Governmental public health agencies at all levels should use existing and emerging tools (including information technologies) for effective management of public health information and for internal and external communication. To be effective, such communication must be culturally appropriate and suitable to the literacy levels of the individuals in the communities they serve.** To build this capacity in the public health workforce, communications skills and competencies should be included in the curricula of all workforce development programs. Communication competencies should include training in risk communication, interpersonal and group methods for gathering and transmitting information, and interfacing with the public about public health information and issues, as well as the interpretation of health-related news. This is addressed in greater detail in a companion report, *Who Will Keep the Public Healthy: Educating Public Health Professionals for the 21st Century* (IOM, 2003).

Information Networks

Information and the systems through which it is produced are critical tools that enable public health agencies to meet their responsibilities for monitoring health status and for identifying health hazards and risks to the populations they serve. Public health agencies also rely on information and information systems to assess communities' resources and their capacity to respond to health needs and problems. Such assessments inform the interventions and policies designed to address the community's health needs (Keppel and Freedman, 1995). It is essential that the governmental public health infrastructure have a system that is capable of supporting the collection, analysis, and application of myriad forms of health-related data and information.

> Without adequate surveillance, local, state, and federal officials cannot know the true scope of existing health problems and may not recognize new diseases until many people have been affected.
>
> Bernice Steinhard
> General Accounting Office

The committee uses the term "information" in its most general form, referring to three distinct terms in information science: data, information, and knowledge. Data are the essential elements of information; that is, data are the measurements and facts about an individual, an environment, or a community. Information is what is generated when data are placed in context via the tool of analysis. When rules are applied to the information, knowledge is generated (Lumpkin, 2001). All of these elements—data, information, and knowledge—are critical products of public health information networks.

Of particular concern for the public health infrastructure are interrelated weaknesses in the nation's disease surveillance systems and inadequate access to information systems and communication tools. The committee emphasizes the need for an integrated information infrastructure to overcome many of these problems.

Surveillance Efforts and Reporting Systems

For communicable diseases, effective epidemiological surveillance can make the difference between the rapid identification and treatment of a few cases of disease and an outbreak that debilitates an entire community. Responsibility for surveillance, one of the most important functions of the public health infrastructure, is shared among federal, state, and local public health agencies. States and localities collect and report data; and federal agencies, especially CDC, in the case of infectious and chronic diseases, provide valuable technical support, training, and grant funding (GAO, 1999a).

The rapid development of new information technology offers the potential for a greatly improved surveillance capacity. For example, it is now possible to engage in real-time data collection via the Internet and through linkages to electronic patient records. New technologies also offer the potential for automated data analyses, such as pattern recognition software that would be able to detect unusual disease patterns. Moreover, new technologies offer new options for disseminating the information produced by surveillance efforts (Baxter et al., 2000). However, the nation's surveillance capacity is weakened by fragmentation and gaps.

Fragmentation of Surveillance Systems

Fragmentation has developed in surveillance systems in part because legal authority for surveillance rests with states and localities and they have not developed uniform standards for data elements, collection procedures, storage, and transmission. The lack of uniformity has made it difficult for states and localities to work collaboratively among themselves or with the private sector to develop more effective surveillance systems. Although *The Future of Public Health* recommended the development of a uniform national health data set (IOM, 1988), progress has been limited.

Requirements under the Health Insurance Portability and Accountability Act (HIPAA; P.L. 104–191) for the development and use of comprehensive new standards for the electronic transmission of health information may result in greater consistency of certain types of data. However, there is uncertainty about the scope of the rules under HIPAA, and state and local health departments must determine what portion of their electronic health information might be subject to the requirements established by HIPAA (ASTHO, 2001a, 2001b).

Another key factor shaping the development of surveillance systems is that, historically, investment in these systems has been largely categorical, resulting in fragmentation of surveillance efforts across the spectrum of infectious disease threats and other programs for other specific diseases and populations. An inventory of public health data projects and systems identified more than 200 separate DHHS data systems in seven broad programmatic areas (Boufford and Lee, 2001). The multiplicity of surveillance systems for food-borne illnesses illustrates the problem (see Box 3–3).

A lack of integration in federal data systems helps drive fragmentation at the state and local levels. Data collected in accordance with the specifications of separate federal programs often cannot be accessed at the local level because of differences in formats, definitions, classification systems, personal identifiers, or sampling strategies (Lumpkin et al., 1995). The fragmentation means that state and local public health agencies inevitably must spend time on duplicative data-reporting activities that drain already scarce staff resources (GAO, 1999a). The current combination of system incompatibility and lack of integration hinders the ability of program managers to know what information exists and how to access that information and hinders the ability of local health agencies to provide integrated care to their communities (Lumpkin et al., 1995). CDC's National Electronic Disease Surveillance System (NEDSS) is working to electronically integrate a number of surveillance activities; details can be found in the discussion of information systems later in this chapter.

Gaps in Surveillance

Existing surveillance activities contain notable gaps. In particular, little information is routinely collected on chronic diseases and conditions, such as asthma and diabetes, even though chronic diseases account for four of every five deaths in the United States and annually cost the nation approximately $325 billion in health care and lost worker productivity (Pew Environmental Health Commission, 2000). Similarly, environmental pollutants and toxins are monitored primarily for the purposes of environmental protection and regulation, but no surveillance and tracking system monitors the health outcomes, such as birth defects and developmental disorders, that are potentially linked to toxic exposures. With an improved awareness of these health risks and a more comprehensive understanding of the health status of the population, public health agencies from the federal to the local level would be able to design better interventions and prevention efforts.

The Pew Environmental Health Commission (1999, 2000) has called for the development of a national health-tracking network to monitor the prevalence of chronic conditions such as asthma and for the development of national birth defects registries. Ideally, these comprehensive disease registries and surveillance networks would be accessible to and used by state and local public health agencies to better understand and monitor the health status of the communities they serve. Additionally, these registries would have the potential to be linked with registries from private health care delivery organizations

BOX 3–3
An Example of Fragmentation in Disease Surveillance Systems

A recent study—based on a survey of public health officials in all 50 states, the District of Columbia, and New York City—of the Centers for Disease Control and Prevention's (CDC's) surveillance for food-borne illness notes that 20 different surveillance systems record information about food-borne illnesses and pathogens (GAO, 2001a). Of these, only four principal systems focus exclusively on food-borne illnesses and cover more than one pathogen:

1. The Foodborne Disease Outbreak Surveillance System (FDOSS) collects nationwide data about the incidence and causes of food-borne outbreaks. It relies on local health officials to take the initiative to report outbreaks to CDC through their state public health officials. CDC and others use this system mainly to maintain awareness of ongoing problems.
2. FoodNet actively collects information in nine geographic areas on nine specific food-borne pathogens, as well as on hemolytic-uremic syndrome (a complication of *Escherichia coli* O157:H7 infection), Guillain-Barré syndrome (a complication of *Campylobacter* infection), and toxoplasmosis. Public health officials who participate in FoodNet receive federal funds from CDC to systematically contact laboratories in their general area and solicit incidence data. This system provides more accurate estimates of the occurrence of food-borne diseases than are otherwise available.
3. PulseNet is used to identify whether separate cases of illness are likely to have originated from the same source. Using this system, public health officials can compare the new patterns to other patterns in the database; matches indicate an outbreak.
4. The Surveillance Outbreak Detection Algorithm (SODA) focuses on *Salmonella* and *Shigella* and uses statistical analyses to compare current data against a historical baseline to detect unusual increases in the incidence of these two pathogens. Increases may indicate an outbreak.

Although these four systems have contributed to improved food safety, the usefulness of the systems is marred both by the untimely release of the surveillance data and by gaps in the collected data. Twenty-six of the General Accounting Office survey respondents said that delays in publishing data from the FDOSS diminished the usefulness of the system. Many also said that rapid release of data from FoodNet, PulseNet, and SODA would make these systems more useful.

CDC attributed the delays in data dissemination to shortages in staffing. Additional staff have been hired since then, and they are training state and local health officials about the reporting needs of both state health departments and CDC (GAO, 2001a). However, CDC also noted that some of the delays in releasing information were due to the occasionally untimely reporting of surveillance data by state and local public health officials. Survey respondents said the problem is caused in part by shortages of trained epidemiologists in state and local health departments and by deficiencies in laboratory capabilities. Survey respondents also noted that the decisions regarding which diseases are tracked are made at the state level, which adds to the variability and incompleteness of the data when they are aggregated at the national level.

continued

BOX 3–3 Continued

To help states address some of these issues and submit more complete information, CDC is providing funds to state and local public health departments to help reduce some of their staffing and technology limitations. Additionally, CDC is entering into cooperative agreements with the Council of State and Territorial Epidemiologists and the Association of Public Health Laboratories to encourage more standardized reporting among states and to assess states' capabilities and capacities to address public health issues, including food-borne disease.

(such as hospitals and managed care organizations) so that more comprehensive disease prevalence estimates could be easily and readily obtained. The Pew Environmental Health Commission reports and recommendations have been endorsed by major public health organizations, including APHA, ASTHO, the Association of Public Health Laboratories, the Council of State and Territorial Epidemiologists (CSTE), NACCHO, and the Public Health Foundation (PHF). The committee strongly supports this recommendation and applauds the U.S. Congress for providing $17.5 million for the development and implementation of a nationwide environmental health-tracking network and capacity development in environmental health in state and local health departments (Conference Report Accompanying H.R. 3061, 2002).

Another gap in the current disease surveillance system is syndrome surveillance, which captures data on the basis of clinical signs and symptoms of illness (e.g., a fever or rash), not just formal diagnoses of specific diseases. Related indicators for such surveillance might be sales of prescription and nonprescription medications. Interest in syndrome surveillance has grown because of its potential value for early detection of disease outbreaks, including those that might result from a bioterrorist act. Such a system depends on the rapid aggregation and assessment of data to permit detection of clinical and geographic patterns.

Although no national syndrome surveillance network is in operation, some state and local public health agencies are beginning to test and implement such systems. For example, New York City has had an active syndrome surveillance system since the 1990s (LLGIS, 2001), and systems are also operating in the Seattle–King County Department of Public Health (Duchin, 2002) and the Idaho Department of Health and Welfare (1999). Syndrome surveillance systems played an important role during the anthrax outbreaks in New York City and in the Washington, D.C., area.

These systems generally require partnerships with practicing physicians, hospital emergency rooms and outpatient departments, community-based clinics, and sometimes neighboring state and county health departments. A system conceived at Sandia National Laboratories (2002),[9] the Rapid Syndrome Validation Project (RSVP), is being developed and tested in a collaborative effort with the New Mexico Health Department, Los Alamos National Laboratory, and the University of New Mexico Health Sciences Center, Department of Emergency Medicine. RSVP incorporates a real-time medical database and allows electronic data linkages with all local health departments throughout the state, the four district offices and their satellites, and the state offices.

At the federal level, CDC's Enhanced Surveillance Project (ESP) is working with state and local health departments and information systems contractors to develop real-time syndrome surveillance and analytical methods (CDC, 2001d). During special events, ESP sites monitor data on emergency department visits at sentinel hospitals. These data are analyzed at CDC and reported back to the health departments for confirmation and appropriate follow-up. ESP has been tested at events such as the Republican and Democratic National Conventions in 2000 and the 2002 Olympic Games in Utah (CDC, 2001d). DOD (2002), through its Global Emerging Infections Surveillance and Response System, is evaluating a system for the rapid identification of disease-related syndromes in patients at military health care facilities in the Washington, D.C., area.

The committee notes that although these syndrome surveillance programs show promise, their widespread effectiveness is still being evaluated and no syndrome surveillance system has identified a potential biological emergency. A forthcoming report (2003) by the IOM Committee on Emerging Microbial Threats to Health in the 21st Century addresses syndrome surveillance in more detail.

Information Systems and Communications Tools

New Systems and Technologies

Several initiatives have emerged to try to resolve the problems of fragmentation and incompatibility in the nation's disease surveillance systems and to gain the benefits of integrated health data networks and communications systems. A key 1995 report, *Integrating Public Health Information and Surveillance Systems*, documented the problems and recommended a framework for leadership on the issue as well as specific steps for achieving the long-term vision of integration of public health information and surveillance systems (CDC, 1995). After publication of that report, CDC estab-

---

[9] Sandia is a multiprogram engineering and science laboratory operated by Sandia Corporation, a Lockheed Martin Company, for the Department of Energy's National Nuclear Security Administration.

lished the Integrated Health Information and Surveillance Systems Board to formulate and enact policy for integrating public health information and surveillance systems, yet it is not clear that it has played this role. If adequately supported, the board could provide an ongoing coordinating mechanism for CDC and ATSDR to lead the integration of public health information systems.

In 1992, CDC developed the Information Network for Public Health Officials (INPHO) in collaboration with state health departments. INPHO was established to foster communication between public and private partners, to make information more accessible, and to allow the rapid and secure exchange of data (GAO, 1999a). By 1997, 14 states had begun INPHO projects, some combining their INPHO resources with other CDC grant funds to build statewide networks linking state and local public health departments. Some states' networks include links to private laboratories. The system has produced measurable benefits in some states. For example, in Washington State, electronic information-sharing systems reduced the passive reporting time from 35 days to 1 day and gave both local authorities and the School of Public Health at the University of Washington access to health data for analysis (Davies and Jernigan, 1998; P. Wahl, personal communication, February 2, 2002).

The recommendations of the 1995 report have also led CDC to develop NEDSS (CDC, 2000b). Although the system is now in the early stages of development, one of its objectives is to electronically integrate a variety of surveillance activities, including the National Electronic Telecommunications System for Surveillance and the reporting systems for HIV/AIDS, tuberculosis, vaccine-preventable diseases, and infectious diseases. It is also intended to facilitate more accurate and timely disease reporting to CDC and state and local public health departments. NEDSS will incorporate data standards, an Internet-based communication infrastructure that is designed according to industry and public policy standards on data access and sharing, confidentiality protection, and burden reduction (CDC, 2000b).

CDC has also developed the Epidemic Information Exchange (Epi-X). This system, which became operational in November 2000, enables secure, web-based communication among federal, state, and local epidemiologists, laboratories, and other members of the public health community and allows them to instantly notify others about urgent public health events and search the Epi-X database for information on outbreaks and unusual health events.

Another initiative, the Health Alert Network, emphasizes the communication capabilities that are necessary for more integrated information systems. It was designed as a system for electronic communication between health departments and CDC, with the Internet used as its backbone (CDC, 2000c). It also supports distance-learning activities and provides health departments at all levels with the capacity to broadcast and receive health alerts (CDC, 2000c). Although parts of this system are still in development, CDC used the Health Alert Network at noon on September 11, 2001, to advise public health officials to begin heightened disease surveillance (NACCHO, 2001b).

In support of these various activities, CDC is adopting information technology standards and procedures to establish a secure data network (SDN). Network development focuses on the technical requirements for maintaining the confidentiality of data and providing a secure method for encrypting and transferring files from state health departments to a CDC program application via the Internet. The SDN not only gives CDC several ways of obtaining data from states, but it also provides a consistent method for authenticating the transmission source and ensuring data integrity (CDC, 2000c). A public health information network is under consideration at CDC to serve as a vehicle, with an effective governance mechanism, to ensure the integration of existing public health information systems within CDC and coordinated development of future ones with state and local public health agencies.

Although the committee applauds the development of these important systems and coordination efforts, it is concerned about the apparent lack of an effective mechanism to ensure their integration or their coordination with future efforts to create a fully developed national health information infrastructure, which we strongly support.

Continuing Problems

Despite these efforts, the public health information infrastructure is not yet fully capable of handling situations for which rapid, clear communication and information transfer are essential. Because the integration of public health data and information networks has not yet been accomplished, state and local public health agencies are still obliged to operate the more than 100 disparate data systems whose lack of integration slows the flow of information in times of crisis. Data and information network integration must also take into account the new data and information systems under development. Many of these new systems have not been fully implemented across the nation or, in the case of Epi-X, have been implemented only at the state level, leaving localities with read-only terminals and other tools that prevent interactive access to information or, even worse, leaving them out of

> Early detection and response is critical, and it all hinges on communications and information technology.
>
> Dr. Paul Wiesner
> DeKalb County,
> Georgia, Board of Health

the information loop entirely (Brewin, 2001). Furthermore, many local public health agencies, especially those in small and remote communities, do not have the resources or technical capacity to handle the implementation of new information technology, which requires expensive and complicated hardware and software. These disparities result in some states and localities having easy access to updated or urgent information, whereas others must continue to rely on the now-antiquated methods of paper-based reports, telephone connections, and the U.S. Postal Service as their primary means of retrieving and reporting information.

These weaknesses were demonstrated clearly during the bioterrorism events of October 2001. Despite the years of warning about the potential for such attacks, only half of the nation's state, local, and territorial public health departments had full-time Internet connectivity when the first anthrax case was reported on October 4. Another 20 percent of state, local, and territorial health agencies lacked e-mail and, therefore, were unable to receive electronic updates regarding the anthrax events (Brewin, 2001). Given that robust and smoothly functioning information and communications networks are the key to defending against a bioterrorist attack, many of the nation's public health agencies were left unprepared.

Since September 11, 2001, public health agencies and officials have repeatedly urged the U.S. Congress to increase the levels of funding devoted to improving the nation's public health information infrastructure. The recommendations in CDC's review of this infrastructure specifically emphasized the need to ensure that health departments at all levels have access to modern means of rapid electronic data exchange and communication (CDC, 2001c). Although the current bioterrorism preparedness appropriations ($40 million) are directed toward the Health Alert Network and Epi-X (CSTE, 2001), these are just two of the systems necessary for enhanced, comprehensive disease surveillance (NACCHO, 2001e). It is possible that additional appropriations for bioterrorism or emergency preparedness may be able to provide more resources for the improvement of the other components of the nation's surveillance and information networks.

Moving Toward a National Health Information Infrastructure

Through the Telecommunications Act of 1993, the nation embarked on an effort to develop a National Information Infrastructure (NII), sometimes called the Information Super Highway (Boufford and Lee, 2001). The National Health Information Infrastructure (NHII) is the health component of this effort. Whereas some parts of the federal government, such as the Department of Commerce and the National Aeronautics and Space Administration, have moved ahead quickly on their NII agendas, the areas of public health, human services related to health, and community health are the least developed aspects of NII.

The National Committee on Vital and Health Statistics (NCVHS), the key external advisory body on data activities to the Secretary of DHHS, has outlined a vision and a process for building NHII. The report *Information for Health: A Strategy for Building the National Health Information Infrastructure* (NCVHS, 2002) presents the core of the vision as the pulling together of many separate initiatives and systems into an integrated data system that will give health officials and others optimal access to the information and knowledge they need to make the best possible health decisions for communities. The report's recommendations are comprehensive, stressing the importance of information flow to the public and across sectors of the public health system and attaching equal importance to consumer, clinical, and population health dimensions (NCVHS, 2002). To ensure that NHII supports all facets of individual health, health care, and community health, it must be developed in a manner that takes into account human factors (e.g., values and relationships), institutional requirements (e.g., practices, laws, and standards), and technological components (e.g., systems and applications).

NHII, when implemented, could have a profound impact on the effectiveness, efficiency, and overall quality of health and health care in the United States. It would allow the public health system and others to address concerns such as public health emergencies, medical errors, and health disparities in a more timely and comprehensive fashion (NCVHS, 2002). The links to data from the health care delivery system are critical to state public health agency efforts to monitor the quality of health care. The community aspects of population health are ripe for development as part of NHII because of the emerging scientific insight into the nature of health and its determinants (see Chapter 2). Better access to information on communities and their subpopulations will help health professionals and others identify various health threats, problems related to social or environmental conditions, and the unique needs of vulnerable populations. More powerful information tools will help identify patterns and trends from isolated events, and the rapid communication afforded by the network will aid in informing and educating individuals and the community at large about critical health issues.

The committee agrees with NCVHS that the nation's public health interest is served by the development of a standardized approach to an information infrastructure and that the development of a comprehensive, integrated system is a federal responsibility. Therefore, **the committee recommends that the Secretary of DHHS provide leadership to facilitate the development and implementation of the National Health Information In-**

frastructure (NHII). Implementation of NHII should take into account, where possible, the findings and recommendations of the National Committee on Vital and Health Statistics (NCVHS) working group on NHII. Congress should consider options for funding the development and deployment of NHII (e.g., in support of clinical care, health information for the public, and public health practice and research) through payment changes, tax credits, subsidized loans, or grants.

In carrying out this responsibility, CDC should ensure that this system is easily accessible and can be used and maintained by public health agencies at the federal, state, and local levels. This system should include the establishment of standards for consistent data collection and transmission practices, the assurance of privacy protections, the capacity for transmission of urgent health alerts across all levels of the public health system, and the implementation of data systems that facilitate reporting, analysis, and dissemination. CDC should work with its public health partners to ensure adequate and ongoing training in the effective use of the techniques that comprise this system. Although this system is critical for the fulfillment of the essential services of public health, it should also be both respectful of the need for privacy protections and mindful of the need for efficient data exchange.

The exact cost of a comprehensive NHII needs to be determined. Estimates by Lee and colleagues (2001) indicate a total need of about $14 billion over 10 years. This would be a combination of federal, state, local, and private-sector funds ramping up to a peak investment of $1.7 billion per year in 2007 and flattening out for the remaining years; the amounts needed to sustain the system after that period were not estimated.

Public Health Laboratories

Public health laboratories are a critical component of the disease surveillance resources of the public health infrastructure, providing essential capacity to detect, identify, and monitor the presence of infectious or toxic agents in populations and the environments in which those populations live. Investigations in these laboratories resulted in the identification of the organisms that cause diphtheria, cholera, tuberculosis, Hansen's disease (leprosy), and typhoid fever, paving the way for the development of vaccines and treatments to prevent and control those diseases (Valdiserri, 1993). Public health laboratories are also described as the safety net between the local water plant and the kitchen tap in many communities (APHL, 2000); they provide laboratory support for epidemiological studies and perform diagnostic tests (such as cytology testing and neonatal screening) that may influence the treatment of individual patients. Moreover, public health laboratories provide leadership to set laboratory regulations and serve as the standard of excellence for local and private laboratory performance (APHL, 2002a).

In 1999, the General Accounting Office (GAO) (1999a) reported that the nation had 158,000 clinical laboratories, of which 90,000 were in physicians' offices. About 10,000 laboratories were in hospitals or were privately operated. Every state public health department operates at least one laboratory, and some local health departments have laboratory facilities. Federal laboratories, such as those operated by CDC, provide testing services and consultation not available at the state level and training in testing methods (GAO, 1999b). CDC's Division of Laboratory Systems supports extramural and intramural research and oversees a laboratory standards program that describes laboratory practices and services and that assesses parameters for measuring and testing quality (CDC, 2001c). Highest priority is given to research on testing of diseases that are of the greatest public health importance (e.g., HIV and tuberculosis) and research to enhance the standards under the Clinical Laboratory Improvement Amendments (CLIA) (e.g., genetic testing and cervical cytology).[10]

GAO (1999a) also recommended that the CDC director lead an effort by federal, state, and local public health officials to establish a consensus on the core laboratory capacities needed at each level of government. This information will aid policy makers in assessing whether existing resources are adequate and evaluating where investments are most needed.

With regard to the financing of state public health laboratories, unpublished survey data from the Association of Public Health Laboratories (APHL) show that in FY 2001, public health laboratories received a median of 50 percent of their funding from states, with a median of 33 percent from fee-for-service funding and about 15 percent from the federal government (S. Becker, Executive Director of APHL, personal communication, June 13, 2002). Although these percentages reflect the funding data obtained by APHL for both FY 1999 and FY 2001, the trend is that state funding for public health laboratories has been decreasing and fee-for-service funding has been increasing, potentially encouraging laboratories to increase their levels of fee-for-service activities. Although federal funding has remained relatively constant, the recent increases in federal funding for bioterrorism

---

[10] CLIA, enacted by Congress in 1988, mandated a broad and wide-ranging change in the regulation of laboratories that perform testing for medical diagnoses. CLIA expanded federal regulatory authority to approximately 170,000 laboratories, most of which were previously unregulated laboratories in physicians' offices. In 1997, these laboratories performed an estimated 8 billion tests at a cost of approximately $30 billion. In June 1991, the Secretary of DHHS delegated responsibility for development and implementation of the scientific and technical aspects of the regulations to CDC. Within CDC, the Division of Laboratory Systems, Public Health Practice Program Office, carries out the responsibility of standards development and laboratory improvement, whereas CMS administers the program (CDC, 2001c).

and emergency preparedness and response are likely to increase the federal contribution to public health laboratories.

GAO (2001b) reported that the nation's laboratories and other parts of the infectious disease surveillance system were not well prepared to detect or respond to a bioterrorist attack because of reductions in laboratory staffing and training that have affected the ability of state and local authorities to identify biological agents. The limitations of existing laboratory capacity were clearly demonstrated by the 1999 outbreak of West Nile virus in New York State. Even with a relatively small outbreak in an area served by one of the nation's largest local public health agencies, the investigations taxed federal, state, and local laboratory resources (GAO, 2001b). Both New York State and CDC laboratories were inundated with requests for testing, and CDC had to process the bulk of the testing because of the limited capacity of the New York State laboratories. Federal officials indicated that if another outbreak had occurred simultaneously, CDC would not have been able to respond (GAO, 2001b).

Many public health laboratories are unable to keep pace with the monitoring and tracking of infectious agents that are already known in communities. Some states do not routinely test for important infectious diseases. For example, although most states conducted surveillance for tuberculosis, *Escherichia coli* O157:H7, pertussis, and cryptosporidiosis, fewer than half of state laboratories tested for penicillin-resistant *Streptococcus pneumoniae* and hepatitis C (GAO, 1999a). Nearly half of the state public health laboratories lacked access to advanced molecular detection systems and other technologies for identifying specific strains of pathogens, information that is valuable to epidemiological investigations to trace the sources of disease outbreaks.

Many state public health directors and epidemiologists report that inadequate staffing and information-sharing problems hinder their ability to generate and use laboratory data for surveillance (GAO, 1999a). A recent study conducted by APHL (2002b) raised concerns about the public health laboratory workforce. The study found that the country is facing an imminent shortage of qualified public health laboratory directors. APHL anticipates 13 vacancies over the next 5 years in state public health laboratory directorships, with a replacement pool that current laboratory directors describe as either inadequate or marginally adequate in size to meet future demands (APHL, 2002b). Moreover, inadequate laboratory staffing is a problem. Although there is great variability in laboratory staffing among the states, states devoted a median of 8 staff per 1 million population to laboratory testing of infectious diseases[11] (GAO, 1999b). Additionally,

---

[11] Individual states reported a range from 1.4 to 89 staff per 1 million population.

according to the American Society for Clinical Pathology, the United States faces a serious shortage of medical laboratory personnel (ASCP, 2000). In state or local laboratories that have few personnel trained to handle the complexity and volume of work associated with bioterrorism scares (e.g., anthrax), there is little capacity to sustain states of "alert" for days or weeks (APHL, 2002b).

Efforts are under way to modernize the manner in which laboratory information is recorded and communicated; these efforts emphasize the use of automated, electronic systems (CDC, 1999). A 1997 meeting of CDC, CSTE, and APHL to design strategies for implementing effective electronic laboratory-based reporting produced a recommendation to base such strategies on the use of Health Level 7 (HL–7), a national standard for communicating clinical health information (CDC, 1997). Other issues discussed at a 1999 meeting included modes of data transmission, data privacy, software development, data quality, data flow, and recommendations concerning leadership and coordination, software tools and technical support, policy development, training and education, and public–private collaborations (CDC, 1999).

In 2001, the Center for Infectious Disease Research and Policy (CIDRAP) and the Working Group on Bioterrorism Preparedness[12] estimated that approximately $200 million was needed as an initial investment to improve state and local preparedness with regard to laboratory capacity. This funding would support

- Further development and implementation of the Laboratory Response Network, which is a multilevel laboratory network composed of federal, state, county, and city public health laboratories designed to receive and analyze specimens from a range of sources;
- Full implementation of the National Laboratory System, which is a communications system designed to rapidly share laboratory information among public health, hospital, and commercial laboratories;
- Integration of chemical terrorism preparedness into laboratory improvements; and
- Improved diagnostic testing and identification of potential agents of bioterrorism by animal and wildlife laboratories and improved communications among human, animal, and wildlife laboratories.

---

[12] CIDRAP was established in September 2001 with the mission of (1) supporting the development of and refining public policies relating to the prevention, control, and treatment of infectious diseases to ensure that they reflect the most current biomedical knowledge, and (2) promoting practices among both health care professionals and the public that aim to reduce illness and death from infectious diseases through provision of accurate, up-to-date information and education.

CDC has initiated a program to develop a cohesive national laboratory system to ensure disease surveillance and the capacity for effective response (CDC, 2001c). Under this initiative, the proposed National System for Laboratory Testing for Public Health seeks to ensure the availability of a consistent public health laboratory capacity (CDC, 2001c). A report on the FY 2002 bioterrorism-related appropriations provided for infrastructure improvements. In FY 2000, CDC awarded approximately $11 million to 48 states and four major urban health departments to improve and upgrade their surveillance and epidemiological capabilities (GAO, 2001b). More recently (2002), bioterrorism-related federal funds ($1 billion) designated to help prepare state infrastructures for bioterrorism and other emergencies have begun to flow to states (http://www.hhs.gov/news/press/2002pres/20020131b.html). The bulk of funds designated for laboratory capacity building (about $40 million) will go to enhance CDC's intramural laboratory capacity.

State public health laboratories, assisted by CDC, are working to deploy more sophisticated laboratory equipment that can help identify suspected bioterrorism attacks quickly and precisely. In addition, CDC is working to validate the use of molecular DNA and antibody tests in potential cases of bioterrorism; setting uniform guidelines for the use of faster, more sensitive instruments; and planning to supply state public health laboratories with identical kits of biological reagents necessary to identify bioterrorism agents. The efforts aim to improve confidence in test results and guarantee that the results can be verified quickly at other laboratories (Hamilton, 2001).

Given the important role of public health laboratories in assuring the health of the population and in protecting the nation's security, the committee believes that federal, state, and local public health agencies should have access to a strong, state-of-the-art public health laboratory system. Furthermore, the committee believes that these public health laboratories are an essential part of a robust and stable surveillance capability necessary to identify emerging threats, natural or intentional, to the health of the public and to track the effectiveness of interventions at multiple levels.

In addition to the overall assessment of the public health system, **the committee recommends that DHHS evaluate the status of the nation's public health laboratory system, including an assessment of the impact of recent increased funding. The evaluation should identify remaining gaps, and funding should be allocated to close them. Working with the states, DHHS should agree on a base funding level that will maintain the enhanced laboratory system and allow the rapid deployment of newly developed technologies.**

Special Role of the Governmental Public Health Infrastructure in Emergency Preparedness and Response

In the wake of the events of September 11, 2001, federal, state, and local public health agencies—and indeed, the nation as a whole—have been grappling with the crucial question of whether the public health system is prepared to cope with future terrorist attacks. Even before the events of 2001, the threat of chemical terrorism had grown more real in the United States because of developments in the mid-1990s such as the discovery of the Iraqi biological weapons program and the release of sarin nerve gas in the Tokyo subway by the Aum Shinrikyo cult

> *With our public health infrastructure in its current shape, trying to detect and respond to a bioterrorism attack is comparable to running O'Hare Airport's air traffic control system with tin cans and string.*
>
> Dr. Michael Osterholm
> University of Minnesota

(Henderson, 1998). Resources put into the improvement of the public health system's ability to respond to bioterrorism will yield benefits that go far beyond that specific concern, but only if adequate funds are made available to strengthen the public health infrastructure's ability to detect and combat natural disease outbreaks, such as *E. coli* and other food-borne pathogens, and to work with other vital partners in the public health system to provide the protection necessary for the assurance of public health.

Readiness of Local Public Health Agencies

Until recently, the degree to which public health departments were actually prepared for bioterrorist attacks or other emergencies was unknown. Determining the level of state and local health departments' emergency preparedness and response capacities is crucial because public health officials are among those, along with firefighters, emergency medical personnel, and local law enforcement personnel, who serve on "rapid response" teams when large-scale emergency situations arise. These health department officials must work closely with federal public health agencies such as CDC and, occasionally, law enforcement agencies (e.g., the FBI and the Department of Justice) to investigate and resolve the various threats to the community's health, regardless of whether the threat is natural in origin (e.g., floods, tornadoes, and earthquakes) or intentional (e.g., bioterrorist attacks).

Two weeks following the attacks on September 11, 2001, NACCHO (2001a) conducted a brief survey to understand the impacts of the events on local health departments and to assess how well those health departments

> The public health system is the vital link in our ability to preserve and protect human life when disaster strikes.
>
> ASTHO (2001c)

would be able to respond in the event of this and other types of emergencies such as biological or chemical threats. Of the 999 NACCHO members contacted, 530 responded within a week. Survey results indicated that local public health officials played a variety of roles in response to the September 11 terrorist events, including communicating with various community-level partners; working with response partners to develop, update, and review emergency response protocols and plans; and providing information to the media and the concerned public. Of the inquiries received by local health officials, most concerned vaccination and the availability of medicines. Other inquiries focused on the degree to which the local community was prepared and what the local public health agency was doing to prepare the community.

An alarming finding was the extent to which the local public health agencies themselves were unprepared for bioterrorist attacks. Of those who responded, only 20 percent indicated that their agency had a comprehensive response plan. Most of the respondents, 56 percent, indicated that their agency's response plan was still under development, and 24 percent indicated that their agency had no plan at all (NACCHO, 2001a). Health officials themselves were also unprepared. When asked how prepared they felt to respond to concerned citizens' inquiries, only 38 percent of health officials stated that they were "pretty well prepared" to respond, whereas another 50 percent of respondents indicated that they were only "somewhat prepared." The remaining respondents (12 percent) felt that they were "not prepared at all" (NACCHO, 2001a).

Survey respondents also reported on the frustrations that they encountered during that time of crisis. For example, the main frustration voiced was the lack or malfunctioning of resources and equipment, including necessary communications tools such as pagers, cell phones, e-mail, and faxes. The second most common frustration was the partial or total lack of communication from federal and state agencies, which was often interpreted as a sign of poor leadership. In fact, some health officials indicated that they had to rely on the news media rather than on local disaster response agencies, state public health departments, or federal agencies to be alerted to and receive updates about the September 11 crisis (NACCHO, 2001a). Other state and local public health officials noted that during the subsequent anthrax outbreaks, staff attention to other public health activities was diverted to responding to the public's concerns and questions, not to mention the investigation of false anthrax reports (California Bay Area Health Officials, personal communication, 2001).

Improving Preparedness

The data from the NACCHO survey paint a disquieting picture of the preparedness of the nation's local health departments and thus the heightened vulnerability of communities. This is hardly surprising news, however, given that state and local public health agencies have been underfunded and understaffed for decades and have less "surge capacity or potential" (i.e., the ability to respond to a sudden influx of demand) than hospitals (Center for Civilian Biodefense Studies, 2001). Several efforts to improve readiness are under way.

In 1999, DHHS created the Bioterrorism Preparedness and Response Initiative, which is aimed at upgrading the nation's public health capacity to respond to bioterrorism and to establish a formal Bioterrorism Preparedness and Response Program.[13] So far the accomplishments that have been under this initiative include creation of a National Pharmaceutical Stockpile Program and operationalization of the Rapid Response and Advanced Technology Laboratory, which is able to identify rapidly biological and chemical agents rarely seen in the United States (CDC, 2001a).

The development of a nationwide, integrated information, communication, and training network (of which the Health Alert Network, NEDSS, and Epi-X should be a part), as recommended by the National Committee on Vital and Health Statistics, will also help strengthen the ability of federal, state, and local public health agencies to share information (CDC, 2001a). External communications systems also must be strengthened to ensure the rapid and effective transfer of information and communication between public health agencies and other frontline emergency responders, including health care providers, law enforcement and emergency response personnel, and government officials (CDC, 2000a). The importance of effective communication in times of crisis cannot be overstated (ASTHO, 2001c).

The Columbia University School of Nursing Center for Health Policy is a CDC-supported project that has specified the competencies in emergency response needed by all public health workers (Columbia Center for Health Policy, 2001). These individual competencies are complementary to the organizational capacities for bioterrorism response developed by CDC (2001b), the standards for state and local public health performance (CDC,

---

[13] At the time that this report was drafted, legislation for a Department of Homeland Security was under debate. The legislation proposes a "single focal point" for managing and overseeing security functions across Congress, federal departments and agencies, state governments, and local governments. Such a department undoubtedly will have direct and indirect implications for governmental public health agencies. However, the evolving nature of this process led the committee not to include a discussion of this work in progress.

2001b), and procedures for state and local public health department leaders to notify CDC in the event of a bioterrorist attack (CDC, 2001a).

It is also vital that health care providers and facilities acknowledge their important role as part of the larger system that assures population health, both in general and in times of crisis. Because frontline health care providers (i.e., those in urgent care and emergency room facilities) are often the first to see unusual illnesses or injuries, they must constantly be vigilant to notice trends that seem out of the ordinary and must report these trends to local public health departments (ASTHO, 1999; CDC, 2000a). Once such observations are reported, public health investigators can provide appropriate follow-up through epidemiological investigations.

Investing in Infrastructure Improvements

If the United States is going to be appropriately prepared for a terrorist attack (biological, chemical, or otherwise), one of the top priorities must be to strengthen the public health infrastructure at all levels so that it is strong enough, flexible enough, and capable enough to respond to emergency situations of this nature (CDC, 2000a).

An estimated initial investment of approximately $400 million is needed to improve state and local preparedness with regard to personnel, training, epidemiology, and surveillance capacity (Center for Infectious Disease Research and Policy and Workgroup on Bioterrorism Preparedness, 2001). This level of investment would cover the integration of bioterrorism preparedness activities into existing communicable disease prevention and control programs such as CDC's emerging infections program, the training of public health practitioners, and the hiring of designated public health veterinarians for states that do not have one. An estimated additional $200 million was also recommended to begin to improve state and local preparedness with regard to information and communication systems (e.g., Health Alert Network, NEDSS, Epi-X, and rapid communication systems). It was also noted that additional funds would be needed to sustain these systems effectively over time.

Progress toward these estimated needs has been addressed by some of the new resources for infrastructure improvement made available through bioterrorism-related appropriations. A report on the FY 2002 appropriations makes reference to infrastructure improvements such as those authorized by the Public Health Improvement Act of 2000 (P.L. 106–505). Furthermore, in 2002, Congress authorized a variety of bioterrorism-related activities in the Public Health Security and Bioterrorism Preparedness and Response Act of 2002 (OMB, 2002) (see Table 3–1).

Following the passage of the Public Health Threats and Emergency Act of 2000, there were plans to develop two separate grant programs—one for

TABLE 3–1   FY 2002 DHHS Bioterrorism Funding

DHHS and Departments of Labor and Education Appropriations for Bioterrorism Preparedness and Response (in millions)	
Agency	FY 2002 Enacted
CDC	181.9
DHHS Office of Emergency Preparedness	62.0
NIH	92.7
Total	336.6

Emergency Supplemental Appropriations: DHHS Funding for Bioterrorism Preparedness and Response (in millions)		
	President's Request	Enacted
National Pharmaceutical Stockpile	643.6	593.0
Smallpox vaccine	509.0	512.0
State and local public health capacity	80.0	865.0
Hospital capacity	50.0	135.0
Metropolitan Medical Response System	50.0	0.0
Office of the Secretary-National Disaster	33.0	55.8
CDC capacity and research	50.0	100.0
CDC environmental hazard control	0.0	7.5
CDC-NIH laboratory security	38.8	71.0
National Institute of Allergy and Infectious Diseases, NIH	0.0	155.0
FDA vaccine approval, food inspections, and security	95.6	151.1
SAMHSA (mental health service for youth)	0.0	10.0
Recovery and response (New York City, New Jersey, Virginia)	45.0	0.0
Emergency health care reimbursement	0.0	140.0
Total	1,595.0	2,795.4

SOURCE: U.S. House of Representatives (2002).

basic public health infrastructure and the other for bioterrorism preparedness. These were subsequently combined with a stronger emphasis on specific preparation for bioterrorism and other such emergencies.

CDC staff (Office of Terrorism Preparedness and Emergency Response) provided information on funding for the state and local public health infrastructure from FY 1999 to FY 2002 as a subset of total appropriations for bioterrorism. Of total appropriations of $124 million (FY 1999), $156 million (FY 2000), and $182 million (FY 2001), $55 million, $57.6 million, and $67.8 million, respectively, were allocated to state and local capacity building prior to the FY 2002 DHHS bioterrorism funding. The bulk of the funding was for the Health Alert Network; and smaller amounts were allocated for public health laboratory infrastructure and other needs, such as staff development and epidemiology and detection systems. For FY 2002, and prior to September 11, 2001, states were to receive $75 million; however, this amount was supplemented with $915 million. The following seven "capacity areas" (along with the estimated funding levels), deemed necessary for bioterrorism preparedness, were identified for allocation of these funds:

1.   Preparedness planning and readiness assessment ($183 million, including $65 million for the pharmaceutical stockpile)
2.   Surveillance and epidemiology capacity ($183 million)
3.   Laboratory capacity, biological agents ($118.9 million)
4.   Laboratory capacity, chemical agents ($0)
5.   Health Alert Network/communication and information technology ($109.8 million)
6.   Communicating health risks and health information dissemination ($46.7 million)
7.   Education and training ($91.5 million)

The total represents about 42 percent of CDC's total appropriations for bioterrorism and emergency preparedness.

Although the overall resources for the improvement of state and local public health department capacities have increased substantially because of these allocations, it should be noted that the local public health infrastructure provides other important functions that are not covered by the improvements made as a result of these appropriations (e.g., conducting active syndrome surveillance, performing on-the-spot epidemiological investigation, developing local-level bioterrorism preparedness plans, and administering mass vaccinations) (NACCHO, 2001c). For these reasons, it is important to ensure that the improvements that will be made to state and local infrastructures are based on comprehensive data about what is needed to ensure the delivery of the 10 essential public health services at the community level. Furthermore, it is important to ensure that funding levels are sustained over time to maintain these

> Can an appropriate balance be struck between responding to the threat of bioterrorism and ensuring an effective public health response to the health problems facing the nation on a daily basis, such as HIV/AIDS and heart disease?
>
> Eileen Salinsky
> National Health Policy Forum

improvements. Most importantly, however, the improvement of public health preparedness capabilities will require the sustained involvement and commitment of policy makers at all levels of government, with ample attention being given to ensuring appropriate accountability (Salinsky, 2002). Doing so is crucial in assuring the safety and preparedness of all of the nation's communities.

FINANCING THE PUBLIC HEALTH INFRASTRUCTURE

State and local governments traditionally have had financial responsibility for basic governmental public health services, such as workforce training, the development of information systems and the organizational capacity to conduct disease surveillance and prevention programs, the management of public health laboratories, the implementation of population-based prevention and health education programs, and other protections such as water and air quality management, waste disposal, and pest control. Yet the federal government also has a financial responsibility for assuring the capacity of the public health infrastructure at the state and local levels. Unlike the areas of medical care and biomedical research, however, the federal government has never made a similar level of investment in the public health infrastructure, such as the clinical laboratories, surveillance systems, or environmental monitoring systems needed to monitor health and health threats at the state and community levels. In the past, in response to perceptions of great national need, substantial federal investments played a crucial role in the development of the hospital industry and of the biomedical research capacity as well as the expansions of medical schools. What a national government pays for is a critical statement about priorities.

Assessing Infrastructure Costs and the Need for Federal Investment

As the committee has noted, there are vast differences across the country in the scope of activities, the resources available, and the organization of the governmental public health infrastructure at the state and local levels and in the sizes of the populations served. This complicates the task of assessing the cost of public health services and the appropriate investment in the governmental infrastructure that delivers these services or ensures that they are provided. In 1997, the DHHS Office of the Assistant Secretary for Planning and Evaluation commissioned the Lewin Group[14] to develop a

---

[14] The Lewin Group is a health and human services consulting firm whose activities include advising public, private, and nonprofit sectors to improve policy, manage and evaluate programs, and maximize performance as well as other issues.

comprehensive data strategy to characterize the state of the nation's public health infrastructure. The report urged a collective effort with ASTHO, NACCHO, and PHF to study the status of the public health infrastructure and respond with a sustained investment plan to address the needs identified (The Lewin Group, 1997).

Assessing the funds and expenditures for the public health infrastructure at the local level is complex. Data from NACCHO (2001d) illustrate some of this complexity. The average annual expenditure of the 630 local public health agencies reporting was $4.5 million (1999 dollars), but 50 percent of these agencies had expenditures of $621,000 or less. By contrast, 25 percent of the agencies serving large populations of 500,000 or more had annual expenditures of more than $46 million. On average, local public health agencies reported receiving 44 percent of their funding from local government, 30 percent from state government (including funds passed through federal programs), 19 percent from reimbursements for services, 3 percent from the federal government, and 4 percent from other sources.

ASTHO, NACCHO, the National Association of Local Boards of Health (NALBOH), and PHF, in various collaborative efforts supported by DHHS, have been exploring ways to measure actual expenditures at the state and local levels for each of the 10 essential public health services (Barry et al., 1998; Public Health Foundation, 2000). Feasibility studies show promise, but no systematic accounting of this sort is being done on a regular basis.

Almost no data are available on how much would be needed to adequately build and sustain the necessary public health infrastructure to support the nationwide provision of the essential public health services at the local level. One jurisdiction—Bergen County, New Jersey—conducted a detailed analysis of the funding needed for the public health infrastructure to be able to meet new state public health practice standards. Its estimate of $5.1 million per year translates into about $6.61 per capita and represents the county's best current judgment of the total, ongoing investment in infrastructure required to support the provision of the 10 essential public health services throughout the county (National Partnership for Social Enterprise, 2002). Various IOM reports (IOM, 1988, 1992, 1997a, 1997b, 2000a) have made a case for sustained action, both domestically and internationally, to strengthen the public health infrastructure. A detailed examination of infrastructure needs specifically in support of the nation's immunization system produced a recommendation for annual federal funding of $200 million for the next 5 years, along with an overall increase in funding from state governments of $100 million (IOM, 2000b). That report also emphasized the importance of stability in infrastructure funding, documenting the adverse impact at the state and local levels of rapid increases followed by rapid decreases in federal funding during the 1990s.

As policy makers and the public health community contemplate substantial increases in funding to improve the ability of the public health system to respond to threats of bioterrorism, the committee urges them to consider the lessons that the experience of the immunization program offers. Congress responded to the national measles outbreak in 1989–1991, in part, by increasing funding for state immunization infrastructure grants from $37 million in 1990 to $261 million in 1995, but the appropriations were reduced by about $80 million in 1996 and had fallen to $111 million by 1999. A variety of barriers (e.g., the requirements of state budget cycles and the administrative constraints of a 1-year grant period) had made it difficult for states to absorb the initial influx of grant funds, but funding was cut just as states had begun to build program capacity (IOM, 2000b). Moreover, the influx of federal funding had led state legislatures to cut state funding for infrastructure activities (Freed et al., 2000). Both stable and sustained funding is needed for the effective performance of the public health infrastructure.

On the basis of available data, the committee was unable to conclude what level of federal funding may be warranted as an ongoing, governmental investment in the development and maintenance of the public health infrastructure to ensure that it can provide the essential public health services to all Americans. It is expected that funding for the Public Health Improvement Act of 2000 will enhance the public health infrastructure, but it is unclear to what extent these additional investments would further improve the ability of the public health infrastructure to meet its broad day-to-day responsibilities for protecting and improving the health of the population. A commitment for sustained public health infrastructure financing (unrelated to bioterrorism-related activities) is clearly needed.

Prior efforts at systematic nationwide studies of financing for public health have failed because of their exclusive focus on the budgets of state and local governmental public health agencies rather than the funding of the public health system, thus preventing appropriate benchmarking for communities that have various approaches to the allocation of roles and responsibilities within the system. For example, in the late 1960s, Congress became increasingly aware of the need for accountability pertaining to state expenditures and performance as the amount of funding allocated to state health departments was increasing under Section 314(d) of the Public Health Service Act. As a result, the PHS agencies allocated funds to create the National Public Health Program Reporting System (NPHPRS). Started in 1970 and operated by the Public Health Foundation, all states routinely participated in this voluntary reporting system. Data were collected and verified for items such as federal and nonfederal expenditures by program areas, the organizational structures of health departments, and revenue amounts and sources. This was the only data source of this type in the nation. While discussions were occurring around health care reform in the early 1990s, PHF worked with state and local public health agencies to improve NPHPRS, using the *Healthy People 2000* objectives as the basis for performance measures and the 10 essential services as the framework for collecting expenditure data. In 1995, PHS discontinued funding because NPHPRS could not provide program management data for federal agencies. Nearly a decade later, no reporting system exists and no data on state public health expenditures and programs are available. Although different methods of categorizing and cataloging expenditures have been studied, the research indicates that use of the 10 essential public health services for collection of expenditure data is feasible, reliable, and beneficial to the public health community. In addition, the National Public Health Performance Standards Program's Local Public Health System Performance Assessment Instrument appears to be effective in assessing the capabilities of local public health agencies to provide essential public health services.

There is still a great need for an expenditure reporting system for public health agencies based on the framework of the essential public health services and consistent with the newly implemented National Public Health Performance Standards Program to produce a needs assessment and expenditures data as a basis for estimating the investments needed. To begin this process, **the committee recommends that DHHS be accountable for assessing the state of the nation's governmental public health infrastructure and its capacity to provide the essential public health services to every community and for reporting that assessment annually to Congress and the nation. The assessment should include a thorough evaluation of federal, state, and local funding for the nation's governmental public health infrastructure and should be conducted in collaboration with state and local officials. The assessment should identify strengths and gaps and serve as the basis for plans to develop a funding and technical assistance plan to assure sustainability. The public availability of these reports will enable state and local public health agencies to use them for continual self-assessment and evaluation.**

Organizational Impact of Federal Grant Funding

The ways in which funds are transmitted have an impact on program effectiveness. At present, most discretionary funding distributed by DHHS to states and some local entities is allocated through block grants, formula grants, and categorical programs. According to the White House's Blueprint for New Beginnings accompanying the FY 2002 budget, DHHS manages hundreds of discrete public health activities. For these activities, states receive about $4 billion in formula grants and about $3 billion through block grants. The Blueprint for New Beginnings (White House, 2001) notes that potential reform of formula and block grant programs is a priority of the administration. The administration is considering increasing state flexibility to address public health needs through expanded transfer authorities and other mechanisms to remove barriers to effective targeting of public health resources at the state and local levels. The Blueprint does not address the need to increase the flexibility of categorical grants.

Formula grants are characterized by the allocation of funds to states in accordance with a distribution formula prescribed by law or administrative regulation. Two examples of formula grants can be found under Title I and Title II of the Ryan White CARE Act. Formula-driven grants have been difficult to modify on the basis of new variables influencing a particular issue or changes in the demographics of affected populations. The political process often prevents formula revisions that would negatively affect significant numbers of states, even if the expressed purposes of funding would be better realized by shifts to more needy populations or to other geographic areas.

Block grant programs are a subset of formula allocation programs in which the recipient has broad discretion in the application of funds received in support of broad program areas (e.g., Prevention and Treatment of Substance Abuse and Preventive Health and Health Services Block Grants). Block grant programs have various reporting requirements.

One of the questions that has been long asked is about the effectiveness of the block grant mechanism in targeting funding to a particular purpose or need. Michael Rich (1993) conducted highly regarded studies of this issue, in the area of funding for the poor. After significant empirical analysis of the distribution of Community Development Block Grants, he drew several broad conclusions about this funding vehicle:

- State and local officials play an important role in determining the degree to which federal grants are used to balance income and resources in resource-poor areas.
- The capacity and will of governments to target federal grant funds to the poor vary widely. Government officials tend to spread benefits widely as opposed to concentrating them where the need is the greatest.
- Strong coalitions are more effective in influencing federal program decisions, including targeting areas of greatest need. However, local coalitions need a strong federal partner to make explicit targeting more acceptable locally.

A literature review of different models for federal funding conducted by the DHHS Office of the Inspector General in 1994 noted that states report that block grants increased administrative efficiency and integration and did not replace state funds.

Categorical grants provide states and other recipients with funding for specific programs. CDC provides a significant amount of funding to state government departments of health through categorical grants (e.g., for HIV/ AIDS prevention, sexually transmitted disease control, tuberculosis control, and chronic disease). They are highly restrictive in terms of how the recipients may use the funding, may add administrative costs and complexities, and may worsen fragmented program management and service delivery, as federal prohibitions against mixing funds create programmatic "stove-pipes." The result can be separation and gaps in services, because even related program areas become insulated and isolated from each other and lack the flexibility to respond to changes at the recipient level. Furthermore, measuring their real effectiveness has been difficult at times because of the large number of individual grants and the lack of resources for effective performance monitoring (Boufford and Lee, 2001).

The DHHS Performance Partnership initiative and the Oregon Option are examples of efforts to use a more performance-oriented approach to categorical funding by integrating multiple categorical programs under larger umbrella categories. Under the Performance Partnership initiative, DHHS and its partners worked together to reach consensus on the results to be achieved by the program and develop performance measures to monitor progress toward the stated results. The Oregon Option tested the proposition that multiple levels of government can align their efforts to achieve results that matter to people. Both initiatives involved signing memoranda of understanding (MOU) that committed them to work cooperatively to both determine the results to be achieved and to get the job done. The question of creating linkages of funding to benefit coalitions demands another role for governments in partnering with key local stakeholders.

This situation should be remedied. Expanded transfer authorities and other mechanisms to remove barriers and facilitate, rather than hinder, the alignment of resources and policy for the actualization of national health objectives should be considered. Thus, **the committee recommends that the federal government and states renew efforts to experiment with clustering or consolidation of categorical grants for the purpose of increasing local flexibility to address priority health concerns and enhance the efficient use of limited resources.**

Financial Implications of a Changing Mission for Governmental Public Health Agencies in Providing Health Care Services

Essential public health service number 7 (see Box 3–1) charges state and local governmental public health agencies to "link people to needed personal health services and assure the provision of health care when otherwise unavailable" (Public Health Functions Steering Committee, 1994). Thus, state and local governmental public health agencies are responsible for providing a safety net to guarantee that personal health care services are available to all members of the communities they serve. As noted earlier, since 1988, state and local governments have turned increasingly to the private sector, particularly managed care organizations, to provide health care services for Medicaid beneficiaries and others, many of whom were once served directly by local public health departments. In addition, an increasing number of employees (approximately 85 percent) (Kuttner, 1999) are covered by private health insurance, reducing their need for services from public health departments. These changes seemed to provide great promise that local public health agencies would be able to shift their focus from the provision of personal health care services to previously neglected population-based public health functions (IOM, 1996). In some states and communities, however, services to Medicaid patients had offered an important revenue stream that subsidized the population health programs of governmental public health agencies (Keane et al., 2001).

Thus, these agencies find themselves in a difficult relationship with managed care plans: on the one hand, encouraging their active partnership in the public health system, while, on the other, competing with them for revenues for some of these services (Lumpkin et al., 1998). A study of state public health agencies found that 16 of 47 states had some kind of collaboration between their public health departments and managed care groups (DHHS, 1999). In most cases, the managed care organizations were contracted to provide direct patient care (e.g., primary care and clinical preventive services). Other studies of this collaboration reported similar findings.

Although there is great potential benefit from collaborations between public health agencies and managed care plans, current economic trends for managed care programs are not optimistic. In 1997, 67 percent of managed care plans sponsored by safety-net providers lost money, and only 8 percent indicated that they broke even (Gray and Rowe, 2000). In recent years, managed care organizations have been withdrawing from collaborative contracts with governmental public health agencies, once again leaving these agencies with the pressure of having to deliver personal health care services including primary care services to the uninsured or vulnerable populations rejected by the medical care system. This instability in service delivery is also contributing to the disruption of individuals' continuity and availability of care (IOM, 2000a).

Of potential assistance to safety-net providers is the reemerging interest in federal support for "a doubling" of community health centers, operated either by traditional governmental public health agencies or by nongovernmental organizations. Congress recently awarded DHHS with funding to add 1,200 new and expanded health center sites over a 5-year period. At the end of 2002, DHHS will have invested $165 million in 260 new and expanded health centers capable of serving an additional 1.25 million people (HRSA, 2002). As these centers redevelop, the lessons of the past must be kept in mind. The allocation of federal and state resources to communities for these facilities and other health-related programs should be coordinated in a process that ensures the involvement and approval (or at least acknowledgment) of local public health agencies. Moreover, coordination with state and local public health authorities and other community resources is essential (IOM, 1988).

The committee finds that, as in 1988, the continued lack of a nationwide strategy to ensure adequate financing of personal medical, preventive, and health promotion services will continue to place undue burdens on the public health system and to fragment the provision of personal health care services to those most in need of comprehensive integrated approaches. Also, if the number of uninsured continues to increase, the diversion of resources urgently needed for population health efforts to the health care assurance component of the governmental public health system may be required.

The recent downturn in in-state revenues due to the national economic slump will exacerbate problems of sustaining the state share of Medicaid funding and lessen the likelihood of increased or, perhaps, even sustained state funding for the governmental public health infrastructure.

Improving the Operation and Management of the Governmental Public Health Infrastructure

Successfully implementing health policy based on multiple determinants of health and their impact on the health of communities and populations will depend on the effective performance of public health agencies at all levels of government. The committee has discussed the need to strengthen specific aspects of the governmental public health infrastructure at the federal, state, and local levels—the competency of the workforce, the integration and enhancement of information and communication networks, and the improvement of the laboratory and organizational capacities to ensure that the essential public health functions are available to all Americans. Another important priority is to improve the management and coordination of the work of public health agencies as they support this goal of protecting and improving the health of the population.

Public Health Performance Standards and the Accreditation of State and Local Health Departments

Performance measurement has become an essential tool for guiding quality improvement efforts and for holding organizations in the public and private sectors accountable for meeting specified responsibilities. The National Public Health Performance Standards Program (NPHPSP), initiated in 1998, is an effort to use the ideas of performance measurement to promote the organization of state and local public health practice around delivery of the essential public health services (see Box 3–4).

In a national partnership, CDC, ASTHO, NACCHO, NALBOH, APHA, and PHF are working together to establish measurable performance standards for state and local public health systems, to develop tools to assess performance against these standards, and to create incentives for states and localities to use such tools. Some of these measures could be used in a "report card" or as standards in a national program that accredits public health agencies.

The performance standards effort is seen as one way to help move the state and local components of the nation's public health system closer to the system envisioned in *The Future of Public Health* (IOM, 1988). Separate sets of tools for governance have been developed and tested. The instruments are available via CDC's NPHPSP website (www.phppo.cdc.gov/nphpsp), the ASTHO website for the state instrument (www.astho.org/phiip/performance.ht-ml) (ASTHO, 2001d), the NACCHO website for the local instrument (www.naccho.org/project48.cfm) (NACCHO, 2001f), and the NALBOH website for the governance instrument (www.nalboh.org/perfstds/perfstds.htm) (NALBOH, 2001). Although the program is aimed at assessing the performance of the public health system as a whole, it recognizes that governmental public health agencies have key responsibilities for leading, coordinating, and supporting the efforts of various contributors.

The interest in measuring the performance of the public health system extends to the possibility of establishing a formal process of accreditation to certify that governmental public health agencies are meeting specified levels of performance. Several states have developed or are developing state-specific performance requirements for local governmental public health agencies, but interest has also emerged in the development of nationally standardized, systematic performance evaluations for state and local public health agencies.

No agreement has been reached on the appropriate criteria or process for accreditation. One of the key challenges is to create a system that is flexible enough to accommodate the wide variety of public health department structures and circumstances across states. Given the resource constraints that state and local governmental public health agencies currently face, it is unclear how performance standards can be met or accreditation

BOX 3–4
The National Public Health Performance Standards Program

Started in 1998, the National Public Health Performance Standards Program (NPHPSP) is a collaborative effort between the Centers for Disease Control and Prevention (CDC) and a variety of national organizations representing state and local public health agencies and other elements of the public health community: the National Association of County and City Health Officials (NACCHO), American Public Health Association, Association of State and Territorial Health Officials, National Association of Local Boards of Health, and Public Health Foundation (Halverson et al., 1998; NACCHO, 2001a). Designed to measure public health practices at the state and local levels, the mission of NPHPSP is to improve quality and performance, increase accountability, and increase the science base for public health practice.

The performance standards are based on the 10 essential public health services, and for each essential service there are model standards (descriptions of and conditions for optimum performance of the public health system) and measures (multiple-choice questions that address components of the model standard). The measurement instruments concentrate on three aspects of the public health system:

1. State-level measures that focus on the state-level public health system and on the agencies and partners that contribute to population health at the state level;
2. Local-level measures that focus on the local public health system and on the entities that contribute to public health within a community; and
3. Governance measures that focus on the governing body or bodies that are ultimately accountable for public health at the local level (including boards of health or county commissioners).

The development of a local-level instrument began in 1998. Since then, the instrument has been tested in local public health agencies throughout Florida, Hawaii, Minnesota, Mississippi, New York, Ohio, and Texas. This testing ensures that the instrument is responsive to the needs of communities, accurately assesses local performance and capacities, and addresses the broad variation in local public health infrastructures across the nation (NACCHO, 2001f). Recent pilot testing of the NPHPSP instruments indicates that the performance standards based on the 10 essential services have validity for measuring local public health performance (Beaulieu and Scutchfield, 2002). The local instruments were developed by the same NACCHO–CDC partnership that developed the community-wide strategic planning tool for improving community health, Mobilizing for Action through Planning and Partnerships (MAPP), as part of the Assessment Protocol for Excellence in Public Health project. The local instrument will be included in the new MAPP tool as a method for assessing the local public health system and identifying areas of improvement.

can be achieved when the resources to provide even the most basic services are often lacking. Linking federal funding to accreditation based on public health performance standards has been proposed, but there may not be adequate incentives for states and localities that do not receive significant portions of their overall funding from federal agencies. The promise of a long-term federal investment at the state and local levels linked to such a system could change the situation considerably.

To address these and other concerns, NACCHO has convened the Voluntary Accreditation Committee, which consists of eight local health officers who are charged with maintaining an ongoing discussion of the advantages and disadvantages of voluntary accreditation of local health departments. They are currently researching lessons that might be learned from other voluntary accreditation efforts, such as those for hospitals, managed care organizations, and law enforcement agencies. The Voluntary Accreditation Committee is also taking into account the work of states such as Florida, Illinois, Michigan, Missouri, Ohio, and Washington that are already active in the development of state-specific accreditation or performance standards for their local public health agencies.

Despite the controversies concerning accreditation, the committee believes that greater accountability is needed on the part of state and local public health agencies with regard to the performance of the core public health functions of assessment, assurance, and policy development and the essential public health services. Furthermore, the committee believes that development of a uniform set of national standards leading to public health agency accreditation could provide such a mechanism, but only if adherence to such standards is linked to a commitment of sustained federal investment in the state and local public health infrastructure to assure that resources are available. Moreover, such a mechanism could serve to increase levels of accountability among state and local elected officials in whose jurisdictions these agencies operate. The breakthrough concepts of NPHPSP provide a way to conceptualize the system as the unit of accreditation and, from there, to evaluate the role of the agencies in facilitating the work of the system.

Accreditation is a useful tool for improving the quality of services provided to the public by setting standards and evaluating performance against those standards. Accreditation mechanisms have helped to ensure the robustness of the health care delivery system (hospitals, clinics, programs) and medical and other educational programs. Accreditation processes also provide information to the public about the quality of the services they receive (e.g., National Committee for Quality Assurance report cards on health plans) (IOM, 2001). Governmental public health agencies currently have no such framework, and the communities they serve have little information on the quality of the services they receive. An accreditation process could provide a structure for establishing quality assurance and improvements in governmental public health agencies. Therefore, **the committee recommends that the Secretary of DHHS appoint a national commission to consider if an accreditation system would be useful for improving and building state and local public health agency capacities. If such a system is deemed useful, the commission should make recommendations on how it would be governed and develop mechanisms (e.g., incentives) to gain state and local government participation in the accreditation effort. Membership on this commission should include representatives from CDC, ASTHO, NACCHO, and nongovernmental organizations.**

This commission should focus on the development of a system that will further the efforts of NPHPSP. The work of this commission should be closely linked to that of the commission whose creation the committee has recommended to examine issues related to the credentialing of public health workers, because it is conceivable that these mechanisms could be linked. In both efforts, the relationship of the official public health agency to its role in the larger public health system will be key to accreditation.

Special Concerns About the Capacity to Meet Local Public Health Needs

In *The Future of Public Health* (1988), the IOM committee concluded that "no community, no matter how small or remote, should be without identifiable and realistic access to the benefits of public health protection, which is possible only through a local component of the public health delivery system" (IOM, 1988: 144). The rationale behind this finding is clear: If a community is going to be able to meet its own health needs, it must have access to an identifiable public health infrastructure to provide the essential public health services. Today, concerns remain about the availability of an adequate local public health infrastructure, particularly in terms of staffing and communications systems, to provide these services.

> Either we are all protected or we are all at risk.
>
> Dr. Jeffrey Koplan,
> Formerly, Centers for Disease
> Control and Prevention

Despite the presence of some 3,000 local public health agencies throughout the country, these agencies are not equally distributed across states or across rural and urban areas. For example, Bergen County, New Jersey, with a population of approximately 884,000 and an area of 234 square miles (Census Bureau, 2001a), is served by a strong county health department, 55 local boards of health, and 22 independent public health agencies that serve different and occasionally overlapping communities (T. Milne,

NACCHO, personal communication, October 31, 2001). By contrast, the state of Maine, with a population of about 1.3 million distributed over 30,862 square miles (Census Bureau, 2001b), has two local public health agencies (T. Milne, NACCHO, personal communication, October 31, 2001). Challenges come from both an abundance of local public health agencies and their scarcity. When multiple public health departments serve the same geographic area, they may experience difficulties coordinating activities and aligning priorities. However, rural areas, with little or no local public health presence, may suffer from inadequate public health capacity or resources to address local needs and a paucity of educational and training support (Johnson and Morris, 2000).

Data from NACCHO (2001e) also point to substantial differences in the workforce available to local public health agencies. NACCHO's 1999–2000 survey found that 50 percent of all local public health agencies responding had 17 or fewer full-time employees or contract staff, but for those serving metropolitan areas, 50 percent had at least 28 full-time employees or contract staff. Some local public health agencies, however, currently have only one half-time employee as their entire public health agency staff. Staffing levels have shown little change over the past decade. A 1997 survey found that the median number of full-time employees was 16 (NACCHO, 1998), and in 1992–1993, NACCHO (2001e) reported that 42 percent of local public health agencies had less than 10 full-time staff members. Given the many responsibilities and wide-ranging duties inherent in the assurance of population health, the committee is concerned that these low numbers do not bode well for the core capacity of some local public health agencies to provide the 10 essential public health services to their communities.

Simply increasing the size of the local public health agency workforce appears problematic, however. The committee is concerned about reports by 68 percent of local public health agencies that budget restrictions prevent them from hiring needed staff, including public health nurses, environmental specialists, health educators, epidemiologists, and administrative personnel (NACCHO, 2001d). In addition, local public health agencies in smaller, nonmetropolitan jurisdictions indicated that they could not hire the necessary staff because of a lack of qualified candidates in their areas and difficulty attracting other candidates to their locations. Only 19 percent of the local public health agencies indicated that they needed new staff because of projected expansions of their programs and services (NACCHO, 2001d).

Many local public health departments also lack even the most basic tools necessary for rapid communication and access to information (GAO, 1999b). For example, a 1999 survey of 1,200 local public health departments found that 19 percent did not have the capacity to send and receive e-mail via the Internet (Fraser, 1999). The most common barriers cited by the departments without Internet access were prohibitive costs (64 percent), the need for hardware (64 percent), and the need for staff training (63 percent). Additionally, only 48 percent of the health departments surveyed indicated that the director had continuous, high-speed Internet access at work, and only 44 percent indicated that the department had broadcast fax capabilities (Fraser, 1999). In all cases, public health agencies in smaller and more remote jurisdictions had the least access to information and communications technologies, even though these agencies may actually have the greatest need for such technologies.

Given the evidence concerning the local public health workforce and communication capacity as well as related observations made throughout this chapter, the committee finds that too little has been done to support and strengthen the local public health infrastructure. Over the past 14 years, governmental public health agencies have made great efforts in response to the recommendations concerning local public health agencies in *The Future of Public Health* (1988) (see Appendix C). Unfortunately, until recently, progress has been slow because of the lack of political and financial support that was needed long ago to fully realize the vision of the 1988 report. Recent increases in infrastructure support in connection with bioterrorism preparedness are somewhat encouraging, but there is concern that such efforts may reinforce the complex problems created by prior categorical funding if excellent specific services (e.g., surveillance are informatics) are built on the foundation of a crumbling infrastructure. For these reasons, the committee believes that every community, no matter how small or remote, should have identifiable and realistic access to the essential public health services, and that it is the responsibility of the states to ensure that such services are available. However, for states to meet this obligation, **the committee recommends that DHHS develop a comprehensive investment plan for a strong governmental national public health infrastructure with a timetable, clear performance measures, and regular progress reports to the public. State and local governments should also provide adequate, consistent, and sustainable funding for the governmental public health infrastructure.** This investment is crucial to assure the preparedness of public health departments and the protection of communities, regardless of their size or location.

Some communities provided comments to the committee noting that a more precise description of an essential minimum level of local official agency capacity would aid their efforts to obtain public health services. In an effort to be responsive to these requests, the committee struggled with the challenge to be more explicit with regard to the level of public health capacity that should be present in these small and remote communities. Not surprisingly, some familiar problems were encountered. For example, there are questions involving the proper definition of a "community" for this purpose and the appropriate response if a community has too small an economic base to sustain a formal public health agency with the necessary presence and capacity to provide public health protections.

The most robust approach to assessing need seems to be the use of a functional analysis based on the ability to provide the essential public health services, as recommended above. The committee recognizes the potential value of a recommendation regarding the development of a formula to determine the "critical mass" of services and population (e.g., a ratio of one of each of the critical professions per 50,000 or 100,000 population), the geographic accessibility of services, and the workforce capacity necessary for the effective development of local public health agencies to serve small or remote communities. Before such a recommendation can be made, however, solid, practice-oriented research must be conducted to provide the evidence on which to base a formula or other criteria.

The committee had hoped to be able to provide specific guidance to assist the nation in its efforts to rebuild and finance its public health infrastructure. However, a comprehensive search of the published literature and extensive information gathering yielded very little firm, generalizable evidence on which to structure public health practice recommendations like those noted. To remedy this situation, **the committee recommends that CDC, in collaboration with the Council on Linkages between Academia and Public Health Practice and other public health system partners, develop a research agenda and estimate the funding needed to build the evidence base that will guide policy making for public health practice.**

Strengthening the Management Capacity of DHHS

From 1993 to 1997, DHHS, like all federal government departments, conducted a reinvention exercise to determine what work it should do and how it could do that work more effectively and responsively. A recent monograph on DHHS and the impact of departmental reinvention efforts in the late 1990s identified two issues of particular significance: (1) the effect of the balance between centralization and decentralization on the management of departmental activities and (2) the relationship of the department with other agencies (Boufford and Lee, 2001).

Centralization versus Decentralization: Models for Managing DHHS

The committee's discussion of key federal functions—policy making, financing, infrastructure development, and the like—illustrate how the problems of fragmentation in federal public health activities affect the functioning of state and local public agencies. Such problems are related to historical patterns and political interests that have shaped federal health structures, but they are not being addressed by the present management structure for health activities in DHHS. The reinvention exercise led to a decision to have each of the PHS agencies report directly to the Secretary of DHHS rather than to the Assistant Secretary for Health. Potential advantages were seen in bringing the agency heads closer to the Secretary and having more than a single voice for health at the decision-making table. Boufford and Lee (2001) found that without a formal mechanism for joint priority setting and routine decision-making across the department, operations became even more decentralized, with staff identifying more with their own agencies or programs than with the department as a whole. The leadership of operating divisions generally prefers to report directly to the Secretary, but division leaders would also welcome a clearly defined structure to formalize coordination, collaboration, and communication among departmental units. Creating a formal mechanism for regular meetings of the heads of operating divisions, as well as meetings with the Secretary, would permit more substantive and forward-looking discussion of priorities and policies and would address the operational challenges of coordination and communication within the department. Such a forum could also provide better oversight and interaction with cross-departmental groups created to address issues identified by the Secretary, such as the Data Council, the Children's Council, and the Environmental Health Policy Committee. A defined charter, staff, and timetable for selected cross-cutting activities would strengthen collaboration across units and produce specific recommendations for action.

Recent decisions by DHHS leadership to recentralize public and legislative affairs functions do not address the fundamental issue of policy and program coordination. There is also tension within DHHS about the role of the regional offices (Boufford and Lee, 2001). Advocates for strong regional offices see them as effective vehicles for communicating DHHS priorities, learning about local needs and circumstances, and developing appropriate responses through the department or by other means. The regional offices are also seen as aids in convening state leadership in health and human services in those regions and in convening local leaders to help them find ways to increase their access to federal programs or to collaborate with others in the public and private sectors to make DHHS programs effective. Although others prefer that DHHS agencies work directly with state and local governments and grantees, such agency-by-agency linkages can add to the fragmentation of efforts to address population health.

If regional offices are to become an integral and valuable part of DHHS, they will require managerial attention and resources for significant staff development or redeployment to obtain the expertise needed in certain program areas (Boufford and Lee, 2001).

Interagency Collaboration

Interagency collaboration at the federal level can be difficult because of the specialized nature of agency structures. Every agency has its traditional role and expectations for performance, its legislative champions, and its special-interest advocates. According to Bardach (1998), barriers to collaboration across agency lines are the fact that collaboration tends to blur an agency's mission and the fact that the agency is politically accountable for pursuing that mission. This historical reality has led to the increasing isolation of cabinet departments and the agencies within those departments from each other and has created real barriers to the programs within agencies that seek to collaborate. This is understandable historically but is clearly dysfunctional in an increasingly complex world where no single agency can do its important work in isolation.

This lack of integration is especially evident in the area of health, where health-related programs are already fragmented within DHHS and are widely distributed across cabinet and subcabinet departments outside DHHS. For example, when EPA became an independent agency, it assumed the regulatory functions of environmental protection, yet the key expertise in the human health effects of environmental hazards remains at DHHS in the National Center for Environmental Health at CDC, ATSDR, the National Institute of Environmental Health Sciences at NIH, and some parts of FDA.

Many agencies not traditionally associated with health issues make policy and manage programs with potential implications for health (see Chapter 2). Greater policy coordination with the Departments of Education, Energy, Treasury, and Labor, to name a few, could enhance the potential to create the societal conditions needed for people to be as healthy as possible. Another area for greater collaboration and coordination is with nongovernmental entities. This can be particularly challenging in the area of health care delivery because of the government's role as regulator and payer. The same holds true at the state level.

The need for effective coordinating structures is very important because most experienced government officials agree that major organizational restructuring is rarely worth the time and political trouble involved (even if it could be achieved), so although it may seem advisable to reunite DHHS and EPA or create a food safety agency independent from portions of FDA, the Department of Agriculture, and EPA, the obstacles are formidable. Bardach (1998) found, however, that various administrative mechanisms could enhance the effectiveness of cross-agency collaboration. These may include formal agreements at the executive level; assignment of personnel, budget, equipment, and space to a collaborative task; delegation and accountability for the relationships relating to the task; and the provision of administrative services to support the work. The success of efforts such as the Presidential

Task Force on Food Safety, the Task Force on Environmental Health Risks and Safety Risks to Children, and the multiagency task force on bioterrorism demonstrate the benefits of cross-agency collaboration.

The committee particularly noted that the lack of coordination between DHHS and other agencies with health-related responsibilities often creates major obstacles to the effective use of federal regulatory and standard-setting powers in health. Inconsistencies between DHHS agencies and other science-based regulatory agencies—for example, between DHHS and EPA—lead to standards on the levels of particular chemicals or toxins hazardous to the health of humans that are different from the levels hazardous to the health of animals and vegetation (Boufford and Lee, 2001). These issues are usually addressed on a case-by-case basis through work groups or crisis management activities. During the Reagan administration, for example, cabinet councils chaired by a designated secretary were used to coordinate efforts across departments. They worked when they were well staffed and participation at the deputy or assistant secretary level was consistent, with secretaries available as needed (Edward Brandt, personal communication, 2001).

A final challenge is the integration of federal standard setting and regulation with the equally varied jurisdictions of state and local health departments or other health-related agencies. Again, creative and sustained mechanisms to develop collaborative relationships and to harmonize regulations within DHHS, across federal agencies, and among federal, state, and local governments are critical to effective action for protecting the population's health.

In June 2001, the Secretary of DHHS established the Advisory Committee on Regulatory Reform. The committee is charged with conducting a department-wide initiative to reduce regulatory burdens in health care and to respond faster to the concerns of health care providers, state and local governments, and individual Americans who are affected by DHHS rules. The Advisory Committee conducted six data-gathering meetings across the country. The committee was expected to present a final report and recommendations in the fall of 2002 for changes in four areas: health care delivery, health systems operations, biomedical and health research, and the development of pharmaceuticals and other products. A review of the report shows that much attention was directed to implementing changes in the health care delivery component of the public health system, with little attention paid to the regulatory inconsistencies, burdens, and inefficiencies in the governmental public health component of the system.

Given these organizational and management findings, **the committee recommends that the Secretary of DHHS review the regulatory authorities of DHHS agencies with health-related responsibilities to reduce overlap and inconsistencies, ensure that the department's management structure is** best suited to coordinate the efforts among agencies within DHHS with health-related responsibilities, and, to the extent possible, simplify relationships with state and local governmental public health agencies. Similar efforts should be made to improve coordination with other federal cabinet agencies performing important public health services, such as the Department of Agriculture and the Environmental Protection Agency.

The committee also notes that the division of authority in the federal government hinders the development of a coherent international health policy. With increasing cross-border flows of people, pharmaceuticals, and food, countries cannot adequately protect their populations through unilateral domestic or foreign policy action; they must collaborate with other countries and within the frameworks of international agreements. This is especially true in matters of health and environment. The World Health Organization (WHO) is a forum for standard setting on issues such as international travel health standards, the quality of pharmaceuticals, and food quality and safety. A lack of funding for research on diseases that disproportionately affect the developing world (the "10/90" gap) (Davey, 2000), the weakness of the research infrastructure in these countries, and the need to address matters of intellectual property involved in making basic drugs available to nations without their own production capacities are only a few of the issues that can benefit from high levels of involvement from developed countries such as the United States, with its wealth and scientific expertise.

At present, the Department of State is the lead U.S. agency on international affairs and pays dues to international agencies like WHO. Because of the importance of health and science to its work, it has recently appointed a deputy assistant secretary for health and science. The funding for U.S. development assistance in health comes through congressional funding to the U.S. Agency for International Development, which funds much of its international health work by contract with DHHS, largely CDC. DHHS has only limited authority from Congress to spend money on international health activities. Coordination across all these agencies is critical to assuring a coordinated strategy for international health. During the Clinton administration, a senior public health officer served on the National Security Council (NSC) as health liaison to the various agencies. In a consultation conducted by IOM, among representatives from the major departments that address international health issues (and others involved in international health policy, from EPA to the Departments of Agriculture and Commerce), all agreed that there was a problem in coordination and clear leadership on international health that prevented effective long-term planning. They agreed that NSC leadership could provide a focal point for such coordination, absent an executive decision to appoint a lead agency

(IOM, 1999). The NSC health liaison position was phased out during the early days of the Bush administration.

In America's *Vital Interest in Global Health,* IOM (1997a) called for better coordination of global health policy within the U.S. government through the use of a Task Force on Global Health. That report also recommended legislative changes to expand international authorities and funding to DHHS "because of its unique scientific and technical expertise" to lead such an effort across the government and to serve as a focal point for links to nongovernmental organizations and academia. This committee concurs with the need for an effective mechanism for coordination of international health policy making and urges the administration and Congress to consider steps to this end such as the appointment of a permanent NSC liaison for international health, the designation of a lead agency for international health or the formation of a formal cross-cabinet body, and the review of Public Health Service Act authorities for DHHS funding of international health initiatives.

Federalism and a National Public Health Policy

The relationships among various levels of government have always been complex and hotly contested. In most spheres of public health (e.g., injury prevention, clean air and water, and infectious disease surveillance and control), federal, state, and local governments all have a presence. As in all essential government endeavors, good communication and cooperation among the various levels of government are vital. Federalism functions as a sorting device for determining which government, federal or state, may legitimately respond to a public health threat. Often, the national and state governments exercise public health powers concurrently, but the Supremacy Clause gives Congress the authority to preempt state public health regulation, even if the state is acting squarely within its police powers (*Gade v. National Solid Waste Management Association,* 505 U.S. 88, 98 [1992]). Federal preemption occurs in many areas of public health regulation, including labeling and advertising of cigarettes, self-insured health care plans, and occupational health and safety.

Although there may be debates over the constitutional roles of the federal and state governments, a more fundamental concern is that each level of government operates effectively in assuring the conditions for the public's health. First, strong public health leadership is essential. This means that where the various levels of government are operating at the same time, clear understanding of who is in charge and who has responsibility for which tasks must exist. During the anthrax outbreak, for example, it was often unclear which level of authority was in charge: the Secretary of DHHS, the local public health commissioners in Florida, New York, and Washington, D.C., or the Department of Justice (FBI). Second, no significant gaps in public health protection should exist. This means that at least one level of government should be actively involved in dealing with important health problems.

Because the major interactions of the federal and state governments in recent years have related to issues of health care financing through the Medicaid program (or through welfare programs), they have tended to focus on arguments over money and degrees of freedom to spend it. States have often been reduced to being just another interest group. If a mechanism could be developed to engage the states as potential partners in a larger national strategy such as the health agenda that clearly depends on collaborative action for success, it could change these relationships.

Direct relationships between the federal government and local governments constitute a complicated issue. In the American system, local governments are the creatures of state governments, from which they get their authority and resources (or the authority to raise revenues). There are more than 90,000 units of local government in the United States; 90 percent have populations of less than 10,000 and 80 percent have populations of less than 5,000 (Cigler, 1998). Their policy-making and managerial capacities are highly variable, as are their capacities and resources in health. It is clear that some units of local government look to the federal government to correct the inequities that they experience at the hands of state governments; others are in tense relations with their state counterparts, and direct federal connections may exacerbate tensions. Ways to manage relationships that engage local governments but that respect the rights of the state governments in terms of their relationships to local governments must be considered in any long-term partnership-building process.

The committee believes that a more comprehensive and coordinated approach to health policy is necessary to improve the alignment of federal, state, and local governmental authorities and financial resources to support effective action in improving population health. This kind of coordination is critical to creating a true public health system from the multiple, often disconnected, and somewhat competitive organizations that must work together to promote and protect the health of the public. As one step toward better coordination, DHHS should be looking to new ways to collaborate more effectively with governmental public health agencies at the state and local levels.

This is not a new problem for DHHS. In 1960, then Surgeon General Leroy Edgar Burney convened an external expert group to "study the present and future mission of the public health service and design the best possible structure to deal with its multiple new functions." It found that PHS needed to develop mechanisms to allow it to work "with, rather than through state agencies" (Study Group on the Mission and Organization of the Public Health Service, 1960). During the Nixon administration, there was similar recognition of the importance of improving relationships between federal, state, and community organizations to serve the populations in greatest need. This led to strengthening of the regional offices of DHHS and establishing an office on intergovernmental affairs. As discussed earlier, the department's policy and structures for dealing with state and local governments have varied over the years, but the mechanisms within the department are weak at present.

One way to achieve better communication is through formal links with the national organizations representing state and local health officials, ASTHO and NACCHO, which often collaborate with the department in activities such as the Healthy People (2010) initiative and the development of National Public Health Performance Standards. The department could also enhance its efforts to seek state and local perspectives on public health policy through the National Governors Association and the U.S. Conference of Mayors, which have staff who work on health issues.

The committee believes that a more formal entity could facilitate the link between the Secretary of DHHS and state public health officers for the purpose of improving communication, coordination, and collaborative action on a national health agenda. In considering the form of such an effort, it is important to recognize that the U.S. health care system is highly devolved, and as noted earlier, historically, the major responsibility for the essential public health services has rested with state governments, but with that responsibility subject to federal regulations and with the public health services partially supported by federal revenues (more revenues are provided for health care delivery than for the public health infrastructure). Because governments have a unique role in assuring the conditions for health of the population and because health is a public good, the high level of interdependence of federal and state governments in achieving national health goals such as those articulated in *Healthy People 2010* (DHHS, 2000) requires effective communication and collaboration.

In a 1997 report on the principles of state–federal relations, the National Governors Association, while noting the importance of state autonomy and the preservation of the ability of the states to address local circumstances, agreed that there was a need for a federal role in certain domestic issues—when issues are national in scope and the national interest is at risk and to help states meet the needs of special populations. It also reaffirmed its support for a federal role in assuring equality of access, addressing the issues beyond the capacities of individual states, and ensuring that all states have the fiscal capacity to meet the requirements of federal goals. It further cites the critical importance of close working relationships with "our federal partners" (NGA, 1997). Although this discussion did not specifically address collaboration in public health, the principles would seem to apply and call for direct interaction between the governmental public health leadership of states and the DHHS rather than through annual meetings of representative organizations or interest groups.

Therefore, the committee recommends that Congress mandate the establishment of a National Public Health Council. This National Public Health Council would bring together the Secretary of DHHS and state health commissioners at least annually to

- Provide a forum for communication and collaboration on action to achieve national health goals as articulated in *Healthy People 2010*;
- Advise the Secretary of DHHS on public health issues;
- Advise the Secretary of DHHS on financing and regulations that affect the governmental public health capacity at the state and local levels;
- Provide a forum for overseeing the development of an incentive-based federal–state-funded system to sustain a governmental public health infrastructure that can assure the availability of essential public health services to every American community and can monitor progress toward this goal (e.g., through report cards);
- Review and evaluate the domestic policies of other cabinet agencies for their impacts on national health outcomes (e.g., through health impact reports) and for their impacts on the reduction and elimination of health disparities; and
- Submit an annual report on their deliberations and recommendations to Congress.

The Council should be chaired by the Secretary of DHHS and cochaired by a state public health director on a rotating basis. An appropriately resourced secretariat should be established in the Office of the Secretary to ensure that the council has access to the information and expertise of all DHHS agencies during its deliberations.

The committee believes that public health exists within a sphere of political and policy-making activity, from which it cannot and should not be separated. Thus, public health must operate within the boundaries of democracy and must take place in a rational, evidence-based political process. Therefore, the proposed Council may change with changes in administration.

CONCLUDING OBSERVATIONS

To most effectively protect and promote the health of the population, the nation's entire governmental public health infrastructure—its human resources, information systems, and organizational capacity—must be revitalized and strengthened. Doing so will require federal, state, and local governmental collaboration to assess the needs in each community and to identify national and local strategies to meet those needs. Furthermore, federal, state, and local governments will need to create innovative financing mechanisms that can add new resources (including those from the private sector) to those already committed by all levels of government to infrastructure development and capacity building and ensure that these investments are sustainable over time. Most importantly, it is the responsibility of the federal government to ensure that these actions at the federal, state, and local levels contribute to the creation and maintenance of a comprehensive, intersectoral public health system that serves to protect and promote the health of Americans.

REFERENCES

Altman LK. 2001. CDC team tackles anthrax. New York Times, October 16.

APHL (Association of Public Health Laboratories). 2000. On the front line: protecting the nation's health. Available online at http://www.phppo.cdc.gov/dls/aphl-ofl.asp. Accessed March 12, 2002.

APHL. 2002a. Advancing the National Electronic Disease Surveillance System: An Essential Role for Public Health Laboratories. Report of the Association of Public Health Laboratories. Washington, DC: APHL.

APHL. 2002b. Who Will Run America's Public Health Labs? Educating Future Laboratory Directors. Report prepared by Schoenfeld E, Banfield-Capers SY, and Mays G for the Association of Public Health Laboratories. February. Washington, DC: APHL.

ASCP (American Society for Clinical Pathologists). 2000. Laboratory workforce shortage stresses need for health professions funding (last updated on April 6, 2000). Available online at http://www.ascp.org. Accessed March 18, 2002.

ASTHO (Association of State and Territorial Health Officials). 1999. Bioterrorism preparedness: medical first response. Testimony of David R. Johnson, MD, MPH, Deputy Director for Public Health and Chief Medical Executive, Michigan Department of Community Health, on behalf of the Association of State and Territorial Health Officials, to the U.S. House of Representatives Subcommittee on National Security, Veterans Affairs, and International Relations, September 22. Available online at http://www.aphl.org/Advocacy/Testimony/index.cfm. Accessed March 12, 2002.

ASTHO. 2001a. HIPAA Issue Brief No. 1, February 1. Covered entities under HIPAA. Available online at http://www.astho.org/phiip/documents.html. Accessed March 12, 2002.

ASTHO. 2001b. HIPAA policy brief, March 28. Available online at http://www.astho.org/phiip/documents.html. Accessed March 12, 2002.

ASTHO. 2001c. Bioterrorism preparedness. Testimony submitted to the U.S. Senate Committee on Appropriations, Subcommittee on Labor, Health and Human Services, and Education, October 3. Washington, DC: ASTHO.

ASTHO. 2001d. Performance assessment and standards, state tool. Available online at http://www.astho.org/phiip/performance.html. Accessed March 12, 2002.

ASTHO. 2002. 2002 salary survey of state and territorial health officials. Available online at http://www.astho.org/about/salary.html. Accessed March 12, 2002.

Bardach, E. 1998. Getting Agencies to Work Together. Washington, DC: Brookings Institution.

Barry MA, Centra L, Pratt E, Brown CK, Giordano L. 1998. Where do the dollars go? Measuring local public health expenditures. Submitted to the Office of Disease Prevention and Health Promotion, Department of Health and Human Services, by NACCHO, NALBOH, and PHF. Available online at www.phf.org. Accessed March 12, 2002.

Baxter R, Rubin R, Steinberg C, Carroll C, Shapiro J, Yang A (for The Lewin Group). 2000. Assessing Core Capacity for Infectious Diseases Surveillance. Final report. Department of Health and Human Services.

Beaulieu J, Scutchfield FD. 2002. Assessment of the validity of the National Public Health Performance Standards: the local public health performance assessment instrument. Public Health Reports 117(1):28–36.

Boufford JI, Lee P. 2001. Health Policies for the 21st Century: Challenges and Recommendations for the U.S. Department of Health and Human Services. New York: Milbank Memorial Fund.

Brewin B. 2001. Anthrax threat exposes IT ills. Computerworld, October 22.

Bureau of the Census. 2001a. State and county quick facts: Bergen County, New Jersey (year 2000 data). Available online at http://quickfacts.census.gov/qfd/states/34/34003.html. Accessed March 12, 2002.

Bureau of the Census. 2001b. State and county quick facts: Maine (year 2000 data). Available online at http://quickfacts.census.gov/ qfd/states/23000.html. Accessed March 12, 2002.

CDC (Centers for Disease Control and Prevention). 1995. Integrating public health information and surveillance systems: report and recommendations, Spring 1995. Available online at www.cdc.gov/od/hissb/docs/katz-0.htm. Accessed March 12, 2002.

CDC. 1997. Electronic reporting of laboratory data for public health. Report and recommendations from the March 24–25 meeting sponsored by the Council of State and Territorial Epidemiologists, Association of State and Territorial Public Health Laboratory Directors, and CDC. Available online at http://www.cdc.gov/od/hissb/act_elr.htm. Accessed March 12, 2002.

CDC. 1998. National Public Health Performance Standards Program. Available online at http://www.phppo.cdc.gov/nphpsp/index.asp. Accessed June 2, 2002.

CDC. 1999. Electronic reporting of laboratory information for public health. Report and recommendations from the January 7–8, 1999, meeting sponsored by the Centers for Disease Control and Prevention, Association of Public Health Laboratories, Council of State and Territorial Epidemiologists, and Association of State and Territorial Health Officials. Available online at http://www.cdc.gov/od/hissb/act_elr.htm. Accessed June 2, 2002.

CDC. 2000a. Biological and chemical terrorism: strategic plan for preparedness and response. Recommendations of the CDC Strategic Planning Workgroup. Morbidity and Mortality Weekly Report 49(RR–4):1–14.

CDC. 2000b. Integration project: National Electronic Disease Surveillance System. Available online at www.cdc.gov/od/hissb/act_int.htm. February 29. Accessed June 2, 2002.

CDC. 2000c. Supporting public health surveillance through the National Electronic Disease Surveillance System (NEDSS). Available online at www.cdc.gov/od/hissb/docs.htm. Accessed June 3, 2002.

CDC. 2000d. Proceedings from the Public Health Workforce Expert Panel Workshop, Pine Mountain, GA, November 1–2. Atlanta, GA: CDC.

CDC. 2001a. Bioterrorism: program in brief, January. Available online at www.cdc.gov/programs. Accessed June 2, 2002.

CDC. 2001b. Public health's infrastructure: a status report. Prepared for the Appropriations Committee of the U.S. Senate, March. Available online at www.phppo.cdc.gov. Accessed June 2, 2002.

CDC. 2001c. Innovations in public health: 2001 program review. Available online at http://www.phppo.cdc.gov/documents/ProgramReview2001.pdf. Accessed June 2, 2002.

CDC. 2001d. Enhanced surveillance project (ESP). Available online at http://www.bt.cdc.gov/episurv/esp.asp. Accessed June 2, 2002.

CDC. 2001e. A Global Life-Long Learning System: Building a Stronger Frontline Against Health Threats. January 5. Atlanta, GA: CDC.

CDC. 2001f. Genomics workforce competencies 2001. Available online at www.cdc.gov/genetics/training/competencies/comps.htm. Accessed June 2, 2002.

CDC. 2002. Programs in brief: chronic disease prevention. Available online at www.cdc.gov/programs/chronic. Accessed March 19, 2003.

CDC and Agency for Toxic Substances Disease Registry (ATSDR). 2001. A Global and National Implementation Plan for Public Health Workforce Development. Draft dated January 5. Atlanta, GA: CDC.

Center for Civilian Biodefense Studies. 2001. Hearing on FEMA's role in managing bioterrorist attacks and the impact of public health concerns on bioterrorism preparedness. Testimony of Tara O'Toole, MD, MPH, Senior Fellow, Center for Civilian Biodefense Studies, the Johns Hopkins University Schools of Public Health and Medicine, to the U.S. Senate Government Affairs Subcommittee on International Security, Proliferation and Federal Services, July 23. Available online at http://www.hopkins-biodefense.org/pages/library/fema.html. Accessed March 12, 2002.

Center for Infectious Disease Research and Policy and Workgroup on Bioterrorism Preparedness. 2001. Preparing a framework for public health action and bioterrorism preparedness: recommendations for federal funding of public health activities. Available online at www.asmusa.org/pasrc/fundingforbwc.htm. Accessed March 12, 2002.

Center for Law and the Public's Health. 2001. The Model State Emergency Health Powers Act: legislative specifications table. December 21. Available online at: http://www.publichealthlaw.net. Accessed March 12, 2002.

Cigler BA. 1998. Emerging trends in state and local relations. In Hanson RL (Ed.). Governing Partners: State–Local Relations in the United States. Boulder, CO: Westview Press.

Columbia Center for Health Policy. 2001. Local public health competency for emergency response. Columbia University School of Nursing, Center for Health Policy, April 2001. Available online at http://cpmcnet.columbia.edu/dept/nursing/institute-centers/chphsr/ERMain.html. Accessed July 18, 2002.

Connolly C. 2001. U.S. officials reorganize strategy on bioterrorism. Washington Post, November 8, p. A01.

Council on Linkages between Academia and Public Health Practice. 2001. Core competencies for public health practice. Available online at http://www.trainingfinder.org/competencies/list.htm. Accessed July 18, 2002.

CSTE (Council of State and Territorial Epidemiologists). 2001. The CSTE Washington Report, Vol. 5 (No. 20), October 24.

Davey S. 2000. The 10/90 Report on Health Research 2000. Geneva: Global Forum for Health Research.

Davies J, Jernigan DB. 1998. Development and evaluation of electronic laboratory-based reporting for infectious diseases surveillance. Paper presented at the International Conference for Emerging Infectious Diseases, Atlanta, GA, March 8–11.

Department of Defense. 2002. Syndromic surveillance: a new way to track emerging infectious diseases. Available online at http://www.geis.ha.osd.mil/getpage.asp?page=Syndromic-Surveillance.htm&action=7&click=KeyPrograms. Accessed March 19, 2002.

DHHS (Department of Health and Human and Services). 1994. Federal Approaches to Funding Public Health Programs: A Literature Review. Document No. OEI-01-94-00/60, August. Washington, DC: DHHS.

DHHS. 2000. Public health infrastructure. In Healthy People 2010. Available online at http://www.health.gov/healthypeople/document/tableofcontents. htm#volume2. Accessed March 19, 2002.

Duchin JS. 2002. Syndromic surveillance for bioterrorism and naturally-occurring communicable disease outbreaks. Presentation slides. Presented at the Asia Pacific Economic Cooperation Forum Network of Networks meeting, Seattle, WA, January 28–30. Available online at www.apec.org/infectious/NoN/Duchin.pdf. Accessed March 18, 2002.

Duffy J. 1990. The Sanitarians: A History of American Public Health. Urbana, IL: University of Chicago Press.

Ferrell JA, Mead PA. 1936. History of county health organizations in the United States 1908–1933. Washington, DC: Government Printing Office.

Forquera R. 2001. Urban Indian health. Issue brief prepared for the Henry J. Kaiser Family Foundation, November. Available online at http://www.kff.org/content/2001/6006/. Accessed March 18, 2002.

Fraser M. 1998. State and Local Health Department Structures Implications for Systems Change. Transformations for Public Health (The Turning Point Newsletter) 1(4).

Fraser MR. 1999. Information technology and local health departments. Presentation to the NACCHO Board Annual Meeting, Dearborn, MI, July 1. Available online at www.naccho.org/GENERAL156.cfm. Accessed March 18, 2002.

Freed GL, Clark SJ, Cowan AE. 2000. State-level perspectives on immunization policies, practices, and program financing in the 1990s. American Journal of Preventive Medicine 19(3 Suppl.):32–44.

GAO (General Accounting Office). 1999a. Emerging infectious diseases: consensus on needed laboratory capacity could strengthen surveillance. Report to the Chairman, U.S. Senate Subcommittee on Public Health, Committee on Health, Education, Labor, and Pensions, February. Document No. GAO/HEHS-99-26. Available online at www.gao.gov. Accessed March 18, 2002.

GAO. 1999b. Emerging infectious diseases: national surveillance system could be strengthened. Testimony of Bernice Steinhardt, Director of Health Services Quality and Public Health Issues, Health, Education, and Human Services Division, U.S. General Accounting Office, to the U.S. Senate Subcommittee on Public Health, Committee on Health, Education, Labor, and Pensions, February 25. Document No. GAO/T-HEHS-99-62. Available online at www.gao.gov. Accessed March 18, 2002.

GAO. 2001a. Food safety: CDC is working to address limitations in several of its foodborne disease surveillance systems. Report to the Chairman, U.S. Senate Committee on Agriculture, Nutrition, and Forestry, September. Document No. GAO-01-973. Available online at www.gao.gov. Accessed March 18, 2002.

GAO. 2001b. Bioterrorism: coordination and preparedness. Testimony of Janet Heinrich, Director, Health Care—Public Health Issues, U.S. General Accounting Office, to the Subcommittee on Government Efficiency, Financial Management, and Intergovernmental Relations, Committee on Government Reform, U.S. House of Representatives, October 5. Document No. GAO-02-129T. Available online at www.gao.gov. Accessed March 18, 2002.

Gostin LO. 2000. Public Health Law: Power, Duty, Restraint. Berkeley: University of California Press.

Gostin LO. 2002. Public Health Law and Ethics. Berkeley, New York: University of California Press and Milbank Memorial Fund.

Gostin LO, Burris S, Lazzarini Z. 1999. The law and the public's health: a study of infectious disease law in the United States. Columbia Law Review 59(1999):35.

Gostin LO, Sapsin JW, Teret S, Burris S, Mair JS, Hodge JG Jr, Vernick JS. 2002. The model state emergency health powers act: planning and response to bioterrorism and naturally occurring infectious diseases. Journal of the American Medical Association 288(5):622–628.

Gray BH, Rowe C. 2000. Safety-net health plans: a status report. Health Affairs 19(1):185–193.

Halverson PK, Nicola RM, Baker EL. 1998. Performance measurement and accreditation of public health organizations: a call to action. Journal of Public Health Management and Practice 4(4):5–7.

Hamilton DP. 2001. Public health labs aim to deploy better tests to identify bioagents. Wall Street Journal, October 11, p. A12.

Health Insurance Portability and Accountability Act of 1996. P.L. 104–191; 110 Statute 1936-2103. Available online at http://aspe.hhs.gov/admnsimp/pl104191.htm. Accessed March 12, 2002.

Henderson DA. 1998. Bioterrorism as a public health threat. Emerging Infectious Diseases 4(3). Available online at www.cdc.gov/ncidod/EID/vol4no3/henderson.htm. Accessed March 12, 2002.

HRSA (Health Resources and Services Administration). 2000. The Public Health Workforce: Enumeration 2000. Prepared for HRSA by Kristine Gebbie, Center for Health Policy, Columbia University School of Nursing, December. Washington, DC: HRSA.

HRSA. 2002. HRSA awards 27 community health center grants to improve access to services: president asks for $114 million increase in program for fiscal year 2003. HRSA press release, March 7, 2002. Available online at http://newsroom.hrsa.gov/releases/2002releases/chcgrants030702.htm. Accessed November 3, 2002.

Idaho Department of Health and Welfare. 1999. Public health in the new millennium: progress, new threats, new partners. Idaho Disease Bulletin 6(6). Available online at http://www2.state.id.us/dhw/cdp/bulletin/db12-99htm. Accessed March 12, 2002.

IHS (Indian Health Service). 2001a. Eligibility. February. Available online at http://info.ihs.gov/TreatiesLaws/Treaties_INDEX.asp. Accessed March 12, 2002.

IHS. 2001b. Indians in urban areas. February. Available online at http://info.ihs.gov/People/People_INDEX.asp. Accessed March 12, 2002.

IHS. 2001c. Tribal self-determination. February. Available online at http://info.ihs.gov/TreatiesLaws/Treaties_INDEX.asp. Accessed March 12, 2002.

IOM (Institute of Medicine). 1988. The Future of Public Health. Washington DC: National Academy Press.

IOM. 1992. Emerging Infections: Microbial Threats to Health. In Lederberg J, Shope RE, Oaks SC, Jr. (Eds.). Washington DC: National Academy Press.

IOM. 1996. Healthy Communities: New Partnerships for the Future of Public Health. Washington, DC: National Academy Press.

IOM. 1997a. America's Vital Interest in Global Health. Washington, DC: National Academy Press.

IOM. 1997b. In Durch JS, Bailey LA, Stoto MA (Eds.). Improving Health in the Community: A Role for Performance Monitoring. Washington DC: National Academy Press.

IOM. 1999. Creating a High Profile for Global Health. Highlights from an Institute of Medicine conference, February 28, 1999. Washington, DC: National Academy Press.

IOM. 2000a. America's Health Care Safety Net: Intact but Endangered. Washington, DC: National Academy Press.

IOM. 2000b. Calling the Shots: Immunization Finance Policies and Practices. Washington, DC: National Academy Press.

IOM. 2001. Crossing the Quality Chasm: A New Health System for the 21st Century. Washington, DC: National Academy Press.

IOM. 2003. Who Will Keep the Public Healthy? Educating Public Health Professionals in the 21st Century. Washington, DC: The National Academies Press.

Johnson R, Morris TF. 2000. Stabilizing the rural public health infrastructure. Publication for the National Advisory Committee on Rural Health, February. Available online at http://www.nal.usda.gov/orhp/nac_rep.htm. Accessed March 12, 2002.

Keane C, Marx J, Ricci E. 2001. Privatization and the scope of public health: a national survey of local health department directors. American Journal of Public Health 91(4): 611–617.

Keppel KG, Freedman MA. 1995. What is assessment? Journal of Public Health Management and Practice 1(2):1–7.

Kuttner R. 1999. The American health care system—employer-sponsored health coverage. New England Journal of Medicine 340(3):248–252.

Larson C, Sweeney C, Christian A, Olson L. 2002. Collaborative Leadership and Health: A Review of the Literature. Seattle, WA: Turning Point National Program Office.

Lee PB, Abramovice BG, Lee PR. 2001. Written supplement to the testimony of Dr. Philip R. Lee to supplement a presentation to the Workgroup on Health Statistics for the 21st Century and the Workgroup on National Health Information Infrastructure of the National Committee on Vital and Health Statistics. Available online at http://ncvhs.hhs.gov/001030h7.htm. Accessed September 23, 2002.

The Lewin Group. 1997. Strategies for obtaining public health infrastructure data at the federal, state and local levels. Prepared for DHHS. Available online at http://aspe.hhs.gov/PIC/pdf/6179.PDF. Accessed November 3, 2002.

LLGIS (Local Leaders for Geographic Information Systems) Consortium. 2001. Bioterrorism in New York. Available online at http://www.llgis.org/pages/news/index.htm. Accessed March 12, 2002.

Lumpkin JR. 2001. Air, water, places, and data—public health in the information age. Journal of Public Health Management and Practice 7(6):22–30.

Lumpkin JR, Atkinson D, Biery R, Cundiff D, McGlothlin M, Novick LF. 1995. The development of integrated public health information systems: a statement by the Joint Council of Governmental Public Health Agencies. Journal of Public Health Management and Practice 1(4):55–59.

Lumpkin JR, Landrum LB, Oldfield A, Kimel P, Jones MC, Moody CM, Turnock BJ. 1998. Impact of Medicaid resources on core public health responsibilities of local health departments in Illinois. Journal of Public Health Management and Practice 4(6):69–78.

Mays GP, Halverson PK, Stevens R. 2001. The contributions of managed care plans to public health practice: evidence from the nation's largest local health departments. Public Health Reports 116(Suppl. I):50–67.

Meit MB. 2001. I'm OK, but I'm not too sure about you: public health at the state and local levels. Journal of Public Health Management and Practice 7(1):vii–viii.

NACCHO (National Association of County and City Health Officials). 1998. Preliminary results from the 1997 Profile of U.S. Local Health Departments. NACCHO Research Brief No. 1., September. Washington, D.C.: NACCHO.

NACCHO. 2001a. Assessment of local bioterrorism and emergency preparedness. NACCHO Research Brief No. 5, October. Available online at www.naccho.org/project48.cfm. Accessed March 12, 2002.

NACCHO. 2001b. Testimony of Rex Archer, director, Kansas City Health Department, Kansas City, Missouri, on behalf of NACCHO before the U.S. Senate Subcommittee on Labor, Health and Human Services, Education and Related Agencies, Committee on Appropriations, October. Available online at http://www.naccho.org/advocacydoc424.cfm. Accessed March 12, 2002.

NACCHO. 2001c. NACCHO statement to the press regarding the administration's bioterrorism emergency funding request, October 18. Available online at www.naccho.org/press40.cfm. Accessed March 12, 2002.

NACCHO. 2001d. Local public health agency infrastructure: a chartbook, October. Available online at www.naccho.org/prod111.cfm. Accessed March 12, 2002.

NACCHO. 2001e. Letter to the president regarding bioterrorism funding, October 18. Available online at www.naccho.org/advocacydoc430.cfm. Accessed September 13, 2002.

NACCHO. 2001f. National Public Health Performance Standards Program (NPHPSP), local instrument. Available online at www.naccho.org/project48.cfm. Accessed March 12, 2002.

NALBOH (National Association of Local Boards of Health). 2001. National Public Health Performance Standards program, governance instrument. Available online at http://www.nalboh.org/perfstds/instrument.htm. Accessed March 12, 2002.

National Partnership for Social Enterprise. 2002. A Business Plan for the Implementation of Practice Standards in Bergen County: A Demonstration Project of the New Jersey Department of Health and Senior Services, December 29, 2001. Bergen County, NJ: Bergen County, Department of Health Services.

NCVHS (National Committee on Vital and Health Statistics). 2002. Information for Health: A Strategy for Building the National Health Information Infrastructure. Report and recommendations from the Work Group on the National Health Information Infrastructure, Washington, DC, November 15, 2001. Available online at http://ncvhs.hhs.gov. Accessed March 12, 2002.

NGA (National Governors Association). 1997. Policy positions. Washington, DC: National Governors Association.

Noren J, Kindig D, Sprenger A. 1998. Challenges to Native American health care. Public Health Reports 113(1):22–33.

NRC (National Research Council). 2002. Making the Nation Safer: The Role of Science and Technology in Countering Terrorism. Washington, DC: The National Academies Press.

OMB (Office of Management and Budget). 2001. Budget summary, FY 2002. Available online at http://www.whitehouse.gov/omb/budget/fy2002/budiv_3.html. Accessed September 18, 2002.

OMB. 2002. Budget of the United States Government, Fiscal Year 2003. Washington, DC: OMB.

Osterholm MT, Schwartz J. 2000. Living Terrors: What America Needs to Know to Survive a Bioterrorist Catastrophe. New York: Delacorte Press.

Pew Environmental Health Commission. 1999. Healthy from the Start: Why America Needs a Better System to Track and Understand Birth Defects and the Environment. Report sponsored by the Pew Environmental Health Commission at the Johns Hopkins School of Hygiene and Public Health, November. Available online at http://pewenvirohealth.jhsph.edu. Accessed September 18, 2002.

Pew Environmental Health Commission. 2000. America's Environmental Health Gap: Why the Country Needs a Nationwide Tracking Network. Report sponsored by the Pew Environmental Health Commission at the Johns Hopkins School of Hygiene and Public Health, November. Available online at http://pewenvirohealth.jhsph.edu. Accessed September 18, 2002.

Pew Health Professions Commission. 1998. Recreating Health Professional Practice for a New Century. San Francisco: Pew Health Professions Commission.

Public Health Foundation. 2000. Statewide public health expenditures: a pilot study in Maryland, March 2000. Available online at http://www.phf.org/Reports.htm. Accessed March 12, 2002.

Public Health Functions Steering Committee. 1994. Public health in America, fall 1994. Available online at www.health.gov/phfunctions/public.htm. Accessed March 12, 2002.

Rich M. 1993. Federal policymaking and the poor: national goals, local choices, and distributional outcomes. Princeton, NJ: Princeton University Press.

Rosen G. A History of Public Health. 1993. Baltimore, MD: Johns Hopkins University Press.

Salinsky E. 2002. Will the nation be ready for the next bioterrorism attack? Mending gaps in the public health infrastructure. National Health Policy Issue Brief No. 776, June 12. Available online at http://www.nhpf.org/ibonline.cfm. Accessed September 18, 2002.

Sandia National Laboratories. 2002. Rapid Syndromic Validation Project (RSVP). Available online at http://www.cmc.sandia.gov/bio/rsvp. Accessed September 18, 2002 .

Study Group on the Mission and Organization of the Public Health Service. 1960. The Hundley Report.

Turnock B. 2000. Public Health: What It Is and How It Works, 2nd ed. Gaithersburg, MD: Aspen Publishers.

U.S. House of Representatives. 2002. House Report 107-350 - Making Appropriations for the Department of Defense for the Fiscal Year Ending September 30, 2002, and for Other Purposes. Available online at: http://thomas.loc.gov. Accessed October 21, 2002.

USPHS (U.S. Public Health Service). 1997. The Public Health Workforce: An Agenda for the 21st Century. Washington, DC: Department of Health and Human Services.

Valdiserri R. 1993. Temples of the future: an historical overview of the laboratory's role in public health practice. Annual Review of Public Health 14:635–648.

Wall S. 1998. Transformations in public health systems. Health Affairs 17(3):64–80.

White House. 2001. A Blueprint For New Beginnings: A Responsible Budget for America's Priorities. Washington, DC: U.S. Government Printing Office. Available online at: http://www.whitehouse.gov/news/usbudget/ blueprint/budtoc.html. Accessed March 18, 2002.

4

The Community

The community stagnates without the impulse of the individual.
The impulse dies away without the sympathy of the community.

William James

This chapter is at the heart of the *Healthy People 2010* vision reiterated by the committee: "healthy people in healthy communities." Communities are both the physical and cultural settings for and—through their residents and community-based organizations—participants in action to promote the public's health. They are also points of convergence for the interests of employers, businesses, and academia; the messages of the media; and the services of governmental public health agencies and the health care delivery system.

This chapter examines the multiple dimensions of community and its critical importance to an effective public health system. This critical role has been a fundamental concept in the international literature on population health for many years. The Health For All initiative, begun by the World Health Organization in the 1970s, called for a strong primary care system to include basic health services, clean water and air, basic sanitation, adequate nutrition, and full engagement with the community served. In the United States, the sophistication of the health care delivery system and the emphasis on individual health have led to the focus of policy and resources on the high-technology and research ends of the health care delivery spectrum and an underestimation or overlooking of the role of the community in achieving health gains. This is changing.

DEFINING THE COMMUNITY

A community can be described as a group of people who share some or all of the following: geographic boundaries; a sense of membership; culture and language; common norms, interests, or values; and common health risks or conditions (IOM, 1995; Jewkes and Murcott, 1996; Ruderman, 2000; Ricketts, 2001). Members of communities typically experience the shared reality of living or working in the same location or environment and so are in a position to influence and be influenced by the social, economic, and physical risk factors in that environment (Roussos and Fawcett, 2000; Kreuter et al., 2001). Although acknowledging the increasing influence of "communities of interaction" such as online groups, this chapter focuses mainly on activities based in geographic communities—neighborhoods, cities, counties, and in a few cases, states—that are critical to creating the conditions for a community to be as healthy as it can be.

Communities consist of individuals and families, as well as the various organizations and associations that make up a community's "civil society": nonprofit, nongovernmental, voluntary, or social entities, including ethnic and cultural groups; advocacy organizations; and the faith community (Salamon et al., 1999; Himmelman et al., 2001). Organizations exist between the level of the individual and that of the community or society. The United States has both a history of individualism and, as de Tocqueville observed in 1831, a rich civic tradition of individuals associating or organizing to accomplish common goals. The public sector at the community level encompasses local government officials and agencies traditionally seen as having health-related responsibilities, as well as many others that have important but sometimes less obvious roles in health but whose policies and objectives may have potential health consequences. The latter may include city councils, public schools, colleges and universities, police and fire departments, zoning boards, housing authorities, parks and recreation agencies, and agricultural development and cooperative extension services. Other members of the community may come from the private sector, including private schools, colleges, and universities; health care providers and payers; and small and large businesses.

A healthy community is a place where people provide leadership in assessing their own resources and needs, where public health and social infrastructure and policies support health, and where essential public health services, including quality health care, are available. In a healthy community, communication and collaboration among various sectors of the community and the contributions of ethnically, socially, and economically diverse community members are valued. In addition, the broad array of determinants of health is considered and addressed, and individuals make informed, positive choices in the context of health-protective and supportive environments, policies, and systems (Goodman et al., 1996; CDC, 1997; Norris and Pittman, 2000).

Health is a "fundamental resource to the individual, the community and to society" (Kickbusch, 1989: 13). When people are healthy, they are better able to work, learn, build a good life, and contribute to society. However, as noted in Chapter 2, the health of neither individuals nor populations occurs in a vacuum. Instead, it is shaped by a wide range of factors, such as income and education, social connectedness, employment, and access to quality health care. Inadequate and dangerous physical environments in homes, schools, neighborhoods, and workplaces and risk factors such as air and water pollution, unsafe food, social isolation, high rates of unemployment, violence, and crime constitute some of the problems experienced by communities. It may seem that these types of problems can be distanced from the concerns of the general population, as if these circumstances affect only certain groups (e.g., those with high blood pressure, smokers, or people who live in specific neighborhoods). In reality, the effects of health risks touch us all in many ways, and actions to address health at the population level benefit everyone in society (Rose, 1992). Moreover, the solutions for assuring population health are not owned by governmental public health agencies; they can be found in communities and in community organizations and partnerships (CDC, 1997; WHO, 1998; Bowles, 1999; Mitchell and Shortell, 2000). Today's health challenges, ranging from jet-setting microbes and soaring obesity rates to emerging environmental risks and bioterrorism, highlight the interconnectedness of people and communities and the need for joint efforts to meet those challenges (McGinnis and Foege, 1993; Ruderman, 2000; Norton et al., 2002).

The linkages among people and communities and people are clearly evident in the processes set into motion by globalization. A local community in many areas of the United States may be a microcosm of the world community, with a complex mix of beliefs, traditions, and languages. Given the rich fabric of most American communities, it has become impossible to consider threats to health someone else's problem. Disease and disability do not differentiate between cultures and ethnic backgrounds—microbes and environmental toxins move easily among and across nations and regions, and no person or community is completely safe unless all are safe.

COMMUNITY-BASED COLLABORATION

Growing Commitment to Collaboration

Although this report defines public health as "what we as a society do collectively to assure the conditions in which people can be healthy" (IOM, 1988: 1), in practice, the community's role in health programs has sometimes been that of passive recipient, beneficiary, or research subject, with active work in public health carried out by experts (e.g., governmental public health agencies) using approaches that are frequently unsuccessful in responding to the complex issues and needs of the community (Schwab and

Syme, 1997). A great deal has changed since the Committee for the Future of Public Health observed that health departments and public health professionals worked largely in isolation, with little in the way of "constituency building, citizen participation, or continuing (as opposed to crisis-driven) communications with elected officials or with the community at large" (IOM, 1988: 5). Today, dialogue and collaboration between local health departments and the communities they serve have become more common in practice and more critical in concept. For example, a recent study of 10 local health departments from different states found that they were substantially involved with community and youth organizations, schools, and the media in the areas of tobacco use prevention, injury prevention, and physical activity promotion (McHugh et al., 2000).

Many communities, through individuals and organizations, have become partners with health departments in health improvement and have even become leaders in spearheading collaborative efforts (Fawcett et al., 1996; Mitchell and Shortell, 2000; Norton et al., 2002). The present committee found during its site visit to the Caring Community Network of the Twin Rivers, a Turning Point site in New Hampshire (see Appendix F), an example of an innovative way to create a local public health system that works effectively despite a limited governmental public health infrastructure. This community, a spread-out cluster of 12 towns, has no health department. Instead, each town has a more or less volunteer health officer, who in some cases is not a health professional. The work of assuring the public's health is carried out through the collaborative efforts of committed individuals and groups, including the local public health officials, health care and mental health services providers, social service and community development organizations, educators, and the chamber of commerce (CCNTR, 2001).

In authentic community-based partnerships, the participation and contributions of various stakeholders are likely to produce benefits in the form of increased effectiveness and productivity by reducing duplication of effort and avoiding the imposition of solutions that are not congruent with the local culture and needs. Community partnerships are also likely to have the benefits of empowering the participants, strengthening social engagement, establishing trust, and ensuring accountability (Israel et al., 1998; Mitchell and Shortell, 2000; Robinson and Elliott, 2000; Steele, 2000; Butterfoss et al., 2001; Chaskin et al., 2001; Lasker et al., 2001; Williams and Yanoshik, 2001; Wolff, 2001a, 2001b).

A variety of vehicles can be used for community collaborations, including coalitions, partnerships, community advisory boards, consumers' rights and advocacy groups, and nonprofit organizations. These groupings can bring together participants from many sectors of a community, including businesses, ethnic groups, faith-based organizations, and various public agencies. The Kansas LEAN (Leadership to Encourage Activity and Nutrition) Coalition is an example of a statewide coalition that began at the local level in 1990. By 1997, it had expanded to include 60 organizations and 100 individuals. The coalition brought together governmental agencies such as the state and local public health departments and state and local extension offices, nonprofit community and professional organizations, and businesses such as supermarkets to prevent chronic disease through dietary change and exercise (Johnston et al., 1996).

Some opportunities for collaboration have less obvious but important health effects, as in the case of community redevelopment efforts. The economic condition of a community has clear implications for health. Higher employment levels, for example, tend to improve not only personal income and access to health insurance but also a community's tax revenues and, thus, its ability to address health threats and to provide opportunities for health improvement. In some communities, local health departments have become partners in efforts to revitalize neighborhoods through the remediation of areas with industrial waste and environmental contamination (NACCHO, 2000a). Empowerment zones and enterprise communities are examples of public–private partnerships with significant government resources requiring collaboration at the local level to improve health in communities. A recent study found that 119 of the 144 national empowerment zones and enterprise communities initiatives had an interest in health issues (PHF, 2000).

Some collaborations come into existence through the independent initiative of communities or community groups, whereas others are created in response to an outside stimulus, such as when government agencies or foundations require the formation of broad partnerships as part of grant processes (Mitchell and Shortell, 2000). The committee is encouraged to see indications that governmental public health agencies, community health centers, hospitals, and health maintenance organizations recognize that community collaboration is a necessity in health improvement (CDC, 1997; Pronk and O'Connor, 1997; Omenn, 1999). Some of the major federal and foundation initiatives that require and support the creation of broad-based community coalitions include Healthy Start, a community-based infant mortality reduction program; Turning Point[1] and Community Voices,[2]

---

[1] Turning Point is a grant program of the W. K. Kellogg and Robert Wood Johnson Foundations that began in 1996 and ended in 2002. The goal of Turning Point has been to "transform and strengthen the public health infrastructure in the United States" by supporting states and local communities to "improve the performance of their public health functions through strategic development and implementation processes" (www.wkkf.org).

[2] Community Voices is a 5-year initiative launched by the W. K. Kellogg Foundation in 1998 in 13 U.S. communities. The goal of Community Voices is to improve health care for the uninsured and underinsured by strengthening and securing the safety net and community support services.

privately funded community public health improvement grant programs; and Center for Substance Abuse Prevention programs, which support community-based substance abuse prevention "systems" that involve community coalitions and intersectoral collaboration (Lasker et al., 2001).

Ingredients for Successful Collaboration

Although collaborations to improve community health have become increasingly common, the committee recognizes that bringing together diverse agendas, institutional cultures and jargon, personalities, and expectations can be complicated, frustrating, and sometimes disappointing. One lesson that has been learned from such experiences, however, is that the community must be engaged before an agenda is set—the active participation of community leaders, members, and organizations is needed in the earliest stages of community-based public health action, if it is not already the force that drives such action (The Lewin Group, 2002). The initial communication and networking necessary to launch a community health improvement project entail frank examination and discussion of motivations, approaches, and goals by all stakeholders. At times, agencies and organizations may seek to implement their own unilateral agendas in communities, driven by scientific, political, economic, or professional interests, with token community involvement and often negative outcomes (Schwab and Syme, 1997; Fawcett, 1999; Norton et al., 2002). Many communities have been "coalitioned to death" without reaping any significant benefits (Himmelman et al., 2001). Such problems illustrate the need for thoughtful, broadly inclusive, well-planned, and realistic community health improvement approaches.

Clearly, community health initiatives involve complex social and relational dynamics, as well as efforts to produce change that require significant investments of time and resources (Wickizer et al., 1998; Kreuter et al., 2000; Sharpe et al., 2000; Shortell, 2000; Rhein et al., 2001). The importance of allotting adequate time to the process of collaborative planning was well illustrated during the committee's site visit to Healthy New Orleans, a Turning Point project in Louisiana (see Appendix F). Healthy New Orleans worked over a period of 2 years to build a partnership of diverse stakeholders. After establishing and clarifying roles and relationships, the partnership was able to develop a plan for community health improvement that was truly a product of community knowledge and effort (Healthy New Orleans, 2001).

The HIV/AIDS movement provides another example of successful collaboration for community action (Stewart and Weinstein, 1997). AIDS volunteerism has uniquely demonstrated the effectiveness of turning people affected by AIDS into experts who both (1) mobilized community building and (2) transformed community attitudes and norms to achieve behavioral change. Communities working on a range of health issues may have much to learn from the example set by the gay and lesbian communities' collaborative action. Yet, although the HIV/AIDS movement has succeeded in mobilizing public opinion and action, more research is needed to show what has worked best in mobilizing action and changing community norms and thus warrants replication (Kegeles and Hart, 1998; Reger et al., 2000).

Research to assess the effectiveness of community collaborations has had somewhat mixed results because of the heterogeneity of communities, the long time lines involved in achieving community health improvement goals, and other complexities inherent in community-driven public health activities (Sharpe et al., 2000; Lasker et al., 2001). However, a growing base of empirical evidence from programs such as Turning Point and Community Voices provides a good road map for communities and their partners. Health improvement and other positive outcomes typically result from collaborations that are sustained over the long term, that institutionalize effective programs and processes, and that mobilize and utilize all available resources to deal with evolving challenges and population health issues (Fawcett et al., 2000b, 2000c).

Success is also more likely with strong community engagement, an awareness of the community's social dynamics, and leadership that reflects the racial and ethnic diversity of the community (CDC, 1997). Other important ingredients include having a clear vision and goals to guide action planning; allotting adequate time and financial, technical, and other supportive resources to collaborations and their health improvement efforts; and recognizing the importance of data collection and dissemination (CDC, 1997; W. K. Kellogg Foundation, 1997; Fawcett et al., 2000c; Roussos and Fawcett, 2000). Success in specific health improvement activities can depend on the use of varied strategies and on their intensity, duration, and penetration into the community (Fawcett et al., 2000b; Wilcox and Knapp, 2000; Lasker et al., 2001; Paine-Andrews, 2002).

Problems arise around leadership, governance, and other management issues, such as planning and evaluation. Inadequate resources of various sorts—insufficient or inadequate funding or data, short time lines, or a lack of technical support—also contribute to problems, as does a lack of broad and authentic community engagement, which may be reflected in narrowly formed partnerships that do not include all the sectors of the community needed for efficient and effective action (Himmelman et al., 2001; Lasker et al., 2001).

Sharing Public Health Governance

Ultimate legal responsibility for safeguarding and promoting the health of the population rests with governmental public health agencies at the federal, state, and local levels (see Chapter 3), but those agencies cannot be effective acting alone. They must be partners in a broader network of individuals and organizations with the potential to act within a public health system. At the local level, in particular, health departments can become the facilitators and supporters of strong local public health systems that are informed by community voices, responsive to community needs, and linked to community assets.

The committee supports a type of shared governance through which the agenda for population health is truly "owned" by the population it serves (Turning Point Community Health Governance Workgroup, 2001a and b; The Lewin Group, 2002). This entails providing opportunities for community input and leadership in planning and in funding decisions. It also requires educating the public about the concepts of public health, including the core functions and essential services (see Chapter 1), to help ensure that public health agencies are accountable to those they serve (Becnel, 2001). An approach used in some communities is governance of the health department by a local board of health, whose members come from various sectors of the community (see Chapter 3). The committee also encourages community involvement in the governance of other health-related activities. For example, a majority of the members of oversight boards for community health centers that receive federal funding (under Section 330 of the Public Health Law) must be community users of those facilities' services.

The Turning Point initiative—which involves 41 communities across 14 states—exemplifies shared governance. The most successful of the Turning Point sites mobilized the community from the earliest stages of assessing needs and setting an agenda for public health system change. These partnerships made community engagement a permanent and ongoing element. In fact, the community's role became institutionalized in the local public health system through formal policies, investments, and programs (The Lewin Group, 2002). This national experiment in transforming local governmental public health agencies (Turning Point Community Health Governance Workgroup, 2001b) suggests that making shared governance a reality requires tools that formalize the governance structure so that it can achieve legitimacy. Also necessary are optimal communication between the community and the governing group and systematic, efficient and flexible management of operations (Turning Point Community Health Governance Workgroup, 2001b). The National Public Health Performance Standards Program[3] includes an evolving set of model standards for the role of a

---

[3] The National Public Health Performance Standards Program is a collaborative effort by the Centers for Disease Control and Prevention, Association of State and Territorial Health Officials, National Association of County and City Health Officials, National Association of Local Boards of Health, American Public Health Association, and Public Health Foundation to develop measurable performance standards to help ensure that state and local public health systems are able to and do deliver the 10 essential public health services (CDC, 2001).

governing body in a local public health system and an instrument for assessing the performance of that governing body (National Association of Local Boards of Health, 2002).

FRAMEWORK FOR COLLABORATIVE
COMMUNITY ACTION ON HEALTH

Once the collaboration has been created, several frameworks are available for use by communities, health departments, and their partners. Some of these models include the Planned Approach to Community Health, Mobilizing for Action through Planning and Partnerships, and the Community Health Improvement Process (Kreuter, 1992; IOM, 1997). The models provide step-by-step guidance for various aspects of the health improvement process, including assessing the health status of the community and the capacity of the local governmental public health agency.

This chapter uses a simple framework provided by Fawcett and colleagues (2000b) to help describe the activities and processes involved in community action on health (CDC, 2002). This framework illustrates five key components of the activities and processes needed in community health action (Figure 4-1). Figure 4-1 illustrates a process that is often cyclical rather than linear, with work on one health improvement initiative leading to subsequent reassessments of a community's health needs and priorities.

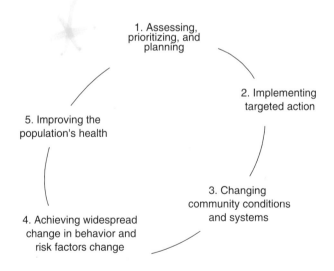

FIGURE 4-1 A framework for collaborative public health action by communities. SOURCES: Fawcett et al. (2000b); CDC (2002).

Although the five components of this particular framework do not necessarily take place in the sequential fashion shown, the diagram reflects the progression of events that has been documented in successful community-based public health initiatives (Fawcett et al., 2000b; Foster-Fishman et al., 2001).

Each step of the framework for collaborative action will be discussed and illustrated with examples from the experience of community health improvement programs and initiatives.

Assessing, Prioritizing, and Planning

The processes of assessing, prioritizing, and planning will help community partnerships formulate a clear statement of goals to guide their work. These collaborative tasks are the first components of community action for health, but they also must be ongoing activities throughout a community's health improvement efforts (IOM, 1996b, 1997; GHCF, 2001). By engaging in these activities, communities come to understand the context, causes, and solutions for various health problems. They include taking inventory of community assets and resources, identifying priorities for community action, and planning the actions to be taken. Community organizing and coalition building are necessary if these activities are to be collaborative.

The Health Action initiative in Monroe County, New York, provides a good example of community involvement in assessing, prioritizing, and planning for health improvement (Milbank Memorial Fund, 1998; Health Action, 2001). Founded in 1995, Health Action is a collaborative of health care providers, hospitals and clinics, the local health department, an urban health commission, a university, the chamber of commerce, a large employers' organization, and a professional association. Between 1998 and 2001, report cards were developed and released for five areas: (1) the health of mothers and children, (2) the health of adolescents, (3) the health of adults, (4) the health of older adults, and (5) environmental health. Focused goals and action plans were developed for each area. For adults and older adults, Health Action selected two goals: to promote healthy behaviors that prevent or delay chronic disease and to promote the use of preventive health services. Health promotion objectives included increasing physical activity and providing nutrition education and weight management, with the aim of decreasing the chronic disease risks posed by overweight and obesity. In 2001, Health Action's Adult/Older Adult coalition began work on a communications campaign supported by program activities (such as workplace fitness) to make Monroe County a more physically active community.

Certain types of quantitative data, such as rates of disease, injury, and death, have usually been available to communities. Other data have become more readily available as more states and local communities, usually with the leadership or support of governmental public health agencies, have begun to conduct systematic assessments of health status and the determinants of health. The availability of data for small areas (at the subcounty level) has been an issue in general for community health programs, and it highlights the need for high-quality, comprehensive assessments of community health to guide action. In 2000, the Health Resources and Services Administration's Community Health Status Indicators (CHSI) Project produced a set of health assessment documents for each of the 3,082 counties in the United States and made them available online (www.communityhealth.hrsa.gov/). The CHSI documents, which used a set of indicators for which comparable data were available for nearly all counties, can serve as a useful starting point for selecting indicators of particular interest to a given community, for making comparisons with other communities throughout the country, or for planning an update of a community's indicators.

A community-based approach to health improvement that considers the broad range of social and environmental determinants of health may call for the use of a variety of indicators, including ones that measure characteristics of the community rather than those of individuals (i.e., community-level indicators). Community report cards and other types of regular assessments should include not only measures directly related to health, such as infant mortality rates and the incidence of infectious diseases, but also measures related to various health determinants (IOM, 1997). Indicators could include local employment rates, housing stocks, and levels of income and education, along with less conventional indicators such as the density of liquor stores; the quality of air and water; the availability of parks and green spaces, housing, and public transportation; and other measures of livability. In addition, qualitative or anecdotal data (e.g., residents' satisfaction with the community, feelings of community cohesion, or informal measures of social capital) may also be an important part of the assessment process.

The interest in community-level indicators is reflected in the work of a panel organized by the Centers for Disease Control and Prevention, which developed indicators for cardiovascular health in three risk areas: diet, physical inactivity, and tobacco use (Cheadle et al., 2000). The community-level indicators for physical inactivity, for example, included "miles of walking trails per capita" and "presence of local policy to include physical education in public K–12 curriculum" (Cheadle et al., 2000: 112). Cross-cutting indicators included the number of media reports that dealt with smoking, nutrition, and physical activity and the number of assessments or screenings within the community for all cardiovascular risk factors. An added benefit of community-level indicators is the fact that they are sometimes easier and less expensive to measure than indicators based on the behaviors or characteristics of individuals, which may require costly household surveys.

The committee notes that new and evolving information and communications technologies are increasingly valuable resources for community-driven public health action (Fawcett et al., 2000a). The University of Kansas Community Tool Box, for example, is an online resource for community-based public health planning and action (http://ctb.lsi.ukans. edu/). The Internet has become instrumental in helping community groups and organizations obtain essential data and information, communicate with partners, and provide technical assistance and support to other collaborations and coalitions in their own community and elsewhere. In recent years, geographic information systems have also become a powerful tool for spatial analysis of diseases, environmental contamination, and social and demographic information (ATSDR, 2000). Some of the governmental jurisdictions (i.e., states) using this technology are able to share vital information with communities and their partners.

Implementing Targeted Action

The second component of community-driven health improvement efforts is implementing targeted action to address high-priority health issues (Fawcett et al., 2000b). As a result of some of the lessons learned in community collaborative action, observers commend the use of multiple strategies, such as education, various forms of communication, political or legal action, and environmental interventions (Fawcett, 1999). Some observers emphasize that community action should focus on changing the community conditions or individual behaviors that affect health risks rather than on only providing health care or other services to individuals (Johnston et al., 1996).

As a result of the sometimes long and often complicated chain of events between program implementation and desired health outcomes, communities are encouraged to focus on proven strategies and best practices to enhance their chances of success (IOM, 1997; Butterfoss et al., 2001). Resources such as *The Guide to Community Preventive Services* (Task Force on Community Preventive Services, 2000), which provides evidence-based evaluations of various interventions, can help communities select appropriate strategies. In some cases, however, coalitions may be justified in selecting interventions that are favored by the community, even if evidence for their effectiveness is weak, to build ownership in community action and to nurture meaningful participation (Himmelman, 2001; W. K. Kellogg Foundation, 2001). The challenge is to achieve a balance between the interrelated efforts to engage coalition involvement and sustain its well-being and to invest in strategies that increase the likelihood of meeting health goals.

The strategies and activities implemented by community partnerships may depend on the particular perspectives and resources brought to the

---

BOX 4-1
Community in Action to Address the Environment

In New York State, the Monroe County Health Department and other public and private community partners formed the Water Education Collaborative to educate citizens about protecting water quality. The Industrial Management Council, the Monroe County Health Department, and the Rochester Institute of Technology are collaborating on a plan to provide environmental health training and technical assistance to small- and medium-size businesses. This will help local businesses develop environmental management systems (environmental monitoring, waste recycling). The Kodak and Xerox corporations, which are headquartered locally, already provide leadership in this area.

SOURCE: Health Action (2001).

---

table by participants. For example, groups that represent the interests of ethnic communities (e.g., National Council of La Raza, Congress of National Black Churches, and Association of Asian Pacific Community Health Organizations) or consumers' rights and advocacy groups can help mobilize communities for action, provide public education, and advocate for policy change to safeguard population health. Businesses may change their practices and policies to address community health concerns and employee health needs (see Box 4–1). Depending on the nature of the business, such changes might include implementing policies to ban smoking in public places, providing health information to employees and customers, or improving compliance with environmental laws and regulations pertaining to air and water quality.

Religious congregations, which are among "the most pervasive voluntary organizations in our society," and other faith-based entities can play a significant role in community health improvement (DHHS, 1999). For instance, the outreach workers of Oakland's Asian Health Services reach Korean groups with information about health care access at church health fairs. Faith-based groups are often community institutions, deeply rooted in neighborhoods, and may play an important role in local public health systems and community-based health improvement initiatives (DHHS, 1999; Lundblad, 1999). This is especially true in many African-American communities. Additionally, faith communities can act as conveners and mobilizers of community residents and others affiliated with them around issues of health policy and interventions for health promotion and disease prevention (e.g., nutrition, fitness, and health screening services) (see Box 4–2).

BOX 4–2
A Project in the Faith Community

Project Joy was conducted by university researchers in collaboration with a local faith community to promote cardiovascular health among church-going African-American women in Baltimore, Maryland (Yanek et al., 2001). Sixteen churches were randomly selected, and 529 female members of those churches received one of three behavioral interventions: an active intervention with a spiritual component, an active intervention without the spiritual component, and a self-help intervention as a control group. The active intervention consisted of weekly sessions on nutrition, including cooking demonstrations and taste tests, and 30 minutes of some moderate aerobic activity, conducted by project educators in collaboration with trained lay leaders from the churches. The spiritual component consisted of religious messages and prayer and gospel music for workout sessions. The control intervention provided only educational material and a hotline for health education consultation.

By the end of the intervention, the two active groups were virtually indistinguishable, because the one without a preplanned spiritual component had created its own. Both of the groups with the active intervention experienced significant improvements, compared with the self-help group, in weight, waist circumference, blood pressure, dietary energy, and total fat and sodium intakes. The input and participation of the community in planning and implementation and a supportive social environment resulted in behavioral changes that led to improved health. Four years after the project began, eight of the nine churches with an active intervention, plus the church that hosted the pilot intervention, continue the weekly support and education sessions—an example of sustained, institutionalized change (Yanek et al., 2001).

Communities can also contribute to the process of health improvement through the efforts of individuals who sometimes become part of the public health workforce. For example, in communities across the United States, health promoters,[4] community health workers, or community outreach workers link community members to systems of care, help to mobilize communities to change the conditions for health, and conduct health education (Ramos et al., 2001). Community workers seem to be most effective when they are selected from among individuals who are respected and trusted by their communities, for example, informal community leaders. In addition to their knowledge of the community's needs, their formal participation in the public health enterprise may also reassure community groups that are wary of gov-

---

[4] In Spanish-speaking communities, they are called *promotores*; if all promoters are women, as is sometimes the case, they are called *promotoras*.

ernment systems or health care providers for political, economic, or other reasons (University of Arizona, 1998; Ramos et al., 2001).

During site visits, the committee observed that community workers are used with apparent success by several projects around the country. In Orange County, California, Latino Health Access, a community-based organization, receives community input, works collaboratively with the local county health department, and manages paid *promotores* who provide education and link community members to services and resources, including those provided by the health department (Bracho, 2000). The Asian Health Services and La Clinica de La Raza in Oakland, California, use the services of staff members from several ethnic communities to conduct culturally and linguistically competent health promotion and health care outreach in those communities (see Appendix F).

Baltimore's Vision for Health Consortium and Men's Health Center (see Appendix F) have community advocates or outreach workers who perform a range of services, including linking uninsured community members to a "medical home," following up with individuals who do not return for test results or treatment, and providing assistance with other referrals and linkages. Denver Health, in Denver, Colorado, also uses the services of community outreach workers to help community members who are uninsured gain access to health care services and to provide health promotion and health education services in the community (see Appendix F). Denver Health's unique public–private public health infrastructure has developed a process for training community outreach workers and integrating them into the public health workforce. Classes and even a degree program are available through local community colleges. In Arizona, a similar *promotora* training program has been created by the Border Health Fronteriza project and is coordinated by the University of Arizona (HRSA, 2001).

Changing Community Conditions and Systems

Changing community conditions and systems is the third component of the framework for community action to improve health. It involves changing aspects of the physical, social, organizational, and even political environments to eliminate or reduce factors that contribute to health problems or to introduce new elements that promote better health. Such changes might include instituting new programs, policies, and practices; changing aspects of the physical or organizational infrastructure in the community; and changing community attitudes and beliefs or social norms (Fawcett et al., 2000b; Mitchell and Shortell, 2000) (see Box 4–3). Some policy changes, for example, are aimed directly at health-related concerns such as improving access to health care or preventing injury and disease through means such as regulation of alcohol and tobacco sales, the institution of require-

---

BOX 4–3
Communities in Action to Address Mental Illness

Communities can be catalysts for a change in societal attitudes toward depression and other mental illnesses—the first step in addressing the stigma attached to these conditions (Corrigan and Penn, 1999; Link et al., 1999; Corrigan et al., 2001). This change may encourage people dealing with mental illness to seek treatment. Through educational efforts, communities can reinforce the public health message that depression and other mental illnesses are real and disabling conditions that can be treated effectively (DHHS, 1999). Communities can also combat the stigma attached to mental illness through sponsorship of low-cost programs that constructively bring the public into contact with people with mental illness.

---

ments for the use of seat belts or bicycle helmets, or the institution of rules and laws on the responsible disposal of hazardous industrial wastes. Various tools can be applied in efforts to achieve changes in community conditions and systems. These can include school and workplace-based educational programs, social marketing, and other social transformation activities. Community groups can also advocate for government bodies to take appropriate actions, such as regulating environmental pollutants. Informed and mobilized communities can help ensure that government agencies enforce such regulations.

The committee found many examples of community-based efforts to modify local conditions as part of a health improvement initiative. These are, in a very real sense, examples of a public health system in action to create conditions in communities for people to choose healthy behaviors. Holder and colleagues (2001), for example, reported on a multilevel intervention in a South Carolina community that was aimed at changing policies and practices through several proven components, including community coalition building and the development and enactment of policies on alcohol outlets. These interventions increased law enforcement as well as the perception in the community that drunk drivers would be caught. In addition, local businesses modified their policies for beverage service, and community groups became mobilized to change the zoning policies that governed the density of alcohol outlets. Following the intervention, rates of crashes related to drunk driving were significantly reduced and binge drinking declined. Holder and colleagues (2001) concluded that education and public awareness about a health problem had to be supplemented with environmental strategies that brought about community and system changes to achieve the health improvement goal of injury reduction.

Kansas LEAN, the state coalition mentioned previously, facilitated a variety of community and system changes aimed at preventing chronic disease through dietary modifications and exercise. The system changes included modifying lunch menus in elementary schools, changing school curricula by adding nutrition education and enhanced exercise activities, supporting the adoption by several employers of a pilot-tested work-site program to lower the intake of dietary fat, working with supermarkets to implement price reductions and shelf prompts for lower-fat foods, and conducting events to promote lean eating in the African-American faith community and among state legislators (Fawcett et al., 1997).

The Healthy Neighborhoods Project (HNP) in western Contra Costa County, California, brought together community residents, the health department, community organizations, and sometimes other partners from the public, private, and civic sectors (Minkler, 2000). Using trained community organizers and neighborhood health advocates, the project conducted a qualitative assessment of the community's health-related needs and capacities. Data on air quality led to changes in areas such as transportation (Minkler, 2000). Another part of the initiative reached recipients of food stamps with information about food and nutrition. HNP also worked with organizers of a local outdoor festival to ban smoking. The activities to change policies related to smoking built on a history of successes, including local collaboration among nonprofit organizations, the health department, and other groups to implement a strong clean-indoor-air policy as well as a tobacco-free youth policy. Today, the Contra Costa County health department provides a real and virtual (online) community gateway for getting involved with existing health-related coalitions, including HNP (Contra Costa Health Services, 2001).

Bias, prejudice, and stereotyping (IOM, 2002) and a sometimes overt lack of cultural competence (see Box 4–4) characterize many institutional and community health settings. Culturally competent public health services are essential for the success of efforts to improve health and eliminate disparities. Staff members present during the committee's site visit to Oakland's Community Voices project considered health care delivery services without cultural competence completely unacceptable, leading to health care encounters that lack basic communication and fail to empower or engage clients in addressing their own health needs (Bayne-Smith, 1996). However, altering discriminatory attitudes and norms, which are sometimes deceptively subtle, and overcoming cultural and linguistic barriers pose significant challenges and require institutional and individual commitments from all entities that are potential partners within the public health system.

Cultural diversity and the knowledge and resources often associated with it are valuable community assets, making communities and systems better equipped to interact appropriately with diverse populations. The

---

BOX 4–4
Working with Communities for Cultural Competence

In 1994 the California Cultural Competency Taskforce defined cultural competence as "appropriate and effective communication which requires the willingness to listen to and learn from members of diverse cultures, and the provision of service and information in appropriate languages, at appropriate comprehension and literacy levels, and in the context of an individual's cultural health beliefs and practices" (Chin, 2000: 26).

Cultural competence entails the provision of services, training, and promotional materials in the context of an individual's or a community's culture and social and historical circumstances and in a range of languages or through interpreters, to whom easy and rapid access is possible (Bayne-Smith, 1996; Chin, 2000).

Office of Minority Health has developed standards for culturally and linguistically appropriate services in health care to provide guidance and tools for health care providers, policy makers, purchasers, patients and advocates, educators, and accreditation or credentialing entities (DHHS, 2001). Standard 12 recommends that health care organizations use a range of mechanisms to "develop participatory, collaborative partnerships with communities" to facilitate the community's involvement in the processes that ensure cultural and linguistic competence (DHHS, 2001).

The process of changing community conditions and systems may also require modification of institutional cultures in terms of attitudes and beliefs about sharing power. This may include changes in attitudes about the role of an empowered citizenry vis-à-vis the role of experts, such as professionals who have traditionally occupied positions of authority (Schwab and Syme, 1997; Bowles, 1999). A participant in the committee's site visit to Healthy New Orleans poignantly summarized an aspect of this tension by asking what it would take before communities could be heard without first having to get the "Ivory Tower Seal of Approval" (personal communication by coalition member to committee members, 2001). Dysfunctional organizational practices may indirectly shape public perceptions and action about health, for example, by discouraging community initiative or by dampening innovation through rigid categorical funding systems.

At the political level, the commitment of elected officials to communitywide health action can have an enormous influence on broadening the impact of a program and increasing the likelihood of sustainability of programs and outcomes. The American Health Decisions network of state organizations has been pioneering new methods of involving the public in community dialogues about health values and trade-off options. The state of Oregon's Health Decisions project in the 1980s may be the most visible example of such an effort. Led by the governor, it involved extensive public education and a long series of statewide public hearings, resulting in the Oregon Health Plan setting priorities for public and private health insurance coverage. The states of Georgia and California have initiated Health Decisions projects, and although mostly focused on health care reform, the model illustrates the power of political commitment in helping to mobilize community engagement on health issues (Kari et al., 1994).

Achieving Widespread Change in Behavior and Risk Factors

Changing individual behavior to avoid health-related risk factors is another stage on the road to health improvement. Behavioral change may sometimes be achieved through interventions, such as health education and counseling, that are aimed directly at individuals, although the evidence base shows that a broad array of interventions go beyond the individual and function at an ecological level (e.g., the neighborhood or the workplace). Efforts to change individual risk must consider the influence of community conditions and systems that affect the population in general (see Box 4–5).

The effective way to approach health improvement from a population health perspective has been to focus on a combination of individual and community factors. For example, Callahan (2000: 164) observed that "people can and do stop smoking on their own, but it is easier for them if their family members and friends don't smoke, if they can't smoke in their workplace, and if the taxes on cigarettes make buying tobacco products exceedingly expensive." Individual behavior and health risks can be shaped by conditions throughout the community, including the workplace, business practices, and neighborhood resources.

Many communities have been motivated to address tobacco-related issues, such as teen smoking, smoking cessation, and advertising for tobacco products, as exemplified by coalitions formed in Florida, Massachusetts, Minnesota, and Missouri to influence policy and public opinion (Heser and Begay, 1997; Fisher et al., 1998; Givel and Glantz, 2000; Johnson, 2000). In St. Louis, Missouri, Neighbors for a Smoke Free North Side took on smoking cessation (Fisher et al., 1998). The project was implemented in three neighborhoods, with four zip code areas in Kansas City, Missouri, serving as comparators. The interventions included media inputs (interviews and stories), billboards, community events, and other health promotion efforts. Unlike the COMMIT (Community Intervention Trial for Smoking Cessation) randomized controlled trials, which, although well designed, had just one modest and partial positive outcome (Susser, 1995), this project found a significant decline in the prevalence of self-reported smoking after the intervention. It also demonstrated an association between its success

BOX 4–5
Ideas for Communities in Action: Obesity

Community-based programs are essential to combating the increasing rates of overweight and obesity in the United States (ACS, 2002). These programs should be culturally specific and relevant to the community being targeted because of cultural differences in foods and in perceptions and attitudes about weight and appearance. For example, in some cultures a heavy child may be viewed as being healthy, whereas a thin child may be considered weak or ill.

The use of a range of strategies, such as social marketing, health education, and policy change, is essential. In addition to traditional methods that have some limited success—such as education about the value of eating well and being active—communities can engage in other activities that change the environments that enable sedentary lifestyles and poor eating choices. They can facilitate exercise by working with community development and planning agencies to make parks and playing fields safe and accessible. Schools can become sites for accessible and affordable community recreation centers. Communities might also develop relationships with farmers to make fresh fruits and vegetables more readily available and affordable through weekly markets. Recently, the Los Angeles Unified School District discontinued soda vending on all school premises in the district, thus removing an element that has been linked to childhood obesity (Wood, 2002). Community restaurants and grocery stores could offer and advertise healthy food choices. Communities could also engage the media and other partners. The recently launched Hearts N' Parks program, sponsored by the National Heart, Lung, and Blood Institute and the National Recreation and Park Association, is getting communities interested and mobilized to become physically active by planning a variety of community and educational activities (NIH, 2001).

and the profound involvement of community members in planning, implementation, and governance of the project (Fisher et al., 1998).

Most community partnerships mentioned in this chapter aimed to change behavior and risk factors for the community as a whole. The activities of Kansas LEAN, for example, focused on modifying the environment to encourage improved dietary choices, such as consumption of foods lower in fat. The coalitions associated with the Healthy New Orleans Turning Point project expressed an understanding of the relationship between health and built environments that are unsafe, unpleasant, or otherwise incompatible with living an active life. They described a vision of improving neighborhoods by adding green spaces to facilitate walking and other activities.

In Contra Costa County, California, observation and statistics indicated that African-American women were less likely to receive breast cancer screening for reasons related to the cost of care and a fear of diagnosis, leading to significantly higher rates of mortality from breast cancer in this group (Ryan, 2001). Such barriers became an overwhelming factor in shaping the health behaviors of affected women. A collaborative health department–community initiative to improve access to breast cancer screening for African-American women helped promote behavioral change that ultimately closed the early diagnosis gap between African-American and white women.

Part of the difficulty of changing behaviors is related to the tension between historical, social, and cultural concepts of responsibilities and rights, such as the question of personal responsibility for poor health (e.g., in relation to lifestyle). The committee has found a growing recognition of and empirical support for the influence of population-level factors on the health risk and health status of individuals and populations. This is reflected in the determinants of health discussion in Chapter 2. Efforts to change health behavior and address risk factors cannot reach optimal effectiveness if they depend solely on one-on-one health education or health promotion interventions (Economos et al., 2001).

Improving the Population's Health

Achieving improvement in the health of the public is the final step in the collaborative framework described in this chapter. Depending on the goals of community interventions, these improvements might take the form of lower rates of obesity, reductions in the number of injuries resulting from drunk driving, or fewer cases of sexually transmitted diseases. Sometimes, however, it can be difficult to directly link the desired health outcomes to a community's health actions. The connecting pathways are frequently long and complex. For example, it takes 20 to 30 years to see lower rates of lung cancer after the percentage of the population that smokes has been reduced. Moreover, the effect of a community's actions can be obscured by other societal (secular) trends that may either reinforce or counteract the desired change (Paine-Andrews et al., 2000a).

Despite the difficulties inherent in evaluating final outcomes, progress can be measured by monitoring changes in indicators that reflect intermediate outcomes of community actions, such as higher rates of screening for breast cancer (decreasing mortality) or an increase in the number of community recreation facilities (decreasing obesity). Although such indicators may not specifically measure health or health-related activities (Ricketts, 2001), intermediate measures of community and system changes can be associated with subsequent changes in health outcomes (Fawcett et al., 1997). For example, the activities of a coalition-driven substance abuse prevention project in Kansas led to changes in community policies, programs, and practices (e.g., enhanced law enforcement) that were ultimately linked to a decline in single-vehicle crashes at night and related reductions in injuries and deaths.

Observable and measurable changes within communities and the systems that provide services and assure health offer not only intermediate measures of progress and coalition performance but also vital feedback for community members. The Healthy People agendas (*Healthy People 2000* and *Healthy People 2010*), which have been adopted to guide national health policy and which have been embraced by 47 states, play an important role in measuring the health status of the national "community." An update of progress in meeting Healthy People 2000 goals indicates that of its 319 indicators (organized by 22 health objectives) 15 percent met the goals, 44 percent are making progress in the correct direction, 18 percent are moving away from the specified target, 9 percent have mixed results, and the progress for the remaining indicators cannot be measured at this time (NCHS, 1999).

EVALUATING AND RESEARCHING COMMUNITY HEALTH IMPROVEMENT

Communities interface with the research community in a variety of ways. Sometimes, community organizations collaborate with academic institutions to conduct needs assessments or monitor and evaluate program effectiveness. In other cases, academic researchers study communities to build an evidence base on the ways in which communities work and what works in communities. In more recent cases, community-based participatory research (see Chapter 8) has come to be a valued area of public health research, and partnerships among community groups and organizations and public health researchers and practitioners have become more common and fruitful (Israel et al., 1998).

The committee agrees with those who argue that communities and community members must, for both practical and ethical reasons, be partners in health improvement interventions and in the research that guides these interventions (Green and Kreuter, 1991; Kretzmann and McKnight, 1993; Blackwell and Colmenar, 2000; Potvin and Richard, 2001; Norton et al., 2002). On a practical level, engaging the community in public health research may help with complicated (and often sensitive) issues such as defining research priorities or interpreting results (Israel et al., 1998). Ethically, it is important to involve the community that is being studied— informed individual consent does not seem sufficient when interventions involve the needs, aspirations, and even the future of communities.

A significant amount of public health research has been conceived and conducted from its inception and at every stage of implementation without the involvement of the community or population most affected. This approach has contributed to community distrust of academic researchers and their projects. Additionally, research undertaken without the involvement

---

BOX 4–6
Community Perspectives on Research

A qualitative study by public health researchers and community members in Seattle, Washington, uncovered mostly negative community perceptions of the research conducted in their communities. Respondents noted a power imbalance between researchers and community members and described researchers as focused solely on community needs and things to be fixed. They also expressed a lack of trust in their relationship with researchers and a perception that researchers did not respect the community and were impatient for results (Sullivan et al., 2001: 137). There is "so much rhetoric around this whole issue of community-based [research], it takes an enormous amount of investment of time and energy and expertise and skill and patience in getting the foundation laid properly. . . . [Y]ou spend . . . three or four years, and a lot of funding institutions would probably go faint at that, but it really does take that kind of effort" (Sullivan et al., 2001: 139).

---

of those most affected not only may make it more difficult to develop and implement effective interventions for improvements in the health of the community but may also raise ethical questions (see Box 4–6). Furthermore, research has typically adhered to a scientific paradigm of objectivity and "universal" truth, whereas the issues, dynamics, and stories of communities are generally local, subjective, and unique (Schwab and Syme, 1997). This tension between the nature of the community and the nature of science may help explain why researching the effectiveness of community coalitions and community intervention has been a complicated endeavor and why investment in community-based research has been limited.

Community-based participatory research seeks to overcome some of the criticisms and distrust of academic research by emphasizing the participation and influence of nonacademic researchers in the process of creating knowledge (Israel et al., 1998). However, community members are frequently skeptical that proposed research efforts will be truly collaborative in nature. The promise of community-based participatory research brings with it the need to establish true partnerships with equal decision-making authority, mutual benefit, and shared responsibility. Major issues that must be confronted in such research include power and control, conflicts over funding, and who will be recognized as the community representative. Additionally, according to Israel and colleagues (1998), "emphasis needs to be placed on developing norms and ways of operating that promote understanding and demonstrate sensitivity and competence in working with diverse cultures." All of these factors lead to the need for a well-developed review of ethical issues involved in community-based research and an ongoing discussion of how to ensure that such research is conducted with the highest regard for those who participate. The committee believes that discussion and debate about the ethics of community-based research are necessary and that creating a forum for such dialogue is important.

Because the community is a complex and dynamic subject, the committee agrees with those who assert that entirely new paradigms of research and analysis must be developed, along with a "postmodern epidemiology" or a "participatory eco-epidemiology" that does not sacrifice rigor but that shares power and involves all local perspectives and opinions (Schwab and Syme, 1997). Collaborative public health research that engages the community at every possible level may mean that research will be applicable and useful to them (Israel et al., 1998; Sullivan et al., 2001). Furthermore, the expertise of local community members and groups would constitute a valuable addition to a research project's assets (Omenn, 1999; Schwab and Syme, 1997).

A social marketing project to improve the health of agricultural workers in Florida provides an example of a fruitful partnership in community-based research (Flocks et al., 2001). Florida nursery and fernery workers, who are primarily Hispanic and Haitian, are exposed through their work to a large volume of pesticides known to be harmful to humans. In 1997, health researchers from the University of Florida entered into a partnership with a union, the Farmworker Association of Florida, and a social marketing firm for a project to help expand existing educational efforts and focus them into an effective, wide-scale intervention. Fernery employees participated at all stages of the research, contributing valuable cultural and occupational insights and information. The process has been lengthy and challenging because of the varied interests of the parties involved (workers, unions, health care providers, industry, academia, government agencies), but the initial work has begun to pay off. More funding has been secured, additional research has been launched, and work has begun on social marketing interventions to change employer practices and worker behaviors and on efforts to address barriers to adequate health care for this vulnerable population of workers exposed to environmental hazards (Flocks et al., 2001; L. Clarke, personal communication, April 9, 2002).

Additional discussion of issues in community-based research and the benefits of academic collaboration with communities appears in Chapter 8, which focuses on the role of academia in the public health system.

SUSTAINING COMMUNITY ACTION ON HEALTH

Assuring the health of communities requires continuous community participation and leadership in the context of a broader partnership with other potential actors in a public health system. Communities can work with health departments, hospitals and other health care providers, and the corporate sector and employers. Communities can also develop the expertise and linkages needed to attract media attention to their efforts and messages.

Although specific programs may end once concrete objectives are achieved, communities and their populations are continually changing, as are their health status and the factors influencing their health. The cross-linkages that are created within communities from the pursuit of one health goal should be sustained and expanded or modified to respond to other persistent or emerging needs.

Under what circumstances are health improvement efforts most likely to continue? Institutional and community memories are replete with examples of community initiatives that came and left without much effect, projects that accomplished little, and great collective disappointments about squandered promises and resources (Mitchell and Shortell, 2000; Lasker et al., 2001). It is important to recognize that opposition and conflict are definite possibilities and to appreciate that small wins along the way in terms of program goals can be important in sustaining interest and commitment (Fawcett, 1999). Success appears to be the result of a synergistic blending of community capacity with the capacity of governmental public health agencies and other partners (NACCHO, 2000a; Becnel, 2001; Lasker et al., 2001; McHugh et al., 2001).

Capacity describes the mix of conditions (e.g., shared values, quality of programs and strategies, program congruence with community needs, and political support) and resources (e.g., knowledge, skills, money, time, and technical assistance) necessary for communities and community coalitions to accomplish and sustain change (Blackwell and Colmenar, 2000; Chaskin et al., 2001; Foster-Fishman et al., 2001; Norton et al., 2002). For example, a community can develop capacity by expanding its knowledge about best practices for organizing coalitions, planning programs, or conducting advocacy. Additionally, governmental public health agencies are increasingly aware of the need to build their own capacity by enhancing their ability to provide technical assistance, training, and support to build capable communities (Howat et al., 2001; Norton et al., 2002). Local health department staff generally possess the knowledge and resources needed in the community's efforts to assess local health status, assets, and needs and to evaluate the outcomes of health initiatives. The fact that communities may rely on health departments to provide technical assistance underscores the need to enhance the skills and knowledge of the public health workforce (discussed in greater detail in the Chapter 8). **The committee recommends that local governmental public health agencies support community-led efforts to inventory resources, assess needs, formulate collaborative responses, and evaluate outcomes for community health improvement and the elimi-**

nation of health disparities. Governmental public health agencies should provide community organizations and coalitions with technical assistance and support in identifying and securing resources as needed and at all phases of the process.

The sustainability of health improvement efforts is reflected in the extent of community change and the degree to which initiatives remain in place after funding ends (Paine-Andrews et al., 2000b). A study of six community initiatives, three for teen pregnancy and three for substance abuse prevention, found that after the end of a 5-year grant period, at least a quarter of the activities initiated in each of the six projects were continuing. These activities included mentoring programs and an annual youth job fair, as well as alternative activities (Paine-Andrews et al., 2000b). Among the strategies for sustainability of initiatives identified by the study were grant writing, making a business plan, and integrating programs or individual program components into the regularly budgeted activities of a partner agency (Paine-Andrews et al., 2000b).

Governmental and private-sector funders can play an essential role in supporting the sustainability of changes in a community's conditions for health. Funders can encourage communities to develop clear goals and to follow practices proven to be effective (W. K. Kellogg Foundation, 1997; Wickizer et al., 1998) (see Box 4–7).

For example, funders can require or support the adoption of specific program elements, such as the development of a business plan, and they can

---

BOX 4–7
Lessons from Turning Point

A review of the Turning Point initiative identified five key lessons for public health policy:

- Recognize the need for direct and explicit support for partnerships;
- Move beyond hierarchical top–down approaches to allow direct investments in communities and responses to community priorities;
- Integrate community-based partnerships into program and funding strategies;
- Broaden the education of the public health workforce to include communication and facilitation skills in nongovernmental and even nonhealth issues; and
- Model interagency and public–private integration at the federal and state levels.

SOURCE: Baxter (2001).

encourage linkages with key local partners, including health departments (Fawcett et al., 2000c; NACCHO, 2000a; Paine-Andrews et al., 2000b; Brunner, 2001). Communicating or even partnering with local health departments may help prevent duplication of effort and may help coordinate activities with multiple participants. In addition, funders must realize that significant community change projects require long-term support and, often, active assistance in identifying continuing sources of financing when the initial grants expire. Because of the time lag between initiation of a community-level intervention and measurable health results, short-term "demonstration project" models are rarely effective and may increase community cynicism about outside partners. **The committee recommends that governmental and private-sector funders of community health initiatives plan their investments with a focus on long-lasting change. Such a focus would include realistic time lines, an emphasis on ongoing community engagement and leadership, and a final goal of institutionalizing effective project components in the local community or public health system as appropriate.**

Given the ever-changing nature of communities, health improvement efforts should be seen as a continuing journey rather than a specific destination.

CONCLUDING OBSERVATIONS

Communities and community organizations can be vital contributors to the resources and capacity of a public health system. A community's right to self-determination, its knowledge of local needs and circumstances, and its human, social, and cultural assets, including the linkages among individuals, businesses, congregations, civic groups, schools, and innumerable others, are all important motivations for community health action. In cases in which community health promotion and protection activities are initiated by a health department or an organization, engaging the community is a primary responsibility. Realizing the vision of *healthy people in healthy communities* is possible only if the community, in its full cultural, social, and economic diversity, is an authentic partner in changing the conditions for health.

REFERENCES

ACS (American Cancer Society). 2002. American communities can change lifestyle habits to prevent cancer. Available online at http://www.cancer.org/docroot/nws/content/ nws_1_1x_american_communities_can_change_lifestyle_habits_to_prevent_cancer.asp.Accessed March 6, 2003.
ATSDR (Agency for Toxic Substances and Disease Registry). 2000. Geographic information systems in public health: proceedings of the third national conference. Available online at www.atsdr.cdc.gov/gis/conference98/index.html. Accessed October 30, 2002.

Baxter RJ. 2001. What Turning Point tells us: implications for national policy. Prepared by The Lewin Group for the W. K. Kellogg Foundation on June 27, 2001. Available online at www.wkkf.org/pubs/Health/TurningPoint/Pub722.pdf. Accessed April 9, 2002.

Bayne-Smith M (Ed.). 1996. Race, Gender, and Health. Thousand Oaks, CA: Sage Publications.

Becnel B. 2001. Community-based public health: lessons on power, policy and grassroots leadership. Community-Based Public Health Policy & Practice, Issue No. 2. A policy brief of Partnership for the Public's Health. Available online at http://www.partnershipph.org/documents/policy/pp1.pdf. Accessed December 18, 2001.

Blackwell AG, Colmenar R. 2000. Community-building: from local wisdom to public policy. Public Health Reports 115(2&3):161–166.

Bowles S. 1999. "Social capital" and community governance. Focus 20(3):6–10.

Bracho A. 2000. An institute of community participation. Adelaide, Australia: Dulwich Centre Publications. Available online at http://www.dulwichcentre.com.au/. Accessed May 2, 2002.

Brunner W. 2001. Community-based public health: a model for local success. Community-Based Public Health Policy and Practice, Issue No. 2. Available online at http://ccpublichealth.org/PDFs/PP1.PDF. Accessed October 31, 2002.

Butterfoss F, Cashman S, Foster-Fishman P, Kegler M, Berkowitz B. 2001. Roundtable discussion and final comments. American Journal of Community Psychology 29(2):229–239.

Callahan D (Ed.). 2000. Promoting Health Behavior: How Much Freedom? Whose Responsiblity? Washington, DC: Georgetown University Press.

CCNTR (Caring Community Network of the Twin Rivers). 2001. Caring Community Network of the Twin Rivers. Available online at www.ccntr.org. Accessed April 7, 2002.

CDC (Centers for Disease Control and Prevention). 1997. Principles of community engagement. CDC/ATSDR Committee on Community Engagement. Atlanta, GA: CDC.

CDC. 2001. National Public Health Performance Standards Program. Available online at www.phppo.cdc.gov/dphs/nphpsp. Accessed October 30, 2001.

CDC. 2002. Syndemics overview: what procedures are available for planning and evaluating initiatives to prevent syndemics? The National Center for Chronic Disease Prevention and Health Promotion Syndemics Prevention Network. Available online at www.cdc.gov/syndemics/overview-planeval.htm. Accessed April 7, 2002.

Chaskin RJ, Brown P, Venkatesh S, Vidal A. 2001. Building Community Capacity. New York: Aldine de Gruyter.

Cheadle A, Sterling TD, Schmid TL, Fawcett SB. 2000. Promising community-level indicators for evaluating cardiovascular health-promotion programs. Health Education Research 15(1):109–116.

Chin JL. 2000. Culturally competent health care. Public Health Reports 115(1):25–33.

Contra Costa Health Services. 2001. The Spectrum of Prevention. Available online at http://ccprevention.org/specrtum.html#top. Accessed April 2, 2002.

Corrigan PW, Penn DL. 1999. Lessons from social psychology on discrediting psychiatric stigma. American Psychologist 54(9):765–776.

Corrigan PW, Green A, Lundin R, Kubiak MA, Penn DL. 2001. Familiarity with and social distance from people who have serious mental illness. Psychiatric Services 52(7):953–958.

DHHS (Department of Health and Human Services). 1999. Engaging faith communities as partners in improving community health. Highlights from a forum sponsored by the CDC/ATSDR and the Carter Center Interfaith Program. Available online at www.phppo.cdc.gov/documents/ faithhealth.pdf. Accessed November 14, 2001.

DHHS. 2001. National standards for culturally and linguistically appropriate services in health care. Prepared for the Office of Minority Health. Available online at www.omhrc.gov/clas. Accessed February 25, 2002.

Economos CD, Brownson RC, DeAngelis MA, Foerster SB, Foreman CT, Tucker C, Gregson J, Kumanyika SK, Pate RR. 2001. What lessons have been learned from other attempts to guide social change? Nutrition Reviews 59(3):S40–S56.

Fawcett SB. 1999. Some lessons on community organization and change. In Rothman J (Ed.). Reflections on Community Organization: Enduring Themes and Critical Issues. Itasca, IL: F. E. Peacock Publishers.

Fawcett SB, Paine-Andrews A, Francisco VT, Schultz JA, Richter KP, Lewis RK, Harris KJ, Williams EL, Berkley JY, Lopez CM, Fisher JL. 1996. Empowering community health initiatives through evaluation, pp. 161–187. In Fetterman DM, Kafterian SJ, Wandersman A (Eds.). Empowerment Evaluation: Knowledge and Tools for Self-Assessment and Accountability. Thousand Oaks, CA: Sage Publications.

Fawcett SB, Lewis RK, Paine-Andrews A, Francisco VT, Richter KP, Williams EL, Copple B. 1997. Evaluating community coalitions for prevention of substance abuse: the case of Project Freedom. Health Education & Behavior 24(6):812–828.

Fawcett SB, Francisco VT, Schultz JA, Berkowitz B, Wolff TJ, Nagy G. 2000a. The Community Tool Box: a web-based resource for building healthier communities. Public Health Reports 115(2&3):274–278.

Fawcett SB, Francisco VT, Hyra D, Paine-Andrews A, Schultz, Roussos S, Fisher JL, Evensen P. 2000b. Building healthy communities. In Tarlov AR, St. Peter RF (Eds.). The Society and Population Health Reader: A State and Community Perspective. New York: The New Press.

Fawcett SB, Francisco VT, Paine-Andrews A, Schultz JA. 2000c. A model memorandum of collaboration: a proposal. Public Health Reports 115(2&3):174–179.

Fisher EB, Auslander WF, Munro JF, Arfken CL, Brownson RC, Owens NW. 1998. Neighbors for a Smoke Free North Side: evaluation of a community organization approach to promoting smoking cessation among African Americans. American Journal of Public Health 88(11):1658–1663.

Flocks J, Clarke L, Albrecht S, Bryant C, Monaghan P, Baker H. 2001. Implementing a community-based special marketing project to improve agricultural worker health. Environmental Health Perspectives 109(Suppl. 3):461–468.

Foster-Fishman PG, Berkowitz SL, Lounsbury DW, Jacobson S, Allen NA. 2001. Building collaborative capacity in community coalitions: a review and integrative framework. American Journal of Community Psychology 29(2):241–261.

Givel MS, Glantz SA. 2000. Failure to defend a successful state tobacco control program: policy lessons from Florida. American Journal of Public Health 90(5):762–767.

Goodman RM, Wandersman A, Chinman M, Imm P, Morrisey E. 1996. An ecological assessment of community based interventions for prevention and health promotion: approaches to measuring community coalitions. American Journal of Community Psychology 24(11):33–61.

Green L, Daniel M, Novick L. 2001. Partnerships and coalitions for community-based research. Public Health Reports 116(Suppl. 1):20–31.

Green LW, Kreuter MM. 1991. Health Promotion Planning: An Educational and Environmental Approach, 2nd ed. Mountain View, CA: Mayfield Publishing Company.

Group Health Community Foundation (GHCF). 2001. Improving everyone's quality of life: a primer on population health. Prepared for California Wellness Foundation's Health Improvement Initiative. Seattle: Group Health Community Foundation.

Health Action. 2001. Health Action priorities for Monroe County. Available online at www.healthaction.org/. Accessed April 2, 2002.

Healthy New Orleans. 2001. Community Public Health System Improvement Plan. Prepared January 2001 as part of the implementation of a Turning Point grant. New Orleans, LA: Healthy New Orleans.

Heser PF, Begay ME. 1997. The campaign to raise the tobacco tax in Massachusetts. American Journal of Public Health 87(6):968–973.

Himmelman AT. 2001. On coalitions and the transformation of power relations: collaborative betterment and collaborative empowerment. American Journal of Community Psychology 29(2):277–284.

Himmelman AT, Johnson D, Kaye G, Salzman P, Wolff T. 2001. Roundtable discussion and final comments. American Journal of Community Psychology 29(2):205–211.

Holder HD, Grenewald PJ, Ponicki WR, Treno AJ, Grube JW, Saltz RF, Voas RB, Reynolds R, Davis J, Sanchez L, Gaumont G, Roeper P. 2001. Effect of community-based interventions on high-risk drinking and alcohol-related injuries. Journal of the American Medical Association 284(18):2341–2347.

Howat P, Cross D, Hall M, Iredell H, Stevenson M, Gibbs S, Officer J, Dillon J. 2001. Community participation in road safety: barriers and enablers. Journal of Community Health 26(4):257–270.

HRSA (Health Resources Services Administration). 2001. Fact sheet: HRSA's Border Health Program. Available online at http://newsroom.hrsa.gov/factsheets/borderhealth2001.htm. Accessed April 5, 2002.

IOM (Institute of Medicine). 1988. The Future of Public Health. Washington, DC: National Academy Press.

IOM. 1995. Assessing the Social and Behavioral Science Base for HIV/AIDS Prevention and Intervention: Workshop Summary and Background Papers. Washington, DC: National Academy Press.

IOM. 1996a. Healthy Communities: New Partnerships for the Future of Public Health. Washington, DC: National Academy Press.

IOM. 1996b. Using Performance Monitoring to Improve Community Health: Exploring the Issues. Washington, DC: National Academy Press.

IOM. 1997. Improving Health in the Community: A Role for Performance Monitoring. Washington, DC: National Academy Press.

IOM. 2001. Health and Behavior: The Interplay of Biological, Behavioral, and Societal Influences. Washington, DC: National Academy Press.

Israel BA, Schulz AJ, Parker EA, Becker AB. 1998. Review of community-based research: assessing partnership approaches to improve public health. Annual Review of Public Health 19:173–202.

Jewkes R, Murcott A. 1996. Meanings of community. Social Science and Medicine 43:555–563.

Johnson DS. 2000. Minnesota Decides: a community blueprint for tobacco reduction. Tobacco Control 9(Suppl. 1):65–67.

Johnston JA, Marmet PF, Coen FS, Fawcett SB, Harris KJ. 1996. Kansas LEAN: an effective coalition for nutrition education and dietary change. Wichita, KS: Society for Nutrition Education.

Kari N, Boyte HC, Jennings B. 1994. Health as a civic question. Prepared for the American Civic Forum. Available online at www.cpn.org/sections/topics/health/. Accessed September 23, 2002.

Kegeles SM, Hart GJ. 1998. Recent HIV-prevention interventions for gay men: individual, small-group and community-based studies. AIDS 12(Suppl. A):S209–S215.

Kickbusch, I. 1989. Good planets are hard to find. WHO–EURO, Healthy Cities Papers, No. 5. Copenhagen: World Health Organization.

Kretzmann JP, McKnight JL. 1993. Building Communities from the Inside Out: A Path Toward Finding and Mobilizing a Community's Assets. Evanston, IL: Institute for Policy Research.

Kreuter MW. 1992. PATCH: its origin, basic concepts, and links to contemporary public health policy. Journal of Health Education 23(3):135–139.

Kreuter MW, Sabol BJ, O'Donovan A, Donovan J, Klein L, Green LW, Vliet M, Bradley T, Campuzano MK, Tarlov AR. 2000. Commentaries from grantmakers on Fawcett et al.'s proposed memorandum of collaboration. Public Health Reports 115:180–190.

Kreuter MW, Lezin NA, Young L, Koplan AN. 2001. Social capital: evaluation implications for community health promotion. In Rootman I, Goodstadt M, Hyndman B, McQueen DV, Potvin L, Springett J, Ziglio E (Eds.). 2001. Evaluation in Health Promotion: Principles and Perspectives, WHO Regional Publications, European Series, No. 92. Copenhagen: World Health Organization.

Lasker RD, Weiss ES, Miller R. 2001. Partnership synergy: a practical framework for studying and strengthening the collaborative advantage. The Milbank Quarterly 79(2):179–205.

The Lewin Group. 2002. Community participation can improve America's public health systems. Prepared for the W. K. Kellogg Foundation. Falls Church, VA: The Lewin Group.

Link BG, Phelan JC, Bresnahan M, Stueve A, Pescosolido BA. 1999. Public conceptions of mental illness: labels, causes, dangerousness, and social distance. American Journal of Public Health 89(9):1328–1333.

Lundblad JA. 1999. Finding our place at the table. Lutheran Partners. Available online at www.elca.org/lp/finding.html. Accessed September 12, 2002.

McGinnis JM, Foege WH. 1993. Actual causes of death in the United States. Journal of the American Medical Association 270(18):2207–2212.

McHugh M, Martinez RM, Kliman R, Roschwalb S. 2001. Health departments forge stronger partnerships. Mathematica Policy Research Inc., Issue Brief No. 5, page 1. Available online at http://www.mathematica-mpr.com/PDFs/PHIssueBr5.pdf. Accessed October 31, 2002.

Milbank Memorial Fund. 1998. Partners in community health: working together for a healthy New York 1998. Prepared by the Milbank Memorial Fund in collaboration with the New York State Community Health Partnership. Available online at www.milbank.org/nypartners/foreword.html. Accessed March 5, 2001.

Minkler M. 2000. Using participatory action research to build health communities. Public Health Reports 115(2&3):191–197.

Mitchell SM, Shortell SM. 2000. The governance and management of effective community health partnerships: a typology for research, policy, and practice. The Milbank Quarterly 78(2):241–289.

NACCHO (National Association of County and City Health Officials) and Centers for Disease Control and Prevention. 1995. 1992–1993 National profile of local health departments. Atlanta, GA: Centers for Disease Control and Prevention.

NACCHO. 2000a. Community revitalization and public health: issues, roles and relationships for local public health agencies. Supported through a cooperative agreement with the Agency for Toxic Substances and Disease Registry, U.S. Public Health Service. Washington, DC: NACCHO.

NACCHO. 2000b. Mobilizing for Action through Planning and Partnerships (MAPP). Available online at http://mapp.naccho.org/lphsa/index.asp. Accessed February 25, 2002.

National Association of Local Boards of Health. 2002. Local Public Health Governance Performance Assessment Instrument. Final version OMB3.0. Bowling Green, OH: National Association of Local Boards of Health. Available online at http://www.nalboh.org/perfstds/perfstds.htm. Accessed June 14, 2002.

NCHS (National Center for Health Statistics). 1999. Healthy People 2000 Review, 1998–1999. Hyatsville, MD: Public Health Service. Available online at www.cdc.gov/nchs/data/hp2000/hp2k99.pdf. Accessed October 30, 2002.

NIH (National Institutes of Health). 2001. Hearts N'Parks: Community Mobilization Guide. A project of the National Heart, Lung and Blood Institute and the National Recreation and Park Association. NIH Publication 01–1655. Rockville, MD: National Institutes of Health.

Norris T, Pittman M. 2000. The Healthy Communities movement and the Coalition for Healthier Cities and Communities. Public Health Reports 115(2&3):118–124.

Norton BL, Burdine JN, LeRoy KR, Felix MRJ, Dorsey AM. 2002. Community capacity: theoretical roots and conceptual challenges. In DiClemente R, Crosby R, Kegler M (Eds.). Emerging Theories in Health Promotion Practice and Research. Hoboken, New Jersey: Jossey-Bass Wiley Publishers.

Omenn GS. 1999. Caring for the community: the role of partnerships. Academic Medicine 74(7):782–789.

Paine-Andrews A, Fisher JL, Campuzano, Fawcett SB, Berkeley-Patton J. 2000a. Promoting sustainability of community health initiatives: an empirical case study. Health Promotion Practice 1(3):248–258.

Paine-Andrews A, Fisher JL, Harris KJ, Lewis RK, Williams EL, Vincent ML, Fawcett SB, Campuzano MK. 2000b. Some experiential lessons in supporting and evaluating community-based initiatives for preventing adolescent pregnancy. Health Promotion Practice 1(1):66–76.

Paine-Andrews A, Fisher JL, Patton JB, Fawcett SB, Williams EL, Lewis RK, Harris KJ. 2002. Analyzing the contribution of community change to population health outcomes in an adolescent pregnancy prevention initiative. Health Education and Behavior 29(2):183–193.

PHF (Public Health Foundation). 2000. EZ/EC Health Planning Capacity Survey: Final Report. Washington, DC: Assistant Secretary for Planning and Evaluation, Department of Health and Human Services.

Potvin L, Richard L. 2001. Evaluating community health promotion programmes. In Rootman I, Goodstadt M, Hyndman B, McQueen DV, Potvin L, Springett J, Ziglio E (Eds.). Evaluation in Health Promotion: Principles and Perspectives. WHO Regional Publications, European Series, No. 92. Copenhagen: World Health Organization. Available online at www.who.dk/docpub/documents/hltprom.htm. Accessed October 5, 2001.

Pronk NP, O'Connor PJ. 1997. Systems approach to population health improvement. Journal of Ambulatory Care Management 20(4):24–31.

Ramos IN, May M, Ramos KS. 2001. Environmental health training of promotoras in colonias along the Texas-Mexico border. American Journal of Public Health 91(4):568–570.

Reger B, Wootan MG, Booth-Butterfield S. 2000. A comparison of different approaches to promote community-wide dietary change. American Journal of Preventive Medicine 18(4):271–275.

Rhein M, Lafronza V, Bhandari E, Hawes J, Hofrichter R, Burke N, Skinner I (Eds.). 2001. Advancing Community Public Health Systems in the 21st Century: Emerging Strategies and Innovations from the Turning Point Experience. Washington, DC: National Association of County and City Health Officials.

Ricketts TC. 2001. Community capacity to improve population health: defining community. Draft report. Princeton, NJ: Robert Wood Johnson Foundation.

Robinson K, Elliott SJ. 2000. The practice of community development approaches in heart health promotion. Health Education Research 15(2):219–231.

Rootman I, Goodstadt M, Hyndman B, McQueen DV, Potvin L, Springett J, Ziglio E (Eds.). 2001. Evaluation in Health Promotion: Principles and Perspectives. WHO Regional Publications, European Series, No. 92. Copenhagen: World Health Organization.

Rose G. 1992. The Strategy of Preventive Medicine. Oxford: Oxford University Press.

Rothman J (Ed.). 1999. Reflections on Community Organization: Enduring Themes and Critical Issues. Itasca, IL: F. E. Peacock Publishers.

Roussos ST, Fawcett SB. 2000. A review of collaborative partnerships as a strategy for improving community health. Annual Review of Public Health 21:369–402.

Ruderman M. 2000. Resource guide to concepts and methods for community-based and collaborative problem-solving. Women's and Children's Health Policy Center, Johns Hopkins University School of Public Health. Available online at www.med.jhu.edu/wchpc/pub/resrcgd.PDF. Accessed November 6, 2001.

Ryan J. 2001. The power of ordinary people. Community-Based Public Health Policy and Practice, Partnership for the Public's Health, Issue No. 1. Available online at www.partnershipph.org/col4/policy/pp1.pdf. Accessed September 12, 2002.

Salamon LM, Anheier HK, List R, Toepler S, Wojciech Sokolowski S, and Associates. 1999. Global Civil Society: Dimensions of the Nonprofit Sector. Baltimore, MD: Johns Hopkins Comparative Nonprofit Sector Project.

Schwab M, Syme SL. 1997. On paradigms, community participation, and the future of public health. American Journal of Public Health 87(12):2049–2051.

Sharpe PA, Greaney ML, Lee PR, Royce SW. 2000. Assets-oriented community assessment. Public Health Reports 115(2&3):205–211.

Shortell SM. 2000. Community health improvement approaches: accounting for the relative lack of impact. Health Services Research 35(3):555–560.

Steele J. 2000. Leading the way with community health partnerships. Healthcare Executive, Sept. /Oct.:20–25.

Stewart E, Weinstein RS. 1997. Volunteer participation in context: motivations and political efficacy within three AIDS organizations. American Journal of Community Psychology 25(6):809–837.

Sullivan M, A Kone, KD Senturia, NJ Chrisman, SJ Ciske, JW Krieger. 2001. Researcher and researched-community perspectives: toward bridging the gap. Health Education and Behavior 28(2):130–149.

Susser M. 1995. The tribulations of trials–interventions in communities. American Journal of Public Health 85(2):156–158.

Task Force on Community Preventive Services. 2000. The guide to community preventive services. Available online at www.thecommunityguide.org/home_f.html. Accessed September 30, 2002.

Turning Point Community Health Governance Workgroup. 2001a. Strengthening and sustaining engagement in community health governance. Background paper prepared for the June 2001 Meeting of the Turning Point Community Health Governance Workgroup, Center for the Advancement of Collaborative Strategies in Health, New York Academy of Medicine. Available online at www.cacsh.org/pdf/EngagementTA.pdf. Accessed January 21, 2002.

Turning Point Community Health Governance Workgroup. 2001b. Using organizational formalization to achieve objectives of public health governance. Background paper prepared for the June 2001 Meeting of the Turning Point Community Health Governance Workgroup, Center for the Advancement of Collaborative Strategies in Health, New York Academy of Medicine. Available online at www.cacsh.org/pdf/orgta.pdf. Accessed January 21, 2002.

University of Arizona. 1998. The National Community Health Advisor Study: Weaving the Future. Final Report. Tucson, AZ: University of Arizona.

WHO (World Health Organization). 1998. Health for All in the 21st Century. Geneva: World Health Organization.

Wickizer TM, Wagner E, Cheadle A, Pearson D, Beery W, Maeser J, Psaty B, VonKorff M, Koepsell T, Diehr P, Perrin EB. 1998. Implementation of the Henry J. Kaiser Family Foundation's Community Health Promotion Grant Program: a process evaluation. The Milbank Quarterly 76(1):121–147.

Wilcox R, Knapp A. 2000. Building communities that create health. Focus on Healthy Communities. Public Health Reports 115(2&3):139–143.

Williams RL, Yanoshik K. 2001. Can you do a community assessment without talking to the community? Journal of Community Health 26(4):233–247.

W. K. Kellogg Foundation. 1997. Sustaining community-based initiatives, Module 1: developing community capacity. An initiative of the W. K. Kellogg Foundation in partnership with the Healthcare Forum. Available online at www.wkkf.org/pubs/Health/Pub656.pdf. Accessed on February 15, 2001.

W. K. Kellogg Foundation. 2001. Community care network. Available online at www.wkkf. org. Accessed November 7, 2001.

Wolff T. 2001a. The future of community coalition building. American Journal of Community Psychology 29(2):263–268.

Wolff T. 2001b. Community coalition building—contemporary practice and research: introduction. American Journal of Community Psychology 29(2):165–172.

Wolkow KE, Ferguson HB. 2001. Community factors in the development of resiliency: considerations and future directions. Community Mental Health Journal 37(6):489–498.

Wood D. 2002. A farewell to fizz from LA lunchrooms. The Christian Science Monitor, August 30, 2002, p. 1.

Yanek LR, Becker DM, Moy TF, Gittelsohn J, Koffman DM. 2001. Project Joy: faith-based cardiovascular health promotion for African American women. Public Health Reports 116(Suppl. 1):68–81.

5

The Health Care Delivery System

For Americans to enjoy optimal health—as individuals and as a population—they must have the benefit of high-quality health care services that are effectively coordinated within a strong public health system. In considering the role of the health care sector in assuring the nation's health, the committee took as its starting point one of the recommendations of the Institute of Medicine (IOM) report *Crossing the Quality Chasm* (2001b: 6): "All health care organizations, professional groups, and private and public purchasers should adopt as their explicit purpose to continually reduce the burden of illness, injury, and disability, and to improve the health and functioning of the people of the United States."

This chapter addresses the issues of access, managing chronic disease, neglected health care services (i.e., clinical preventive services, oral, and mental health care and substance abuse services), and the capacity of the health care delivery system to better serve the population in terms of cultural competence, quality, the workforce, financing, information technology, and emergency preparedness. In addition, the chapter discusses the responsibility of the health care system to recognize and play its appropriate role within the intersectoral public health system, particularly as it collaborates with the governmental public health agencies.

The health care sector in the United States consists of an array of clinicians, hospitals and other health care facilities, insurance plans, and purchasers of health care services, all operating in various configurations of groups, networks, and independent practices. Some are based in the public sector; others operate in the private sector as either for-profit or not-for-profit entities. The health care sector also includes regulators, some voluntary and others governmental. Although these various individuals and organizations are generally referred to collectively as "the health care delivery system," the phrase suggests an order, integration, and accountability that do not exist. Communication, collaboration, or systems planning among these various entities is limited and is almost incidental to their operations. For convenience, however, the committee uses the common terminology of health care delivery system.

As described in *Crossing the Quality Chasm* (IOM, 2001b) and other literature, this health care system is faced with serious quality and cost challenges. To support the system, the United States spends more per capita on health care than any other country ($4,637 in 2000) (Reinhardt et al., 2002). In the aggregate, these per capita expenditures account for 13.2 percent of the U.S. gross domestic product, about $1.3 trillion (Levit et al., 2002). As the committee observed in Chapter 1, American medicine and the basic and clinical research that inform its practice are generally acknowledged as the best in the world. Yet the nation's substantial health-related spending has not produced superlative health outcomes for its people. Fundamental flaws in the systems that finance, organize, and deliver health care work to undermine the organizational structure necessary to ensure the effective translation of scientific discoveries into routine patient care, and many parts of the health care delivery system are economically vulnerable. Insurance plans and providers scramble to adapt and survive in a rapidly evolving and highly competitive market; and the variations among health insurance plans—whether public or private—in eligibility, benefits, cost sharing, plan restrictions, reimbursement policies, and other attributes create confusion, inequity, and excessive administrative burdens for both providers of care and consumers.

Because of its history, structure, and particularly the highly competitive market in health services that has evolved since the collapse of health care reform efforts in the early 1990s, the health care delivery system often does not interact effectively with other components of the public health system described in this report, in particular, the governmental public health agencies. Health care's structure and incentives are technology and procedure driven and do not support time for the inquiry and reflection, communication, and external relationship building typically needed for effective disease prevention and health promotion. State health departments often have legal authority to regulate the entry of providers and purchasers of health care into the market and to set insurance reimbursement rates for public and, less often, private providers and purchasers. They may control the ability of providers to acquire desired technology and perform complex, costly procedures that are important to the hospital but increase demands on state revenues. Finally, virtually all states have the legal responsibility to monitor the quality of health services provided in the public and private sectors. Many health care providers argue that such regulation adds to their costs, and high-profile problems can create additional tensions that impede collaboration between the state public health agency and the health care delivery system.

Furthermore, when the delivery of health care through the private sector falters, the responsibility for providing some level of basic health care services to the poor and other special populations falls to governmental public health agencies as one of their essential public health services, as discussed in Chapter 1. In many jurisdictions, this default is already occurring, consuming resources and impairing the ability of governmental public health agencies to perform other essential tasks.

Although this committee was not constituted to investigate or make recommendations regarding the serious economic and structural problems confronting the health care system in the United States, it concluded that it must examine certain issues having serious implications for the public health system's effectiveness in promoting the nation's health. Drawing heavily on the work of other IOM committees, this chapter examines the influence that health insurance exerts on access to health care and on the range of care available, as well as the shortcomings in the quality of services provided, some of the constraints on the capacity of the health care system to provide high-quality care, and the need for better collaboration within the public health system, especially among governmental public health agencies and the organizations in the personal health care delivery system.

ACCESS TO HEALTH CARE

Health care is not the only, or even the strongest, determinant of health, but it is very important. For most Americans, having health insurance—under a private plan or through a publicly financed program—is a threshold requirement for routine access to health care. "Health insurance coverage is associated with better health outcomes for adults. It is also associated with having a regular source of care and with greater and more appropriate use of health services. These factors, in turn, improve the likelihood of disease screening and early detection, the management of chronic illness, and the effective treatment of acute conditions," IOM notes in a recent report (IOM, 2002a: 6).

Private insurance is predominantly purchased through employment-based groups and to a lesser extent through individual policies (Mills, 2002). Publicly funded insurance is provided primarily through seven government programs (see Table 5–1). Medicare provides coverage to 13.5 percent of the population, whereas Medicaid covers 11.2 percent of the population (Mills, 2002). Additionally, public funding supports directly

TABLE 5-1   Government Health Programs

Program	Year	Enrollment	Expenditures
Medicare	2001	40 million aged and disabled individuals[a]	$242.4 billion[b]
Medicaid	2002	47 million low-income individuals[b]	$247 billion (federal, $147 billion; state, $100 billion)[b]
SCHIP	2001	4.6 million low-income children[c]	$4.6 billion[c]
VHA	2001	4.3 million veterans[d]	$21 billion[d]
IHS	2001	1.5 million American Indians and Alaska Natives[e]	$3.2 billion[e]
DOD TRICARE	2001	8.4 million active-duty members of the military[f]	$14.2 billion[f]
FEHBP	2000	9 million federal employees, dependents, and retirees[g]	$20 billion[g]

NOTE: VHA = Veterans Health Administration; IHS = Indian Health Service; DOD = Department of Defense; FEHBP = Federal Employees Health Benefits Program.
SOURCES: [a]Boards of Trustees (2002). [b]Smith et al. (2002); CMS (2002a); CMS (2002c). [c]CMS (2002a); CMS (2002a); CMS (2002c). [d]GAO (2001b). [e]IHS (2002a, 2002b). [f]Department of Defense (2002). [g]OPM (2001); Office of the President (2001). [h]DHHS (2002).

delivered health care (through community health centers and other health centers qualified for Medicaid reimbursement) accessed by 11 percent of the nation's uninsured, who constitute 41 percent of patients at such health centers (Markus et al., 2002). Because the largest public programs are directed to the aged, disabled, and low-income populations, they cover a disproportionate share of the chronically ill and disabled. However, they are also enormously important for children. In early 2001, Medicaid and the State Children's Health Insurance Program (SCHIP) provided health care coverage to 23.1 percent of the children in the United States, and this figure had risen to 27.7 percent according to data from the first-quarter estimates in the National Health Interview Survey (NCHS, 2002).

Being uninsured, although not the only barrier to obtaining health care, is by all indications the most significant one. The fact that more than 41 million people—more than 80 percent of whom are members of working families—are uninsured is the strongest possible indictment of the nation's health care delivery system. Those without health insurance or without insurance for particular types of services face serious, sometimes insurmountable barriers to necessary and appropriate care.

Adults without health insurance are far more likely to go without health care that they believe they need than are adults with health insurance of any kind (Lurie et al., 1984, 1986; Berk and Schur, 1998; Burstin et al., 1998; Baker et al., 2000; Kasper et al., 2000; Schoen and DesRoches, 2000). Children without health insurance may be compromised in ways that will diminish their health and productivity throughout their lives.

When individuals cannot access mainstream health care services, they often seek care from the so-called safety-net providers. These providers include institutions and professionals that by mandate or mission deliver a large amount of care to uninsured and other vulnerable populations. People turn to safety-net providers for a variety of reasons: some because they lack health insurance and others because there are no other providers in the area where they live or because language and cultural differences make them uncomfortable with mainstream care. Safety-net providers are also more likely to offer outreach and enabling services (e.g., transportation and child care) to help overcome barriers that may not be directly related to the health care system itself.

In this section, the committee reviews concerns about the barriers to health care that are raised by the lack of health insurance and by threats to the nation's safety-net providers.

The Uninsured and the Underinsured

The persistently large proportion of the American population that is uninsured—about one in five working-age adults and one in seven children—is the most visible and troubling sign of the nation's failure to assure access to health care. Yet the public and many elected officials seem almost willfully ignorant of the magnitude, persistence, and implications of this problem. Surveys conducted over the past two decades show a consistent underestimation of the number of uninsured and of trends in insurance coverage over time (Blendon et al., 2001). The facts about uninsurance in America are sobering (see Box 5–1). By almost any metric, uninsured adults suffer worse health status and live shorter lives than insured adults (IOM, 2002a).

Because insurance status affects access to secure and continuous care, it also affects health, leading to an estimated 18,000 premature deaths annually (IOM, 2002a). Having a regular source of care improves chances of receiving personal preventive care and screening services and improves the management of chronic disease. When risk factors, such as high blood pressure, can be identified and treated, the chances of developing conditions such as heart disease can be reduced. Similarly, if diseases can be detected and treated when they are still in their early stages, subsequent rates of morbidity and mortality can often be reduced. Without insurance, the chances of early detection and treatment of risk factors or disease are low.

BOX 5–1
Findings from *Coverage Matters*

In its report *Coverage Matters,* **the IOM Committee on the Consequences of Uninsurance (IOM, 2001a) found the following:**

- Forty-two million people in the United States lacked health insurance coverage in 1999 (Mills, 2000). This number represented about 15 percent of the total population of 274 million persons at that time and 17 percent of the population younger than 65 years of age; 10 million of the uninsured are children under the age of 18 (about 14 percent of all children), and about 32 million are adults between the ages of 18 and 65 (about 19 percent of all adults in this age group).
- Nearly 3 out of every 10 Americans, more than 70 million people, lacked health insurance for at least a month over a 36-month period. These numbers are greater than the combined populations of Texas, California, and Connecticut.
- More than 80 percent of uninsured children and adults under the age of 65 lived in working families. Contrary to popular belief, recent immigrants accounted for a relatively small proportion of the uninsured (less than one in five).
- Insurance status is a powerful determinant of access to care: people without insurance generally have reduced access. Research consistently finds that persons without insurance are less likely to have any physician visits within a year, have fewer visits annually, and are less likely to have a regular source of care. Children without insurance are three times more likely than children with Medicaid coverage to have no regular source of care.
- The uninsured were less likely to receive health care services, even for serious conditions. Research consistently finds that persons without insurance are less likely to have any physician visits within a year, have fewer visits annually, and are less likely to have a regular source of care (15 percent of uninsured children do not have a regular provider, whereas just 5 percent of children with Medicaid do not have a regular provider), and uninsured adults are more than three times as likely to lack a regular source of care.

However, even when the uninsured receive care, they fare less well than the insured. The IOM Committee on the Consequences of Uninsurance found that "[u]ninsured adults receive health services that are less adequate and appropriate than those received by patients who have either public or private health insurance, and they have poorer clinical outcomes and poorer overall health than do adults with private health insurance" (IOM, 2002a: 87). For example, Hadley and colleagues (1991) found that uninsured adult hospital inpatients had a significantly higher risk of dying in the hospital than their privately insured counterparts. Emergency and trauma care were also found to vary for insured and uninsured patients. Uninsured persons with traumatic injuries were less likely to be admitted to the hospital, received fewer services when admitted, and were more likely to die than insured trauma victims (Hadley et al., 1991).

For children, too, being uninsured tends to reduce access to health care and is associated with poorer health. The 1998 IOM report *America's Children: Health Insurance and Access to Care* found that uninsured children "are more likely to be sick as newborns, less likely to be immunized as preschoolers, less likely to receive medical treatment when they are injured, and less likely to receive treatment for illness such as acute or recurrent ear infections, asthma and tooth decay" (IOM, 1998: 3). That report emphasized that untreated health problems can affect children's physical and emotional growth, development, and overall health and well-being. Untreated ear infections, for example, can have permanent consequences of hearing loss or deafness.

Even when insured, limitations on coverage may still impede people's access to care. Many people who are counted as insured have very limited benefits and are exposed to high out-of-pocket expenses or service restrictions. Three areas in which benefits are frequently circumscribed under both public and private insurance plans are preventive services, behavioral health care (treatment of mental illness and addictive disorders), and oral health care. When offered, coverage for these services often carries limits that are unrelated to treatment needs and are stricter than those for other types of care (King, 2000). Cost-sharing requirements for these services may also be higher than those for other commonly covered services. (Additional discussion of these and other "neglected" forms of care appears later in this chapter.)

Access to care for the insured can also be affected by requirements for cost sharing and copayments. Cost sharing is an effective means to reduce the use of health care for trivial or self-limited conditions. Numerous studies, starting with the RAND Health Insurance Experiment, show that copayments also reduce the use of preventive and primary care services by the poor, although not by higher-income groups (Solanki et al., 2000). The same effects have been shown for the use of behavioral health care services (Wells et al., 2000).

As a result of the nation's increased awareness of bioterrorist threats, there are concerns about the implications of copayments and other financial barriers to health care. Cost sharing may discourage early care seeking, impeding infectious disease surveillance, delaying timely diagnosis and treatment, and posing a threat to the health of the public. The committee encourages health care policy makers in the public and private sectors to reexamine these issues in light of the concerns about bioterrorism.

This committee was not constituted to make specific recommendations about health insurance. The issues are complex, and the failures of health care reform efforts over the past 30 years testify to the difficulty of crafting a solution. However, the committee finds that both the scale of the problem and the strong evidence of adverse health effects from being uninsured or underinsured make a compelling case that the health of the American people as a whole is compromised by the absence of insurance coverage for so many. Assuring the health of the population in the twenty-first century requires finding a means to guarantee insurance coverage for every person living in this country.

Adequate population health cannot be achieved without making comprehensive and affordable health care available to every person residing in the United States. It is the responsibility of the federal government to lead a national effort to examine the options available to achieve stable health care coverage of individuals and families and to assure the implementation of plans to achieve that result.

✗ Safety-Net Providers ✗

Absent the availability of health insurance, the role of the safety-net provider is critically important. Increasing their numbers and assuring their viability can, to some degree, improve the availability of care. The IOM Committee on the Changing Market, Managed Care and the Future Viability of Safety Net Providers defined safety-net providers as "[t]hose providers that organize and deliver a significant level of health care and other health-related services to uninsured, Medicaid, and other vulnerable patients" (IOM, 2000a: 21). That committee further identified core safety-net providers as having two distinguishing characteristics: "(1) by legal mandate or explicitly adopted mission they maintain an 'open door,' offering access to services to patients regardless of their ability to pay; and (2) a substantial share of their patient mix is uninsured, Medicaid, and other vulnerable patients" (IOM, 2000a: 3).

The organization and delivery of safety-net services vary widely from state to state and community to community (Baxter and Mechanic, 1997). The safety net consists of public hospital systems; academic health centers; community health centers or clinics funded by federal, state, and local governmental public health agencies (see Chapter 3); and local health departments themselves (although systematic data on the extent of health department services are lacking) (IOM, 2000a). A recent study of changes in the capacities and roles of local health departments as safety-net providers found, however, that more than a quarter of the health departments surveyed were the sole safety-net providers in their jurisdictions and that this was more likely to be the case in smaller jurisdictions (Keane et al., 2001).

Safety-net service providers, which include local and state governmental agencies, contribute to the public health system in multiple ways. Services provided by state and local governments often include mental health hospitals and outpatient clinics, substance abuse treatment programs, maternal and child health services, and clinics for the homeless. In addition, an estimated 1,300 public hospitals nationwide (Legnini et al., 1999) provide free care to those without insurance or resources to pay. A survey of 69 hospitals belonging to the National Association of Public Hospitals indicated that in 1997, public hospitals provided more than 23 percent of the nation's uncompensated hospital care (measured as the sum of bad debt and charity care) (IOM, 2000a). These demands can overwhelm the traditional population-oriented mission of the governmental public health agencies. Furthermore, changes in the funding streams or reimbursement policies for any of these programs or increases in demand for free or subsidized care that inevitably occur in periods of economic downturn create crises for safety-net providers, including those operated by state and local governments (see the section Collaboration with Governmental Public Health Agencies later in this chapter for additional discussion).

The IOM committee that produced the report *America's Health Care Safety Net: Intact but Endangered* (IOM, 2000a: 205–206) had the following findings:

> Despite today's robust economy, safety net providers—especially core safety net providers—are being buffeted by the cumulative and concurrent effects of major health policy and market changes. The convergence and potentially adverse consequences of these new and powerful dynamics lead the committee to be highly concerned about the future viability of the safety net. Although safety net providers have proven to be both resilient and resourceful, the committee believes that many providers may be unable to survive the current environment. Taken alone, the growth in Medicaid managed care enrollment; the retrenchment or elimination of key direct and indirect subsidies that providers have relied upon to help finance uncompensated care; and the continued growth in the number of uninsured people would make it difficult for many safety net providers to survive. Taken together, these trends are beginning to place unparalleled strain on the health care safety net in many parts of the country. . . . The committee believes that the effects of these combined forces and dynamics demand the immediate attention of public policy officials. (IOM, 2000a: 206)

The committee fully endorses the recommendations from *America's Health Care Safety Net: Intact but Endangered* (IOM, 2000a), aimed at ensuring the continued viability of the health care safety net (see Box 5–2).

BOX 5–2
Recommendations Concerning Safety-Net Services

1. Federal and state policy makers should explicitly take into account and address the full impact (both intended and unintended) of changes in Medicaid policies on the viability of safety-net providers and the populations they serve.

2. All federal programs and policies targeted to support the safety net and the populations it serves should be reviewed for their effectiveness in meeting the needs of the uninsured.

3. Concerted efforts should be directed to improving this nation's capacity and ability to monitor the changing structure, capacity, and financial stability of the safety net to meet the health care needs of the uninsured and other vulnerable populations.

4. Given the growing number of uninsured people, the adverse effects of Medicaid managed care on safety-net provider revenues, and the absence of concerted public policies directed at increasing the rate of insurance coverage, the committee believes that a new targeted federal initiative should be established to help support core safety-net providers that care for a disproportionate number of uninsured and other vulnerable people.

SOURCE: IOM (2000a).

NEGLECTED CARE

The committee is concerned that the specific types of care that are important for population health—clinical preventive services, mental health care, treatment for substance abuse, and oral health care—are less available because of the current organization and financing of health care services. Many forms of publicly or privately purchased health insurance provide limited coverage, and sometimes no coverage, for these services.

Clinical Preventive Services

The evidence that insurance makes a difference in health outcomes is well documented for preventive, screening, and chronic disease care (IOM, 2002b). Clinical preventive services are the "medical procedures, tests or counseling that health professionals deliver in a clinical setting to prevent disease and promote health, as opposed to interventions that respond to patient symptoms or complaints" (Partnership for Prevention, 1999: 3). Such services include immunizations and screening tests, as well as counseling aimed at changing the personal health behaviors of patients long before clinical disease develops. The importance of counseling and behavioral interventions is evident, given the influence on health of factors such as tobacco, alcohol, and illicit drug use; unsafe sexual behavior; and lack of exercise and poor diets. These risk behaviors are estimated to account for more than half of all premature deaths; smoking alone contributes to one out of five deaths (McGinnis and Foege, 1993).

Coverage of clinical preventive services has increased steadily over the past decade. In 1988, about three-quarters of adults with employment-based health insurance had a benefit package that included adult physical examinations. Two years later, the proportion had risen to 90 percent (Rice et al., 1998; Kaiser Family Foundation and Health Research and Educational Trust, 2000). The type of health plan is the most important predictor of coverage (RWJF, 2001). The use of financial incentives and data-driven performance measurement strategies to improve physicians' delivery of services such as immunizations (IOM, 2002c) may account for the fact that managed care plans tend to offer the most comprehensive coverage of clinical preventive services and traditional indemnity plans tend to offer the least comprehensive coverage.

Although the trend toward inclusion of clinical preventive services is positive, such benefits are still limited in scope and are not well correlated with evidence regarding the effectiveness of individual services. The U.S. Preventive Services Task Force (USPSTF), a panel of experts convened by the U.S. Public Health Service, has endorsed a core set of clinical preventive services for asymptomatic individuals with no known risk factors. In the committee's view, this guidance to clinicians on the services that should be offered to specific patients should also inform the design of insurance plans for coverage of age-appropriate services. However, the USPSTF recommendations have had relatively little influence on the design of insurance benefits, and recommended counseling and screening services are often not covered and, consequently, not used (Partnership for Prevention, 2001) (see Box 5–3). As might be expected, though, adults without health insurance are the least likely to receive recommended preventive and screening services or to receive them at the recommended frequencies (Ayanian et al., 2000).

Having any health insurance, even without coverage for any preventive services, increases the probability that an individual will receive appropriate preventive care (Hayward et al., 1988; Woolhandler and Himmelstein, 1988; Hsia et al., 2000). Studies of the use of preventive services by Hispanics and African Americans find that health insurance is strongly associated with the increased receipt of preventive services (Solis et al., 1990; Mandelblatt et al., 1999; Zambrana et al., 1999; Wagner and Guendelman, 2000; Breen et al., 2001; O'Malley et al., 2001). However, the higher rates of uninsurance among racial and ethnic minorities contribute significantly

---

BOX 5–3
Partnership for Prevention Survey of Employer Support for Preventive Services

- Counseling to address serious health risks—tobacco use, physical inactivity, risky drinking, poor nutrition—is least likely to be covered by an employer-sponsored health plan. The U.S. Preventive Services Task Force calls these interventions "vitally important."
- Nearly 90 percent of employers' most popular plans cover well-baby care, whereas less than half cover contraceptive devices or drugs to prevent unwanted births. Yet about half of all pregnancies and nearly a third of all births each year are unintended.
- One out of five employer-sponsored plans does not cover childhood immunizations, and one out of four does not cover adolescent immunizations although these are among the most cost-effective preventive services.

SOURCE: IOM (2000a).

---

to their reduced overall likelihood of receiving clinical preventive services and to their poorer clinical outcomes (Haas and Adler, 2001). For example, African Americans and members of other minority groups who are diagnosed with cancer are more likely to be diagnosed at advanced stages of disease than are whites (Farley and Flannery, 1989; Mandelblatt et al., 1991, 1996; Wells and Horm, 1992).

Medicare Coverage of Preventive Services

Preventive services are important for older adults, for whom they can reduce premature morbidity and mortality, help preserve function, and enhance quality of life. Unfortunately, the Medicare program was not designed with a focus on prevention, and the process for adding preventive services to the Medicare benefit package is complex and difficult. Unlike forms of treatment that are incorporated into the payment system on a relatively routine basis as they come into general use, preventive services are subject to a greater degree of scrutiny and a demand for a higher level of effectiveness, and there is no routine process for making such assessments. Box 5–4 lists the preventive services currently covered by Medicare.

The level of use of preventive services among older adults has been relatively low (CDC, 1998). This may reflect the limited range of benefits covered by Medicare, as well as other barriers such as copayments, participants' unfamiliarity with the services, or the failure of physicians to recom-

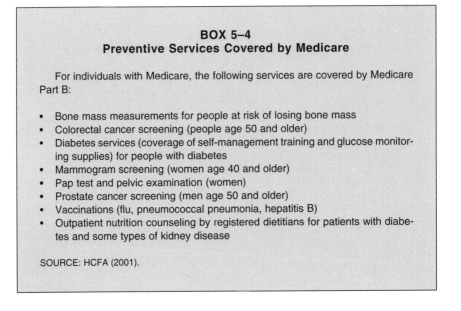

BOX 5–4
Preventive Services Covered by Medicare

For individuals with Medicare, the following services are covered by Medicare Part B:

- Bone mass measurements for people at risk of losing bone mass
- Colorectal cancer screening (people age 50 and older)
- Diabetes services (coverage of self-management training and glucose monitoring supplies) for people with diabetes
- Mammogram screening (women age 40 and older)
- Pap test and pelvic examination (women)
- Prostate cancer screening (men age 50 and older)
- Vaccinations (flu, pneumococcal pneumonia, hepatitis B)
- Outpatient nutrition counseling by registered dietitians for patients with diabetes and some types of kidney disease

SOURCE: HCFA (2001).

mend them. Cardiovascular disease and diabetes exemplify the problem. Although cardiovascular disease is the leading cause of death and diabetes is one of the most significant chronic diseases affecting Medicare beneficiaries, physicians cannot screen for lipids disorders or diabetes unless the patient agrees to pay out-of-pocket for the tests.

Medicaid Coverage of Preventive Services

Medicaid benefits vary by state in terms of both the individuals who are eligible for coverage and the actual services for which coverage is provided. The exception is preventive services for children. In 1976, the U.S. Congress added the Early and Periodic Screening, Diagnosis, and Treatment (EPSDT) program to the federal Medicaid program. This entitled poor children to a comprehensive package of preventive health care and medically necessary diagnostic and treatment services. In 1996, 22.9 million children (20 percent of the nation's children) were eligible for EPSDT benefits. Given its potential to reach such a high proportion of the nation's neediest children, the program could have a very positive, widespread impact on children's health. Unfortunately, data on the program's progress are incomplete and inconsistent across the country, despite federal requirements for state reports (GAO, 2001a). However, some studies have demonstrated that EPSDT has never been fully implemented, and the percentage of children receiving preventive care through it remains low for reasons ranging from systemic state or local deficiencies (e.g., a lack of mechanisms for follow-up, issues related to managed care contracting, and confusing program requirements) to barriers at the personal level (e.g., transportation and language) (GAO, 2001a; Strasz et al., 2002). Of the 22.9 million children eligible for EPSDT in 1996, only 37 percent received a medical screening procedure through the program (Olson, 1998) (see Box 5–5). Additionally, data show that as many as 50 percent of children who have an EPSDT visit are identified as requiring medical attention, but if they are referred for follow-up care, only one-third to two-thirds go for their referral visit (Rosenbach and Gavin, 1998).

Mental Health Care

The Surgeon General's report on mental illness (DHHS, 1999) estimates that more than one in five adults are affected by mental disorders in any given year (see Box 5–6) and 5.4 percent of all adults have a serious mental illness. Data for children are less reliable, but the overall prevalence of mental disorders is also estimated to be about 20 percent (DHHS, 1999). Mental disorders are a major public health issue because they affect such a large proportion of the population, have implications for other health problems, and impose high costs, both financial and emotional, on affected individuals and their families. The cost to society is also high, with indirect costs from lost productivity for affected individuals and their caretakers estimated at $79 billion in 1990, the last year for which estimates are available (Rice and Miller, 1996).

For the most prevalent mental health disorders such as depression and anxiety, receipt of appropriate care is associated with improved functional outcomes at 2 years (Sturm et al., 1995), but the majority of individuals suffering from mental illness are not treated for their condition (DHHS, 1999). Access to care is constrained by limitations on insurance coverage that are greater than those imposed for other diseases. Annual and lifetime coverage limits are frequently less, and mental health coverage often has more hidden costs in the forms of copayments and higher deductibles (Zuvekas et al., 1998). Table 5–2 shows the distribution of sources of payment for treatment for mental health and addictive disorders in 1996. Additionally, those with no insurance all year paid nearly 60 percent of costs out-of-pocket, whereas those with some private insurance paid 40 percent of costs out-of-pocket in 1996 (Zuvekas, 2001).

Adults' use of mental health services in both the general and the specialty mental health sectors correlates highly with health insurance coverage (Cooper-Patrick et al., 1999; Wang et al., 2000; Young et al., 2001), and health insurance coverage specifically for mental health services is associated with an increased likelihood of receiving such care (Wang et al.,

BOX 5–5
Children's Preventive Health Care under Medicaid

Number of eligible children. Between 1991 and 1996, the number of children eligible for the Early and Periodic Screening, Diagnosis, and Treatment (EPSDT) program increased by roughly 5.7 million, with the highest number (23.5 million children) occurring in 1995. The number of eligible children fell by more than half a million between 1995 and 1996.

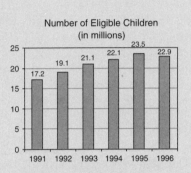

Number of Eligible Children
(in millions)

Medical screening. Of the 22.9 million children eligible for the EPSDT program in 1996, only 37 percent received a medical screen through the EPSDT program. The medical screening rate is not adjusted according to the federal periodicity schedule or the average period of eligibility, but instead reports the percentage of children who were eligible for any period of time during fiscal year 1996 and who received one or more medical screens. Young children were significantly more likely to be screened: 76 percent of infants under age 1 were screened in 1996, whereas 18 percent of adolescents ages 15 to 20 were screened in 1996.

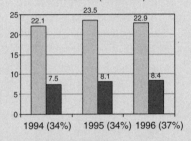

Number of Eligible Children vs. Number Receiving One or More Medical Screening Procedures (in Millions)

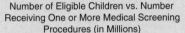

☐ Number of eligible children

■ Number of children receiving one or more medical screening procedures

The participant rate. The participant rate—the number of children screened compared to the number of children expected to be screened, based on the federal periodicity schedule and the average period of eligibility—increased from 51 percent in 1994 to 56 percent in 1996. In 1990, the Health Care Financing Administration established a participant rate goal of 80 percent, to be achieved by fiscal year 1995. As of fiscal year 1996, only nine states reported meeting or exceeding the federally established goal.

SOURCE: Adapted from Olson et al. (1998).

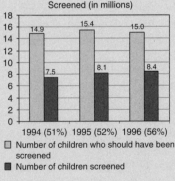

Number of Children Expected to Be Screened vs. Number of Children Screened (in millions)

☐ Number of children who should have been screened

■ Number of children screened

BOX 5–6
Facts About Mental Illness

- About 40 million people (more than one in five) ages 18 to 64 are estimated to have a single mental disorder of any severity or both a mental and an addictive disorder in a given year (Regier et al., 1993; Kessler et al., 1994).
- The most common conditions fall into the broad categories of schizophrenia, affective disorders (including major depression and bipolar or manic-depressive illness), and anxiety disorders (e.g., panic disorder, obsessive-compulsive disorder, posttraumatic stress disorder, and phobia).
- Schizophrenia affects at least an estimated 2 million Americans in any year (Regier et al., 1993), whereas the most prevalent affective disorder, major depression, has been reported to occur in 6.5 percent of women and 3.3 percent of men in any year (DHHS, 2000a). Manic-depressive illness is reported to exist in 1 percent of adults. Anxiety disorders affect an estimated 19 million Americans annually (DHHS, 2000a).
- Only 25 percent of people who have a mental disorder obtain diagnosis and treatment from the health care system, in contrast to 60 to 80 percent of those with heart disease (DHHS, 2000a).
- Evidence-based practice guidelines for depression endorse antidepressant medications and cognitive-behavioral or interpersonal psychotherapies (AHCPR, 1993; Department of Veterans Affairs, 1993; Schulberg et al., 1999).

SOURCE: IOM (2002b).

2000; Young et al., 2000). Recent studies have shown impressive results for treatment of depression in primary care settings (Sturm and Wells, 2000; Schoenbaum et al., 2001). The provision of such services is cost-effective and comparable to the cost-effectiveness of other common procedures. However, reimbursement policies for primary care do not support the services necessary to provide evidence-based care for depression (Wells et al., 2000; Schoenbaum et al., 2001).

Adults with either no insurance coverage or coverage that excludes or limits extended treatment of mental illness receive less appropriate care and may experience delays in receiving services until they gain public insurance (Rabinowitz et al., 2001). Adults with mental disorders are also more likely to lose health insurance coverage within a year following their diagnosis than those without a mental disorder (Sturm and Wells, 2000).

The limited and unstable nature of insurance for treatment of mental illness has several implications for governmental public health agencies because the severely mentally ill are likely to end up receiving care in publicly funded safety-net programs (Rabinowitz et al., 2001). Funding to support the public mental health system comes from reimbursements for

TABLE 5–2   Distribution (percent) of Sources of Payment for Mental Health/Substance Abuse Treatment, by Type of Use, 1996

Payment Source	Total	Ambulatory Care	Psychotropic Medications	Inpatient Care
Total				
Out-of-pocket	23.0	32.4	39.1**	_a
Private	39.4	34.3	42.1**	43.8
Medicaid	19.6	19.5	16.2*	21.7
Medicare	14.3**	7.4**	_a	30.0*
Other public	2.0**	3.7**	1.7**	_a
Other	_a	_a	_a	_a

aRelative standard error is too large to support reliable estimation.
*p < .10
** p < .05
SOURCE: Zuvekas (2001), based on the 1996 Medical Expenditure Panel Survey.

services provided to Medicare and Medicaid participants, from federal block grants to states, and from state and local funds that support community-based programs and hospital care. Taken in the aggregate, these funding streams are neither adequate nor reliable enough to meet the needs of individuals with serious mental disorders (IOM, 2000a). As with other forms of safety-net care, the urgency of providing treatment to the severely mentally ill erodes funds available for prevention purposes.

Treatment for Substance Abuse

In the United States, more than 18 million people who use alcohol and nearly 5 million who use illicit drugs need substance abuse treatment (SAMHSA, 2001). Substance abuse, like mental illness, exacts enormous social costs across all segments of society. The total social costs of alcohol abuse alone were estimated at $177.3 billion in 1997 (Coffey et al., 2001). In that same year, $6.4 billion was spent on treatment. Total spending on drug abuse treatment equaled $5.5 billion in that year, compared with estimated social costs of drug abuse of $116.9 billion.

Most recipients (87 percent) of specialty treatment for alcohol or drug abuse receive it in outpatient settings (RWJF, 2001), but overall, less than one-fourth of those who need treatment get it. Barriers to treatment include stigma, lack of available treatment facilities, unwillingness to admit that treatment is needed, and inability to pay for care. Public sources provide more than two-thirds of the funding for alcohol and drug treatment facilities. Half of such funds come from dedicated funding at the federal, state, and local levels in the form of various block grants to state safety-net programs.

Medicaid and Medicare cover 21 percent of treatment, private insurance covers 14 percent, and 10 percent is paid directly by patients as out-of-pocket costs. Another 5 percent is covered through various charitable sources.

Insurance policies held by many individuals constrain the use of substance abuse services by the exclusion of benefits for such services and by the use of annual and lifetime limits on benefits and other controls on service utilization. Between 1987 and 1997, private insurance for substance abuse services fell 0.2 percent per year on average (inflation adjusted). Over the same period, out-of-pocket payments for specific types of substance abuse treatment increased (Coffey et al., 2001). However, the high out-of-pocket costs faced by individuals who pay for their own treatment discourage many who need care from seeking it.

Oral Health Care

Like mental illness and addiction disorders, oral health has been neglected in the health care delivery system. The consequences in terms of individual and population health are significant—oral health is a matter of public health concern because it affects a large proportion of the population and is linked with overall health status (see Box 5–7). Oral diseases are causally related to a range of significant health problems and chronic diseases, as well as individuals' ability to succeed in school, work, and the community (DHHS, 2000b). The effects of oral diseases are cumulative and influence aspects of life as fundamental as the foods people can eat, their ability to communicate effectively, and their social acceptability. The problems in the way the health care delivery system relates to oral health include lack of dental coverage and low coverage payments, the separation of medicine and dentistry in training and practice, and the high proportion of the population that lacks any dental insurance. The committee focused on the problem of insurance and access to care.

According to the Department of Health and Human Services (DHHS) Office of Health Promotion and Disease Prevention, more than 150 million Americans have limited or no dental insurance, nearly four times the number who lack insurance for medical care (cited by Allukian, 1999). As with other types of health services, insurance is a strong predictor of access to and use of dental services, and minorities and low-income populations are much less likely to have dental insurance or to receive dental care.

Individuals and families living below the poverty level experience more dental decay than higher-income groups, and their cavities are less likely to be treated (GAO, 2000). More than a third of poor children (ages 2 to 9) have one or more primary teeth with untreated decay, compared with 17.3 percent of nonpoor children (DHHS, 2000b). Mexican-American adults and children are more likely to have untreated decayed teeth than any other

---

BOX 5-7
Oral Health as a Component of Total Health

When people think about the components of good health, they often forget about the importance of good oral health. This oversight is often reflected by health insurance coverage restrictions that exclude oral health care.

Oral health is important because the condition of the mouth is often indicative of the condition of the body as a whole. More than 90 percent of systemic diseases have oral manifestations. These diseases include immune deficiency (e.g., HIV/AIDS), viral diseases (e.g., herpes and mumps), cancer and leukemia, diabetes, heart disease, kidney disease, anemia, hemophilia and other bleeding disorders, adrenal gland disorders, and inflammatory bowel disease (Bajuscak, 1999; Glick, 1999). Also, poor oral health can lead to poor general health. Infections in the mouth can enter the bloodstream and affect the functioning of major organs (e.g., bacterial endocarditis, in which infection causes the lining of the heart and the heart valves to become inflamed) (Meadows, 1999). Poor oral care can also contribute to oral cancer, and untreated tooth decay can lead to tooth abscess, tooth loss, and—in the worst cases—serious destruction of the jawbone (Meadows, 1999).

For these reasons, oral health must recognized as an important component of assuring individual and population health. The awareness that the mouth may be a mirror to the body can help to prevent illness, diagnose serious conditions early, and maintain optimum overall health (Glick, 1999).

---

population group. Poor Mexican-American children ages 2 to 9 have the highest proportion of untreated decayed teeth (70.5 percent), followed by poor non-Hispanic African-American children (67.4 percent). The pattern for adults is similar (DHHS, 2000b: 63–64).

Medicare excludes coverage of routine dental care, and many state Medicaid programs do not provide dental coverage for eligible children or adults. According to a report of the Surgeon General, fewer than one in five Medicaid-covered children received a single dental visit in a recent year-long study period (DHHS, 2000b). Low-income Hispanic children and adults are less likely to be eligible for Medicaid than other groups, so even the limited Medicaid benefits are unlikely to be available to them. The forecast for major oral health problems among the nation's fastest-growing population group, Hispanics, is especially alarming.

The committee found that preventive, oral health, mental health, and substance abuse treatment services must be considered part of the comprehensive spectrum of care necessary to help assure maximum health. Therefore, **the committee recommends that all public and privately funded insurance plans include age-appropriate preventive services as recommended by** the U.S. Preventive Services Task Force and provide evidence-based coverage of oral health, mental health, and substance abuse treatment services.

PROBLEMS IN QUALITY OF CARE

Crossing the Quality Chasm (IOM, 2001b) examined health system failures that compromise the quality of care provided to all Americans. As noted, it is often the responsibility of state departments of health to monitor providers and levy sanctions when quality problems are identified. This adds to potential tensions with the public health system. Two particular quality problems have special significance in terms of assuring the health of the population: disparities in the quality of care provided to racial and ethnic minorities and inadequate management of chronic diseases. As the American population grows both older and more racially and ethnically diverse and as rates of chronic disease increase, important vulnerabilities in the health care delivery system are compromising individual and population health (Murray and Lopez, 1996; Hetzel and Smith, 2001).

Disparities in Health Care

A principal finding from *Crossing the Quality Chasm* (IOM, 2001b: 53) is that "the quality of care should not differ because of such characteristics as gender, race, age, ethnicity, income, education, disability, sexual orientation, or place of residence." Disparities in health care are defined as "racial or ethnic differences in the quality of health care that are not due to access-related factors or clinical needs, preferences and appropriateness of intervention" (IOM, 2002b: 4).

Evidence shows that racial and ethnic minorities do not receive the same quality of care afforded white Americans. These findings are consistent across a range of illnesses and health care services and remain even after adjustment for socioeconomic differences and other factors that are related to access to health care (IOM, 2002b). Furthermore, poor-quality health care is an important independent variable contributing to lower health status for minorities (IOM, 2002b). For example, racial differences in cervical cancer deaths have increased over time, despite the greater use of screening tests by minority women (Mitchell and McCormack, 1997). The lower quality of care also compounds the adverse health effects of other disadvantages faced by minorities, including lower incomes and education, less healthy living environments, and a greater likelihood of being uninsured.

As discussed in *Unequal Treatment* (IOM, 2002b), the factors that may produce disparities in health care include the role of bias, discrimination, and stereotyping at the individual (provider and patient), institution, and health system levels. The report found that aspects of the health care system—its organization, financing, and availability of services—may have adverse effects specifically for racial and ethnic minorities. For example, time pressures on physicians hamper their ability to accurately assess presenting symptoms, especially when cultural or language barriers are present. Nearly 14 million people in the United States are not proficient in English.

Changes in the financing and delivery of health care services, such as the emphasis on cost controls and the almost complete conversion to managed care for the delivery of services under Medicaid, may be especially problematic for racial and ethnic minorities. The disruption of traditional community-based care and the displacement of providers who are familiar with the language, culture, and values of ethnic communities create barriers to effective care (Leigh et al., 1999). In addition, segmentation of health care plans was found to play a significant role in producing poorer care for racial and ethnic minorities because they are more likely than whites to be enrolled in "lower-end" health plans (IOM, 2002b). Such plans are characterized by higher per capita resource constraints and stricter limits on covered services (Phillips et al., 2000). Fragmentation of health plans along socioeconomic lines engenders different clinical cultures, with different practice norms (Bloche, 2001).

The committee encourages the health care system and policy makers in the public and private sectors to give careful consideration to the interventions that are identified in *Unequal Treatment* (IOM, 2002b) and aimed at eliminating racial and ethnic disparities in health care (see Box 5–8).

Care for Chronic Conditions

Americans now live longer. A child born today can expect to live more than 75 years, and advances in medicine have also extended the life spans of earlier generations. As detailed in Chapter 1, the result is that individuals over age 65 constitute an increasingly large proportion of the U.S. population—13 percent today, increasing to 20 percent over the next decade. Embedded in these demographic changes is a dramatic increase in the prevalence of chronic conditions. Chronic conditions, defined as illnesses that last longer than 3 months and that are not self-limiting, affect nearly half of the U.S. population. An estimated 100 million Americans have one or more chronic conditions, and that number is estimated to reach 134 million by 2020 (Pew Environmental Health Commission, 2001). Nearly half of those with a chronic illness have more than one such condition (IOM, 2001a). Additionally, disabling chronic conditions affect all age groups, but about two-thirds are found in individuals over age 65. With the projected growth in the number of people over age 65 increasing from 13 percent of the

---

BOX 5–8
Legal, Regulatory, and Policy Interventions to Eliminate Racial and Ethnic Disparities in Health Care

- Avoid fragmentation of health plans along socioeconomic lines.
- Strengthen the stability of patient–provider relationships in publicly funded health plans.
- Increase the proportion of underrepresented U.S. racial and ethnic minorities among health professionals.
- Apply the same managed care protections to publicly funded health maintenance organization (HMO) enrollees that apply to private HMO enrollees.
- Provide greater resources to the Department of Health and Human Services Office of Civil Rights to enforce civil rights laws.
- Promote the consistency and equity of care through the use of evidence-based guidelines.
- Structure payment systems to ensure an adequate supply of services to minority patients and limit provider incentives that may promote disparities.
- Enhance patient–provider communications and trust by providing financial incentives for practices that reduce barriers and encourage evidence-based practice.
- Support the use of interpretation services where community need exists.
- Support the use of community health workers.
- Implement multidisciplinary treatment and preventive care teams.
- Implement patient education programs to increase patients' knowledge of how to best access care and participate in treatment decisions.
- Integrate cross-cultural education into the training of all current and future health care professionals.
- Collect and report data on health care access and utilization by patients' race, ethnicity, socioeconomic status, and, where possible, primary language.

SOURCE: IOM (2002c).

---

population to 20 percent, the need for care for chronic conditions will also continue to grow.

As detailed in *Crossing the Quality Chasm* (IOM, 2001b: 27), effective health care for chronic disease management is a collaborative process, involving the "definition of clinical problems in terms that both patients and providers understand; joint development of a care plan with goals, targets, and implementation strategies; provision of self-management training and support services; and active, sustained follow-up using visits, telephone calls, e-mail, and Web-based monitoring and decision support systems."

The current health care system does not meet the challenge of providing clinically appropriate and cost-effective care for the chronically ill. *Crossing the Quality Chasm* (IOM, 2001b: 28) found that "the prevailing model of health care delivery is complicated, comprising layers of processes and handoffs that patients and families find bewildering and clinicians view as wasteful . . . a nightmare to navigate." Although this reality is a challenge for anyone seeking care, the effects become especially damaging for those with chronic conditions. Wagner and colleagues (1996) identified five elements required to improve outcomes for chronically ill patients:

1. Evidence-based planned care.
2. Reorganization of practices to meet the needs of patients who require more time, a broad array of resources, and closer follow-up.
3. Systematic attention to patients' need for information and behavioral change.
4. Ready access to necessary clinical expertise.
5. Supportive information systems.

The health care delivery system as it exists today cannot deliver those elements. Recent surveys have found that less than half of U.S. patients with hypertension, depression, diabetes, and asthma are receiving appropriate treatments (Wagner et al., 2001). Delivery of high-quality care to chronically ill patients is especially challenging in a decentralized and fragmented system, characterized by small practices (AMA, 1998). Smaller practices have great difficulty in organizing the array of services and support needed to efficiently manage chronic disease. The result is poor disease management and a high level of wasted resources. As the proportion of old and very old increases, the system-wide impact in terms of cost and increased disability may well overwhelm the human and financial resources available to care for chronically ill patients.

CAPACITY OF THE HEALTH CARE SYSTEM
TO SERVE THE POPULATION

The resources of the health care delivery system are not balanced well enough to provide patient-centered care, to address the complex health care demands of an aging population, to absorb normal spikes in demand for urgent care, and to manage a large-scale emergency such as that posed by a terrorist attack. The relentless focus on controlling costs over the past decade has squeezed a great deal of excess capacity out of the health care system, particularly the hospital system. It has also reduced the time that physicians spend with patients and the quality of the clinical encounter. At the same time, the design of insurance plans (in both the public and the private sectors) does not support the integrated disease management protocols needed to treat chronic disease or the data gathering and analysis needed for both disease management and population-level health. Underlying all of these problems is the absence of a national health information infrastructure to support research, clinical medicine, and population-level health.

Shortages of Health Care Professionals

The committee took special note of certain shortages of health care professionals, because these shortages are having a significant adverse effect on the quality of health care. The committee's particular concerns are the underrepresentation of racial and ethnic minorities in all health professions and the shortage of nurses, especially registered nurses (RNs) practicing in hospitals.

However, the focus on these two health care professional shortage areas does not suggest the absence of problems in other fields. Acute shortages of primary care physicians exist in many geographic areas, in certain medical specialties, and in disciplines such as pharmacy and dentistry, to name two. In addition, a growing consensus suggests that major reforms are needed in the education and training of all health professionals. To deliver the type of health care envisioned in *Crossing the Quality Chasm* (IOM, 2001b), health care professionals must be trained to work in teams, to utilize information technology effectively, and to develop the competencies necessary to deliver care to an increasingly diverse population. Health professions education is not currently organized to produce these results.

Underrepresentation of Racial and Ethnic Minorities

In 2000, 9 percent of physicians and 12.3 percent of RNs were from racial and ethnic minority groups (AAMC, 2000). By comparison, racial and ethnic minorities account for more than one-quarter of the nation's population. Among physicians, about 3 percent are African American, 2.2 percent are Hispanic, and 3.6 percent are Asian (AAMC, 2000). The 2000 National Sample Survey of Registered Nurses reported that 5 percent of RNs are African American, 2 percent are Hispanic, and 3.5 percent are Asian (Spratley et al., 2000). The severe underrepresentation of racial and ethnic minorities in the health professions affects access to care for minority populations, the quality of care they receive, and the level of confidence that minority patients have in the health care system.

A consistent body of research indicates that African-American and Hispanic physicians are more likely to provide services in minority and underserved communities and are more likely to treat patients who are poor, Medicaid eligible, and sicker (IOM, 2001c). Some studies indicate that, on average, minority physicians treat four to five times more minority patients than do white physicians, and studies of recent minority medical school graduates indicate that they have a greater preference to serve in minority and underserved areas. Although more research is needed to examine the impact of minority health care professionals on the level of access and quality of care, for some minority patients, having a minority physician results in better communication, greater patient satisfaction with care, and greater use of preventive services (IOM, 2002b). Although evidence has not established that increasing the numbers of minority physicians or improving cultural competence per se influences patient outcomes, existing research supports clear policies to increase the proportion of medical students drawn from minority groups.

Hospital Nursing Shortage

RNs work in a variety of settings, ranging from governmental public health agency clinics to hospitals and nursing homes. The majority, however, work in hospitals, although the proportion dropped from 68 percent in 1968 to 59 percent in 2000 (Spratley et al., 2000). Hospitals are facing shortages of RNs, in addition to shortages of pharmacists, laboratory technologists, and radiological technologists. A recent national hospital survey (AHA, 2001b) found that of 168,000 vacant positions, 126,000 were for RN positions. Hospital vacancy rates for RN positions averaged 11 percent across the country, ranging from about 10 percent to more than 20 percent in some states. Nationally, more than one in seven hospitals report a severe shortage of RNs, with more than 20 percent of RN positions vacant. In general, hospitals in rural areas report the highest percentage of vacant positions. The current shortage of RNs, particularly for hospital practice, is a matter of national concern because nursing care is critical to the operation and quality of care in hospitals (Aiken et al., 1994, 2001). In a study analyzing more than 5 million patient discharges from 799 hospitals in 11 states, Needleman and colleagues (2001) consistently found that higher RN staffing levels were associated with a 3 to 12 percent reduction in indicators—including lower rates of urinary tract infections, pneumonia, shock, and upper gastrointestinal bleeding and shorter lengths of stay—that reflect better inpatient care.

The shortage of hospital-based nurses reflects several factors, including the aging of the population, declining nursing school enrollment numbers (Sherer, 2001), the aging of the nursing workforce (the average age increased from 43.1 years in 1992 to 45.2 years in 2000) (Spratley et al., 2000), and dissatisfaction among nurses with the hospital work environment. Furthermore, nurses have available other professional opportunities, and women, who once formed the bulk of the nursing workforce, now have alternate career prospects. These trends do not appear to be a temporary, cyclical phenomenon. The aging of the population means an increase in the number of patients who require skilled care for chronic diseases and age-related conditions, but the growth in the pool of nursing professionals is not keeping pace with the growth in the patient population.

Although some of this increase is to be expected because of the overall aging of the U.S. labor force, the proportion of workers who are age 35 and older is increasing more for RNs than for all other occupations (IOM, 1996). An aging workforce may have implications for patient care if older RNs have less ability to perform certain physical tasks (HRSA, 2001). The shortage of RNs poses a serious threat to the health care delivery system, and to hospitals in particular.

Hospitals and the Capacity for Emergency Response

Hospitals contribute in various ways to assuring the health of the public, particularly by providing acute care services, educating health professionals, serving as a site for research, organizing community health promotion and disease prevention activities, and acting as safety-net providers. However, hospitals play a uniquely important role by serving as the primary source of emergency and highly specialized care such as that in intensive care units (ICUs) and centers for cardiac care and burn treatment.

Recent changes in the structure of the hospital industry, the reimbursement of hospitals by public- and private-sector insurance programs, and nursing shortages have raised questions about the ability of hospitals to carry out these roles. Although the terrorist incidents in the fall of 2001 did not directly test the ability of hospitals to respond to a medical crisis, they drew particular attention to hospitals' limited "surge capacity"—the ability to absorb a large influx of severely injured patients—in their emergency departments and specialty units.

During the 1990s, the spread of managed care practices contributed to reductions in overall hospital admissions, in the length of hospital stays, and in emergency department visits. As a result of decreasing demand for hospital services and a changing financial environment, hospitals in many parts of the country reduced the number of patient beds, eliminated certain services, or even closed (McManus, 2001). The American Hospital Association (AHA, 2001a) reports that from 1994 to 1999, the number of emergency departments in the nation decreased by 8.1 percent (see Table 5–3). Over the same period, medical and surgical bed capacities were reduced by 17.7 percent, ICU bed capacities were reduced by 2.8 percent, and specialty bed (including burn bed) capacities were reduced by 3.4 percent. Although these reductions may have improved the efficiencies of hospitals, they have important implications for the capacity of the health care system to respond to public health emergencies.

Crowding in hospital emergency departments has been recognized as a

TABLE 5-3   Change in Hospital Capacity, 1994–1999

Component	1994	1999	Percent Change, 1994–1999
Emergency departments	4,547	4,177	–8.1
Medical/surgical beds	533,848	439,426	–17.7
ICU beds	72,229	70,215	–2.8
Special care beds[a]	15,373	14,848	–3.4
Total inpatient beds[b]	621,450	524,489	15.6

[a]Burn care beds and other special care beds intended for care that is less intensive than that provided in an ICU and more intensive than that provided in an acute care area.

[b]Total of medical and surgical beds, ICU beds, and special care beds.

SOURCE: Brewster et al. (2001), citing the American Hospital Association (2001a).

nationwide problem for more than a decade (Andrulis et al., 1991; Brewster et al., 2001; McManus, 2001; Viccellio, 2001). According to the American Hospital Association (2001a), the demand for emergency department care increased by 15 percent between 1990 and 1999. In a random survey of emergency department directors in 1998 and 1999, 91 percent of the 575 respondents reported overcrowding problems (Derlet et al., 2001). The overcrowding was severe, resulting in delays in testing and treatment that compromised patient outcomes. The emergency departments of hospitals in many areas of New York City routinely operated at 100 percent capacity (Brewster et al., 2001). Patients regularly spent significant portions of their admission on gurneys in a hallway.

One consequence of this crowding is the periodic closure of emergency departments and the diversion of ambulances to other facilities. Ambulance diversions have been found to impede access to emergency services in metropolitan areas in at least 22 states (U.S. House of Representatives, 2001); at least 75 million Americans are estimated to reside in areas affected by ambulance diversions. Looking at 12 communities, Brewster and colleagues (2001) found that on average in 2001, two hospitals in Boston closed their emergency departments each day and the Cleveland Clinic emergency departments were closed to patients arriving by ambulance for an average of nearly 12 hours a day.

The increase in demand for emergency care is attributed to several factors (Brewster et al., 2001). In particular, managed care rules have changed to allow increased coverage of care provided in emergency departments. Hospitals are in better compliance with the federal Emergency Medical Treatment and Labor Act, which requires emergency departments to treat patients without regard for their ability to pay. In addition, uninsured patients are making greater use of emergency departments for nonurgent care.

Access to Primary Care

The adequacy of hospital capacity cannot be assessed without considering the system inefficiencies that characterize current insurance and care delivery arrangements. These include the demands placed on hospital emergency and outpatient departments by the uninsured and those without access to a primary care provider. The unique characteristic of primary care is the role it plays as a regular or usual source of care for patients and their families. Good primary care assures continuity for the patient across levels of care, comprehensiveness of services according to the level of health or illness, and better coordination of these services over time (Starfield, 1998).

Defining the right level of immediate and standby capacity for emergency and inpatient care depends in part on the adequacy and effectiveness of general outpatient and primary care. For example, chronic conditions like asthma and diabetes often can be managed effectively on an outpatient basis, but if the conditions are poorly managed by patients or their health care providers, emergency or inpatient care may be necessary. Billings and colleagues (1993) demonstrated strong links between hospital admission rates for such conditions and the socioeconomic and insurance status of the population in an area. For example, admission rates for asthma were 6.4 percent higher in low-income areas than in higher-income areas, with more than 70 percent of the variation explained by household income (Billings et al., 1993). Differences in disease prevalence accounted for only a small portion of the differences in hospitalization rates among low- and high-income areas.

Although Billings and colleagues did not draw conclusions about the causal pathways leading to these higher admission rates, it is likely that the contributing factors include those discussed in this chapter, such as a lack of insurance or a regular source of care and the assignment of Medicaid populations to lower-cost health plans. A follow-up analysis found the situation to be growing worse for low-income populations, as economic pressures, including lower reimbursements rates, higher practice costs, and limitations on payment for diagnostic tests, squeeze providers who have historically delivered care to academic health centers' low-income populations (Billings et al., 1996). Bindman and colleagues (1995) similarly concluded that at the community level, "there is a strong positive association between health care access and preventable hospitalization rates, suggesting that these rates can serve as an indication of access to care." It would be a costly mistake to create additional emergency and inpatient capacity before decompressing demand by improving access to primary care services. Good primary care is associated with better birth weights (Politzer et al., 2001), lower smoking rates, less obesity, and higher rates of seat belt use (Shi et al., 1999) and is a major determinant of receiving preventive services such as blood pressure screening, clinical breast exams, and Pap smears (Bindman et al., 1996). Geographically, areas with higher primary care physician-to-population ratios experience lower total health care costs (Welch et al., 1993; Mark et al., 1996; Franks and Fiscella, 1998; Starfield and Shi, 2002). Additionally, there is evidence that primary care is associated with reduced disparities in health; areas of high income inequality that also had good primary care were less likely to report fair or poor self-rated health (Starfield, 2002). The link between the availability of primary care and better health is also supported by international evidence, which shows that nations that value primary care are likely to have lower mortality rates (all causes; all causes, premature; and cause specific), even when controlling for macro- and micro-level characteristics (e.g., gross domestic product and per capita income) (Macinko et al., in press).

The Unfulfilled Potential of Managed Care

Although Billings and colleagues focused on the preventable demands for hospital care among low-income and uninsured populations, *Closing the Quality Chasm* (IOM, 2001b) makes clear that the misuse of services also characterizes disease management among insured chronically ill patients.

In the early 1990s, managed care became a common feature of the health care delivery system in the United States. In theory, managed care offers the promise of a population-based approach that can emphasize regular preventive care and other services aimed at keeping a defined group as healthy as possible. These benefits are most easily achieved under a fully capitated, group practice model: patients enroll with a health care organization that is paid a certain amount per member per month to provide all necessary or indicated services to the enrolled population, and physicians are paid a monthly fee or are salaried, which separates payment from the provision of individual services. This model allows a relatively stable enrolled population for whom benefits and services can be customized; knowledge of the global budget within which care is to be delivered; and a salaried workforce in which health care providers have an incentive to keep patients healthy and reduce unnecessary use of services but also have a culture in which they monitor each others' practices and quality of care. For the patient, the model provides comprehensive care, an emphasis on prevention, and low out-of-pocket costs. Kaiser Permanente Medical Group pioneered the model more than 50 years ago on the basis of early experiences providing health care programs for employees of Kaiser industrial companies (e.g., construction, shipyards, steel mills) in the late 1930s and 1940s.[1]

An important opportunity was lost when insurance companies, health plans and health providers, and the state and federal governments saw managed care primarily as a cost-containment mechanism rather than a population-based approach to delivering comprehensive and effective health care services. Reimbursement rate reductions, restrictions on care and choice of physician, and other aspects of plan management disaffected millions of Americans from the basic concept of managed care. Furthermore, rapid turnover in enrollment, particularly in Medicaid managed care, ruined economic incentives for plans to view their enrollees as a long-term investment. This loss of trust in the idea of managed care is also the loss of a great opportunity to improve quality and restrain costs. Loosely affiliated physician networks have no ability to identify their populations and develop programs specifically based on the epidemiology of the defined group. There is little ability to use data systems, shared protocols, or peer pressure to improve quality and reduce variations in health care practices.

Managed care is undergoing rapid changes, some of which are likely to further undermine its viability. Consumer demands for more choice and greater flexibility are weakening restrictions on access to providers and limitations on services. Physicians are proving more aggressive and successful in their negotiations with plans to decrease constraints, and to date, most employers have been willing to accept the higher costs that result. Employer acceptance may change in the face of double-digit insurance premium increases.

Predicting the next configuration of insurance and plan delivery systems is dangerous in a system undergoing such rapid transition. A number of major insurance plans have announced that they will begin to offer defined-contribution options.[2] This may be attractive to employers, whose liability will be defined by a specific premium amount rather than by a specified set of benefits. Consumers will be expected to shop for their own care with a medical spending account coupled with catastrophic benefits for very large expenses. This could significantly undermine the current

---

[1] Group Health of Puget Sound and the Health Insurance Plan of New York were also pioneers in group model health maintenance organizations.

[2] Defined-contribution health care benefits are a new way for employers to provide health care coverage to their employees, while no longer acting as brokers between employees and insurance companies contracted to provide benefits. An employer may choose from several different ways to put money into a health benefits account for each employee and offer the employee a menu of coverage options, with different funding levels and employee financial responsibility for each.

pooling of risk and create incentives for overuse of high-technology services once a deductible for catastrophic benefits has been met. However, such plans have yet to assume a significant role in the insurance market, and few employers offer them as an alternative.

Information Technology

The development of enhanced information technology and its use in hospitals, individual provider practices, and other segments of the health care delivery system are essential for improving the quality of care. Better information technology can also support patients and family caregivers in crucial health decisions, strengthen both personal and population-based prevention efforts, and enhance participation in and coordination with public health activities. (See Chapter 3 for a discussion of the information technology needs of the governmental public health infrastructure.)

Crossing the Quality Chasm (IOM, 2001b) formulated the case that information technology is critical to the redesign of the health care system to achieve a substantial improvement in the quality of care. A strong clinical information infrastructure is a prerequisite to reengineering processes of care; coordinating patient care across providers, plans, and settings and over time; supporting the operation of multidisciplinary teams and the application of clinical support tools; and facilitating the use of performance and outcome measures for quality improvement and accountability.

From the provider perspective, better information systems and more extensive use of information technology could dramatically improve care by offering ready access to complete and accurate patient data and to a variety of information resources and tools—clinical guidelines, decision-support systems, digital prescription-writing programs, and public health data and alerts, for example—that can enhance the quality of clinical decision making. Computer-based systems for the entry of physician orders have been found to have sizable benefits in enhancing patient safety (Bates et al., 1998, 2001; Schiff et al., 2000).

Despite profound growth in clinical knowledge and medical technology, the health care delivery system has been relatively untouched by the revolution in information technology that has transformed other sectors of society and the economy. Many health care settings lack basic computer systems to provide clinical information or support clinical decision making. Even where electronic medical record systems are being implemented, most of those systems remain proprietary products of individual institutions and health plans that are based on standards of specific vendors.

The development and application of interoperable systems and secure information-sharing practices are essential to gain greater benefits from information technology. At present, only a few institutions have had the resources to build integrated information systems that meet the needs of diverse specialties and environments. Those efforts illustrate both the costs involved in developing health information systems and some of the benefits that might be expected. Kaiser Permanente, for example, is investing $2 billion in a web-based system encompassing all of the critical features needed to provide patient-centered, high-quality care: a nationwide clinical information system, a means for patients to communicate with doctors and nurses to seek medical advice, access by clinicians to clinical guidelines and other knowledge resources, and computerized order entry (Krall, 1998).

So far, however, adoption of even common and less costly information technologies has been limited. Only a small fraction of physicians offer e-mail interaction (13 percent, in a 2001 poll), a simple and convenient tool for efficient communication with their patients (Harris Interactive, 2001). Some of the documented reasons for the low level of physician–patient e-mail communication include concerns about lack of reimbursement for this type of service and concerns about confidentiality and liability. These legitimate issues are slowly being addressed in policy and practice, but there is a long way to go if this form of communication is to achieve its potential for improving interactions between patients and providers.

Enhanced information technology also promises to aid patients and the public in other ways. The Internet already offers a wealth of information and access to the most current evidence to help individuals maintain their own health and manage disease. In addition, support groups and interactive programs offer additional approaches to empower consumers. Personalized systems for comprehensive home care may improve outcomes and reduce costs. Medicare's pilot project IdeaTel—Informatics for Diabetes Education and Telemedicine—offers web-based home systems to rural and inner-city diabetics to support home monitoring, customized information, and secure links to providers and to the patients' own medical records (www.dmi.columbia.edu/ideatel/info.html).

Other efforts to build a personal health record (PHR) created or cocreated and controlled by the individual—and instantly available to support treatment in any setting—suggest that the PHR may provide a comprehensive, accurate, and continuous record to support health and health care across the life span (Jones et al., 1999).

A sophisticated health information infrastructure is also important to support public health monitoring and disease surveillance activities. Systems and protocols for linking health care providers and governmental public health agencies are vital for detecting emerging health threats and supporting appropriate decisions by all parties. The committee cautions, however, that systems dedicated to a single use, such as bioterrorism, will not be optimal; systems designed to be comprehensive and flexible will be of greater overall value. Ultimately, such systems should also allow the public to contribute and receive information to get the most complete database possible.

For information technology to transform the health sector as it has banking and other forms of commerce that depend on the accurate, secure exchange of large amounts of information, action must be taken at the national level to develop the National Health Information Infrastructure (NHII) (NRC, 2000). The committee endorses the call by the National Committee on Vital and Health Statistics (NCVHS) (2002) for the nation to build a twenty-first century health support system—a comprehensive, knowledge-based system capable of providing information to all who need it to make sound decisions about health. Such a system can help realize the public interest related to quality improvement in health care and to disease prevention and health promotion for the population as a whole. The rapid development and widespread implementation of an extensive set of standards for technology and information exchange among providers, governmental public health agencies, and individuals are critical.

Nevertheless, as the NCVHS report describes, neither the opportunities nor the barriers to the development of the NHII are related solely to information technology. To realize the full potential of the NHII, supportive changes in the social, economic, and legal infrastructures are also required. Policies promoting the portability and continuity of personal health information are essential. Values, practices, relationships, laws, and investment and reimbursement policies must support the creation and use of data and information systems that are consistent with the vision for the NHII (see Chapter 3 for an additional discussion and recommendation).

COLLABORATION WITH GOVERNMENTAL PUBLIC HEALTH AGENCIES

The activities and interests of the health care delivery system and the governmental public health agencies clearly overlap in certain areas, but there is relatively little collaboration between them. In addition, the authority of state health departments in quality monitoring, licensure, and rate setting can cause serious tensions between them and health care organizations. The committee discusses the extent of this separation and the particular need for better collaboration, especially in regard to assuring access to health care services, disease surveillance activities, and partnerships toward broader health promotion efforts.

The Emergence of Separate Systems

Within the public health system in the United States, collaboration between the health care sector and governmental public health agencies is generally weak. This reflects the divergence and separate development of two distinct sectors following the Second World War. Lasker and colleagues observed, "[t]he dominant, highly respected medical sector focused on individual patients, emphasizing technologically sophisticated diagnosis and treatment and biological mechanisms of disease. The considerably smaller, less well-appreciated public health sector concentrated on populations, prevention, nonbiological determinants of health, and safety-net primary care" (Lasker et al., 1997: 274). As disciplines and professional fields, medicine and public health evolved with minimal levels of interaction, and often without recognition of the lost opportunities to improve the health of individuals and the population. The health care and governmental public health sectors are also very unequal in terms of their resources, prestige, and influence on public policy.

The failure to collaborate characterizes not only the interactions between governmental public health agencies and the organizations and individuals involved in the financing and delivery of health care in the private sector but also financing within the federal government. Within the Department of Health and Human Services (DHHS), the Centers for Medicare and Medicaid Services (CMS) administer the two public insurance programs with little interaction or joint planning with agencies of the U.S. Public Health Service (PHS). Even the congressional authorizing committees for these activities are separate. For example, the Substance Abuse and Mental Health Services Administration, a PHS agency, administers block grants to states to augment funding for mental health and substance abuse programs, neither of which is well supported under Medicaid. Until recently, the Medicaid waiver program, administered by CMS on behalf of the Secretary of Health and Human Services, did not provide protection of reimbursement rates for clinics within the safety-net system. At the same time, the Health Resources and Services Administration, the PHS agency charged with funding federally qualified safety-net clinics for the poor, and the Indian Health Service were both seeking funds to support the increasing deficits of these clinics due to the growing number of uninsured individuals and the low rates of reimbursement for Medicaid clinics.

The operational separation of public health and health care financing programs mirrors the cultural differences that characterize medicine and public health. American fascination with technology, science, and medical interventions and a relatively poor understanding of the determinants of health (see Chapter 2) or of the workings of the governmental public health agencies also contribute to the lower status, fewer resources, and limited influence of public health. The committee views these status and resource differences as barriers to mutually respectful collaboration and to achieving the shared vision of healthy people in healthy communities. The committee also urges greater efforts on the part of the health care

delivery system to meet its public health responsibilities and greater efforts on the part of governmental public health agencies to reach out to
health care providers and purchasers and engage them more fully in the
public health system.

The Role of Governmental Public Health Agencies
as Health Care Providers

Public health departments have always differed greatly in regard to the
delivery of health care services, based on the availability of such services in
the community and other reasons (Moos and Miller, 1981). Some provide
no personal health care services at all, whereas others provide some assort-
ment of primary health care and safety-net services. In general, however,
there has been a decrease in the number of local governmental public health
agencies involved in direct service provision. In a recent survey of public
health agencies, primary care or direct medical care services were the least
common services provided (NACCHO, 2001). Despite this, 28 percent of
local public health departments report that they are the sole safety-net
providers in their communities (Keane et al., 2001).

During the 1990s, Medicaid shifted from a fee-for-service program to a
managed care model. This change has been a challenge to the multiple roles
of public health departments as community-based primary health care providers, safety-net providers, and providers of population-based or traditional public health services. The challenge has been both financial and
organizational. First, managed care plans reimburse safety-net providers
less generously than fee-for-service Medicaid providers do (under Medicaid, federally qualified health centers benefited from a federal requirement
for full-cost reimbursement), and they impose administrative and service
restrictions that result in reduced overall rates of compensation (IOM,
2000a). In many states and localities, these changes have decreased the
revenue available to public health departments and public clinics and hospitals. In many cases, funds were no longer available for population-based
essential public health services or had to be diverted to the more visibly
urgent need of keeping clinics and hospitals open (CDC, 1997). The result
of this interplay is that many governmental public health agencies have
found themselves in a strained relationship with managed care organizations: on the one hand, encouraging their active partnership in an
intersectoral public health system and, on the other, competing with them
for revenues (Lumpkin et al., 1998). Second, the shift of Medicaid services
to a managed care environment led some public health departments to scale
down or dismantle their infrastructure for the delivery of direct medical
care. The recent trend of the exit of managed care from the Medicaid
market has left some people without a medical home and, in cases of

changes in eligibility, has left some people uninsured. This problem may be most acute in rural areas, where public health departments are often the sole safety-net providers (Johnson and Morris, 1998).

One strategy to help lessen the negative impacts of changes in health care financing undertaken by some public health departments has been the development of formal relationships (e.g., negotiating and implementing memoranda of agreement) with local managed care organizations that provide Medicaid and, in some cases, safety-net services. Such arrangements have made possible some level of integration of health care and public health services, enhanced information exchange and continuity of care, and allowed public health departments to be reimbursed for the provision of some of the services that are covered by the benefits packages of managed care plans (Martinez and Closter, 1998). At this time, governmental public health agencies are still called on to play a role in assurance broader than that which may be compatible with their other responsibilities to population health. However, closer integration between these governmental public health agencies and the health care delivery system can help address the needs of the uninsured and underinsured. Denver Health, in Colorado, provides an intriguing example of a hybrid, integrated public–private health system (Mays et al., 2000). Denver Health is the local (county and city) public health authority, as well as a managed care organization and hospital service. Although changes in the Medicaid program continue to challenge Denver Health, it continues to balance its broad responsibilities to the public's health with its role and capacity as a large health care provider.

Disease Surveillance and Reporting

Disease surveillance and reporting provide a classic exemplar of essential collaboration between the health care system and the governmental public health agencies. The latter rely on health care providers and laboratories to supply the data that are the basis for disease surveillance. For instance, in the fall of 2001, reports from physicians who diagnosed the first cases of anthrax were essential in recognizing and responding to the bioterrorism attack.

States mandate the reporting of various infectious diseases (e.g., AIDS, hepatitis B, measles, rabies, and tuberculosis) and submit data to federal disease surveillance systems (CDC, 1999). Governmental public health agencies also depend on astute clinicians to inform them of sentinel cases of recognized diseases that represent a special threat to the public's health and of unusual cases, sometimes without a confirmed diagnosis, that may represent a newly emerging infection, such as Legionnaires' disease or West Nile virus in North America. Other types of public health surveillance activities, such as registries for cancer cases and for childhood immunizations, also depend on reporting from the health care system.

Effective surveillance requires timely, accurate, and complete reports from health care providers. In the case of infectious diseases, if all systems work effectively, the necessary information regarding the diagnosis for a patient with a reportable disease is transmitted to the state or local public health department by a physician or laboratory. For unusual or particularly serious conditions, public health officials offer guidance on treatment options and control measures and monitor the community for any additional reports of similar illness. For diseases like tuberculosis and sexually transmitted diseases, public health agencies facilitate active tracking and prophylactic treatment of persons exposed to an infected individual. Disease reporting requirements vary from state to state, although most states include diseases identified by the Centers for Disease Control and Prevention (CDC) as part of the National Notifiable Disease Reporting System.

Disease reporting is not complete, however. For diseases under national surveillance, from 6 to 90 percent of cases are reported, depending on the disease (Teutsch and Churchill, 1994; Thacker and Stroup, 1994). Incomplete reporting may reflect a lack of understanding by some health care providers of the role of the governmental public health agencies in infectious disease monitoring and control. In some instances, physicians and laboratories may be unaware of the requirement to report the occurrence of a notifiable disease or may underestimate the importance of such a requirement. The difficulty of reporting in a busy practice is also a barrier.

Notifiable disease reporting systems within public health departments with strong liaisons with the health care community are important in the detection and recognition of bioterrorism events. However, this valuable tool has not been well supported and, as noted earlier, suffers from issues of lack of timeliness and incomplete reporting, as well as complex or unclear reporting procedures and limited feedback from governmental public health agencies on how data are used (Baxter et al., 2000; Stagg Elliott, 2002). Health care delivery systems may fear that the data will be used to measure performance, and concerns about patient confidentiality can also contribute to a reluctance to report some diagnoses. New federal regulations regarding the confidentiality of medical records, required by the Health Insurance Portability and Accountability Act (P.L. 104–191) have generated enormous uncertainty and apprehension among health care providers and health systems regarding the sharing of individual clinical data.

Health care providers may also reduce their use of laboratory tests to confirm a diagnosis. This may be because of cost concerns or insurance plan restrictions or simply professional judgment that the test is unnecessary for appropriate clinical care. However, when fewer diagnostic tests are performed for self-limiting illnesses like diarrhea, there may be delays in recognizing a disease outbreak. Reduced use of laboratory testing prevents the analyses of pathogenic isolates needed for disease tracking, testing of new pathogens, and determining the levels of susceptibility to antimicrobial agents.

Other changes in the health care delivery system also raise concerns about the infectious disease surveillance system. As patterns of health care delivery change, old reporting systems are undermined, but the opportunities offered by new types of care systems and technologies have not been realized. For example, traditional patterns of reporting may be lost as health care delivery shifts from inpatient to outpatient settings. Hospital-based epidemiological reporting systems no longer capture many diagnoses now made and treated on an outpatient basis. This would not be a problem if health care systems used currently available information technologies, including electronic medical records and internal disease surveillance systems.

Better information systems that allow the rapid and continuous exchange of clinical information among health care providers and with public health agencies have the potential to improve disease surveillance as well as aid in clinical decision making while avoiding the use of unnecessary diagnostic tests. With such a system, a physician seeing an influx of patients with severe sore throats could use information on the current community prevalence of confirmed streptococcal pharyngitis and the antibiotic sensitivities of the cultured organisms to choose appropriate medications. From a public health perspective, such a system would permit continuous analysis of data from a number of clinical sites, enabling rapid recognition and response to new disease patterns in the community (see Chapter 3 for a discussion of syndrome surveillance). For example, toxic or infectious exposures could be tracked more easily if the characteristics of every patient encounter were integrated into one system and if everyone had unimpeded access to systems of care that could generate such data.

A CDC-funded project of the Massachusetts Department of Public Health and the Harvard Vanguard Medical Associates (a large multispecialty group) offers a glimpse of the benefits to be gained through collaboration between health care delivery systems and governmental public health agencies and specifically through the effective use of medical information systems (Lazarus et al., 2002). The Harvard Vanguard electronic medical system is queried each night for specific diagnoses assigned during the preceding day in the course of routine care. Diagnoses of interest are grouped into syndromes, and rates of new episodes are computed for all of eastern Massachusetts and each census tract. Expected numbers of new episodes are obtained from a generalized linear mixed model that uses data from 1996 to 1999. These expected numbers allow estimates of the probability of observing specific numbers of cases, either overall or in specific census tracts, and the rapid identification of an unusual cluster of events. The value of this type of real-time monitoring of unusual disease outbreaks is obvious for early identification of bioterrorism attacks as well as for improvements in clinical care and population health.

Sentinel Surveillance

Reports of sentinel events have proved useful for the monitoring of many diseases, but such reports may be serendipitous and generated because of close clustering, unusual morbidity and mortality, novel clinical features, or the chance availability of medical expertise. Sentinel networks that specifically link groups of participating health care providers or health care delivery systems to a central data-receiving and -processing center have been particularly helpful in monitoring specific infections or designated classes of infections. Examples of such networks are the National Nosocomial Infections Surveillance system and the National Molecular Subtyping Network for Foodborne Disease Surveillance (PulseNet). More recently, CDC has implemented a strategy directed to the identification of emerging infectious diseases in collaboration with many public health partners. The Emerging Infections Program (EIP) is a collaboration among CDC, state public health departments, and other public health partners for the purpose of conducting population-based surveillance and research on infectious diseases. At present, nine states (California, Colorado, Connecticut, Georgia, Maryland, Minnesota, New York, Oregon, and Tennessee) act as a national resource for the surveillance, prevention, and control of emerging infectious diseases (CDC, 2002). The EIP sites have performed investigations of meningococcal and streptococcal diseases and have established surveillance for unexplained deaths and severe illnesses as an attempt to identify diseases and infectious agents, known and unknown, that can lead to severe illness or death (CDC, 2002).

Preparing Health Care Professionals

Academic health centers (AHCs) serve as a critical interface with governmental public health agencies in several ways. First, as noted earlier, AHCs are an important part of the safety-net system in most urban areas. Second, they are the principal providers of specialized services and serve as regional referral centers for smaller towns or cities and rural areas. Both in normal periods and especially when confronted with either natural disasters or terrorist events, the specialized care units are an essential resource for public health. Moreover, they are also primary loci for research and training. AHCs also have a unique and special set of values that they bring to health care that transcend the discrete functions they perform.

The environment in which AHCs operate has changed substantially over the past decade. The advent of managed care plans that seek services from the lowest-cost appropriate provider and changes in federal (Medicare) reimbursement policies that reduced subsidies for costs associated with AHCs' missions in education, research, and patient care have created considerable pressure on academic institutions to increase efficiency and control costs. At the same time, advances in information technology and the explosion of knowledge from biomedical research have enormous implications for the role of AHCs in the health care system and in population health. Scientific and technological advances will permit clinical care to intervene early in a disease process by identifying and modifying personal risk. The burgeoning knowledge base will require different educational approaches to use the continuously expanding evidence base, with an emphasis on continuing education and lifetime learning.

These changes may result in a broader mission for AHCs that explicitly includes improving the public's health, generating and disseminating knowledge, advancing e-health approaches (i.e., that utilize the Internet and electronic communication technologies), providing education to current health professionals, providing community service and outreach, and delivering care that has the attributes necessary for practice. The ability of academic medicine to evolve into a broader mission will depend on changes in payment systems that may be difficult to achieve and on internal changes within AHCs that may be equally difficult.

Governmental public health agencies may also play an important role in preventive medicine and public health education. Health departments, for example, provide unique venues for the training of nurses, physicians, and other health care professionals in the basics of community-based health care and gain an understanding of population-level approaches to health improvement. Furthermore, public health students and preventive medicine residents gain practical experience in health department rotations, where they participate in program planning and evaluation and learn about assessing a community's health care needs and implementing strategies that change the conditions for health.

COLLABORATION WITH OTHER
PUBLIC HEALTH SYSTEM ACTORS

In addition to the linkages between the health care delivery system and governmental public health agencies, health care providers also interface with other actors in the public health system, such as communities, the media, and businesses and employers.

Relationships between the health care sector—hospitals, community health centers, and other health care providers—and the community are not new and have gained increased recognition for the value they bring to health care operations, their potential for enhancing provider accountability (VHA and HRET, 2000), the knowledge and empowerment they help to create in communities, and their potential for promoting health.

The recent trend among universities to assess their level of involvement in their communities and to develop programs focused on "service learning," and such public service oriented academic work includes AHCs. Calleson and colleagues (2002) surveyed the executives and staff of eight AHCs around the country and found that community–campus partnerships can strengthen the traditional mission of AHCs. The involvement of AHCs in the communities is also likely to increase in the coming years. The AHCs surveyed listed several factors that facilitated the development of relationships with communities and community organizations, including the request of the communities themselves and the growing population health orientation of the health care sector. Furthermore, non-academic community health centers also frequently have close ties to their communities, collaborating to assess local health needs, providing needed services, and supporting community efforts with research expertise and technical assistance in planning and evaluation. Many hospitals participate in broad community-based efforts to achieve some of the conditions necessary for health, for instance, collaborating with community development corporations to contribute financial, human, and technical resources (U.S. Department of Housing and Urban Development, 2002). Montefiore Medical Center in the Bronx, New York, for example, has partnered with a local nonprofit organization to develop low- and moderate-income housing and to establish a neighborhood kindergarten (Seedco and N-PAC, 2002). Additionally, Montefiore Medical Center partners with local high schools to develop health care professions education programs intended to create new career options and improve the likelihood inner-city youth will stay in school (Montefiore Medical Center, 2001). Hospitals are also employers, and in the case of two Lawndale, Illinois, hospitals, collaboration with the local development corporation and other neighborhood organizations in 1999 made affordable local housing available to employees, helping to facilitate community development (University of Illinois, 1999). In Providence, Rhode Island, a community partnership of nonprofit and independent hospitals and colleges works to improve children's quality of life by providing school-based health services, innovative and enhanced education through teacher and staff training, and support to improve home environments through housing advocacy (Health & Education Leadership for Providence, 2001; Providence Public School District, 2002).

Many hospitals and health care systems have seen the value of going beyond the needs of the individuals who enter the health care system to engage in broader community health action, even within the constraints of the current environment. The National Community Care Network Demonstration Program, sponsored by the Hospital Research and Education Trust (HRET), reports on hospitals across the country that are supporting activities beyond the delivery of medical care to improve health status and quality of life in local communities. Some of the motivation comes from the increasing pressure on nonprofit hospitals to justify their tax-exempt status through the provision of services that benefit the community, largely the provision of charity care; yet, many are seeing that investments in community health improvement are greater in value than the provision of medical care for preventable diseases (Barnett and Torres, 2001).

Vignettes drawn from the experience of American Hospital Association NOVA Award recipients illustrate the importance of investing in overall community health (AHA, 2002). For example, in 1994, Parkland Health and Hospital System in Dallas noted that injury rates in the community were three times the national average and that trauma admissions had jumped 38 percent in one year (53 percent of that care is uncompensated). As a result, the organization decided to convene the county's leading trauma care providers, police, and civic groups to investigate and solve the problem. With start-up funding from a local foundation, its own fundraising, and annual corporate sponsorships ranging from $35,000 to $150,000 from local hospitals and businesses, the coalition launched a Safe Communities initiative with a 52-member community advisory panel. Coalition members decided to tackle, in order, injuries caused by car accidents, violence, falls, and burns, through 11 initiatives involving more than 80 community organizations and agencies. Over a 2-week period, there was a 13 percent reduction in trauma admissions from car crashes due to a public awareness campaign and police initiative (AHA, 2002).

A 1998 finalist for the Foster G. McGaw Prize for Excellence in Community Service co-sponsored by AHA, the Franklin Community Health Network (FCHN) in Farmington, Maine, took the lead in developing a coalition and providing seed money to start a Rural Schools Equity Campaign (AHA, 2002). With high levels of youth involvement, and media cooperation, the campaign led to the legislative reformulation of property taxes to increase funding for rural schools in FCHN's service area by $1.3 million. In a further example, the Crozer-Keystone Health System that serves Chester, Pennsylvania, was declared a distressed municipality by the state in 1994. Although at the time the health system had been increasing its health care outreach programs, it realized it had to look at "root causes." As the largest employer in Chester, the system organized Community Connections, a mosaic of health, economic, and social programs and services developed in partnership with 20 other organizations, a local university, and governmental agencies. Programs included attracting other businesses to Chester, setting up a business incubator building, and colocating multiple health and social programs to facilitate "one-stop shopping." The effort has had a major stabilizing effect on Chester, and although overall health indicators are still behind state averages for chronic diseases, they are improving. Immunization rates have improved from 36 to 99 percent, and teen pregnancy is down to 31 per 1,000 from 44 per 1,000.

Under the guidance of an external review panel, HRET and the Voluntary Hospital Association of America (VHA) Health Foundation reviewed the experiences of recipients of the Foster G. McGaw Prize[3] from 1986 to 1998 and VHA Community Health Improvement Leadership Awards from 1996 to 1998. Fifteen of 20 winners participated in a study, which included a self-assessment of changes since the time of the award and in-depth interviews with chief executive officers, trustees, and those leading the initiative. Although this survey serves only as an illustration of what may be possible, several elements appeared supportive of a sustained commitment to efforts at community health improvement. These included

- Committing leadership at multiple levels through the top leadership to sustain changes;
- Developing community partnerships to develop champions outside the organization;
- Protecting funding and leadership of community health initiatives while integrating community health values into the culture of the parent organization;
- Linking community work with clinical work (mission alignment);
- Building an evidence base through evaluation and ongoing measurement of community health indicators; and
- Exploring external revenue streams and advocating for changes in current health care financing and funding for such efforts (VHA Health Foundation and HRET, 2000).

Boufford (1999) has suggested a Community Health Improvement Strategy that identifies a number of steps that provider organizations can take in such community-based efforts (see Box 5–9). However, payment systems are critical to encourage and sustain these network initiatives, and current reimbursement policies in public and private insurance are not designed to support population-focused care in a noncapitated system.

The health care sector can also develop linkages with the media to help ensure the accuracy of health information, communicate risk, and facilitate the public understanding of health care. For example, health care organiza-

---

[3] The Foster G. McGaw Prize for Excellence in Community Service is awarded by the American Hospital Association to recognize hospitals that have distinguished themselves through efforts to improve the health and well-being of everyone in their communities.

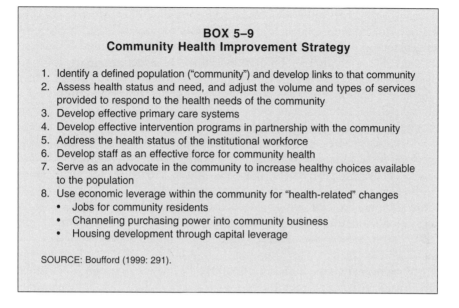

BOX 5–9
Community Health Improvement Strategy

1. Identify a defined population ("community") and develop links to that community
2. Assess health status and need, and adjust the volume and types of services provided to respond to the health needs of the community
3. Develop effective primary care systems
4. Develop effective intervention programs in partnership with the community
5. Address the health status of the institutional workforce
6. Develop staff as an effective force for community health
7. Serve as an advocate in the community to increase healthy choices available to the population
8. Use economic leverage within the community for "health-related" changes
   • Jobs for community residents
   • Channeling purchasing power into community business
   • Housing development through capital leverage

SOURCE: Boufford (1999: 291).

tions may use the media to disseminate health care information to their market areas, as demonstrated by the Minneapolis Allina Health System in its collaboration with a local television station and a health care news provider (Rees, 1999). Additionally, the media may be a powerful tool for familiarizing the public with health and health care issues and a conduit for raising important questions, stimulating public interest, or even influencing the public's health behaviors. For example, the popular prime time television show *ER* frequently serves as a platform for health information, with episodes exploring topics such as childhood immunizations, contraception, and violence (Brodie et al., 2001; also see Chapter 7).

Businesses and employers most commonly interface with the health care sector in purchasing and designing employee health benefits, with goals such as the inclusion of comprehensive preventive health care services. However, there are examples of wide-reaching business–health care linkages, such as the efforts to ensure quality of care and enhanced consumer choice undertaken by the Pacific Business Group on Health (see Chapter 6). Chapter 4 provides additional examples of fruitful community partnerships involving the health care sector.

IMPLICATIONS OF GROWING HEALTH CARE COSTS

As the committee has noted, health-related (mostly health care-related) spending in the United States amounted to $1.3 trillion in 2000, about 13.2

percent of the gross domestic product (Levit et al., 2002). After a period of stability in the mid-1990s, health care costs are again rising because of several factors (Heffler et al., 2002). Prescription drug spending, in particular, has increased sharply, and increased by 17.3 percent from 1999 to 2000 (HCFA, 2002). This increase comes from the growth of the older population and the proportion of the overall population with chronic conditions, along with the introduction of new and more expensive drugs, many of which are used to treat chronic conditions. In addition, spending for hospital services increased by 5.1 percent between 1999 and 2000, reaching $412 billion, and the cost of nursing home and home health care increased by 3.3 percent (Levit et al., 2002). However, the increase in health spending also reflects the success of federal and state efforts to enroll more low-income children in Medicaid and the State Children's Health Insurance Program, increased enrollment in Medicare as the population ages, and some erosion of unpopular cost-control features imposed by managed care plans.

With the economic downturn in 2001, the growth in health care spending creates added financial burdens for everyone, including individuals seeking care or insurance coverage, employers offering health insurance benefits, and governments at the federal, state, and local levels managing publicly funded insurance programs (Fronstin, 2002; Trude et al., 2002). Substantial increases in health insurance premiums are a clear indication of these economic stresses. For example, the California Public Employees' Retirement System, which is the nation's second largest public purchaser of employee health benefits, recently announced that health insurance premiums would increase by 25 percent (Connoly, 2002). States are experiencing serious pressures from growth in Medicaid spending, which increased by about 13 percent from 2001 to 2002, following a 10.6 percent increase in 2001 (NASBO, 2002a). With revenues increasing by only about 5 percent in the same period, Medicaid now accounts for more than 20 percent of total state spending (NASBO, 2002b).

The growing cost of health care has obvious implications for the nation's readiness to address the problems discussed in this chapter. Providing coverage to the uninsured, improving coverage for certain types of care, strengthening the emergency response and surge capacity in the hospital sector, and investing in information systems that can improve the quality of individual care and population-based disease surveillance will all require significant new resources from the public and private sectors. Although these steps can be expected to improve the nation's health and may even reduce costs over time, the initial investment will be substantial. The committee is concerned that with the escalation of expenditures, going in large measure toward maintaining current services, it will be difficult to identify the necessary public- and private-sector resources that will be needed for new activities.

The committee recommends that bold, large-scale demonstrations be funded by the federal government and other major investors in health care to test radical new approaches to increase the efficiency and effectiveness of health care financing and delivery systems. The experiments should effectively link delivery systems with other components of the public health system and focus on improving population health while eliminating disparities. The demonstrations should be supported by adequate resources to enable innovative ideas to be fairly tested.

CONCLUDING OBSERVATIONS

This chapter has outlined the main areas in which the health care delivery system and the governmental public health agencies interface. These areas include the regulatory and quality monitoring functions performed by governmental agencies, disease surveillance and reporting by health care providers, and the provision of safety-net services. Although assurance is a core function of public health, governmental public health agencies often do more than assure that people can access health care services; public health departments may become providers of last resort in areas where no other services are available for low-income, uninsured populations and when managed care services to Medicaid and uninsured populations are discontinued. These circumstances force public health departments to provide personal health care services instead of using their resources and population-level approaches to guide and support community efforts to change the conditions for health. Closer collaboration and integration between governmental public health agencies and the health care delivery system may enhance the capacities of both to improve population health and may support the efforts of other public health system actors.

REFERENCES

AAMC (Association of American Medical Colleges). 2000. Minority Graduates of US Medical Schools: Trends, 1950–1998. Washington, DC: Association of American Medical Colleges.

AHA (American Hospital Association). 2001a. Emergency departments—an essential access point to care. AHA TrendWatch 3(1).

AHA. 2001b. The health care workforce shortage and its implication for America's hospitals. AHA Workforce Survey Results. Available online at www.aha.org/workforce/resources. Accessed April 9, 2002.

AHA. 2002. Nova Award Winners 1994–200. Available online at www.hospitalconnect.com/aha/awards-events/awards/novaaward.html. Accessed October 7, 2002.

AHCPR (Agency for Health Care Policy and Research). 1993. Depression in Primary Care: Treatment of Major Depression. Rockville, MD: Department of Health and Human Services.

Aiken L, Clarke S, Sloane D, Sochalski J, Busse R, Clarke H, Giovannetti P, Hunt J, Rafferty A, Shamian J. 2001. Nurses' report on hospital care in five countries. Health Affairs 20(3):43–53.

Aiken LH, Smith HL, Lake ET. 1994. Lower Medicare mortality among a set of hospitals known for good nursing care. Medical Care 32:771–787.

Allukian M. 1999. Dental insurance is essential, but not enough. In Closing the Gap, a newsletter. July. Washington, DC: Office of Minority Health, Department of Health and Human Services.

American Medical Association. 1998. Socioeconomic characteristics of medical practice 1997/ 98. Chicago: American Medical Association.

Andrulis DP, Kellermann A, Hintz EA, Hackman BB, Weslowski VB. 1991. Emergency departments and crowding in United States teaching hospitals. Annals of Emergency Medicine 20(9):980–986.

Ayanian JZ, Weissman JS, Schneider EC, Ginsburg JA, Zaslavsky AM. 2000. Unmet health needs of uninsured adults in the United States. Journal of the American Medical Association 284:2061–2069.

Bajuscak R. 1999. Warning signs in the mouth. In Closing the Gap, a newsletter. July. Washington, DC: Office of Minority Health, Department of Health and Human Services.

Baker DW, Shapiro MF, Schur CL. 2000. Health insurance and access to care for symptomatic conditions. Archives of Internal Medicine 160(9):1269–1274.

Barnett K, Torres G. 2001. Beyond the Medical Model: Hospitals Improve Community Building. Community Care Network (CCN) Briefings, Fall 2001. Chicago, IL: Hospital Research and Education Trust, American Hospital Association.

Bates D, Cohen M, Leape LL, Overhage JM, Shabot MM, Seridan T. 2001. Reducing the frequency of errors in medicine using information technology. Journal of the American Medical Informatics Association 8(4):299–308.

Bates DW, Leape LL, Culled DJ, Laird N, Petersen LA, Teito JM, Burdick E, Hickey M, Kleefield S, Shea B, Vander Vliet M, Seger DL. 1998. Effect of computerized physician order entry and a team intervention on prevention of serious medication errors. Journal of the American Medical Association 280(15):1311–1316.

Baxter R, Mechanic RE. 1997. The status of local health care safety-nets. Health Affairs 16(4):7–23.

Baxter R, Rubin R, Steinberg C, Carroll C, Shapiro J, Yang A. 2000. Assessing Core Capacity for Infectious Diseases Surveillance. Final Report prepared for the Office of the Assistant Secretary for Planning and Evaluation. Falls Church, VA: The Lewin Group, Inc.

Berk ML, Schur C. 1998. Access to care: how much difference does Medicaid make? Health Affairs 17:169–108.

Billings J, Zeitel L, Lukomnik J, Carey TS, Blank AE, Newman L. 1993. Impact of socioeconomic status on hospital use in New York City. Health Affairs 12(1):162–173.

Billings J, Anderson G, Newman L. 1996. Recent findings on preventable hospitalizations. Health Affairs 15(3):239–249.

Bindman AB, Grumbach K, Osmond D, Komaromy M, Vranizan K, Lurie N, Billings J, Stewart A. 1995. Preventable hospitalizations and access to health care. Journal of the American Medical Association 274:305–311.

Blendon RJ, Scoles K, DesRoches C, Young JT, Herrmann MJ, Schmidt JL, Kim M. 2001. Americans' health priorities: curing cancer and controlling costs. Health Affairs 20(6):222–232.

Bloche MG. 2001. Race and discretion in American medicine. Yale Journal of Health Policy, Law and Ethics 1:95–131.

Boards of Trustees, Federal Hospital Insurance and Federal Supplementary Medical Insurance Trust Funds. 2002. 2002 Annual Report of the Boards of Trustees of the Federal Hospital Insurance and Federal Supplementary Medical Insurance Trust Funds. Available online at http://cms.hhs.gov/publications/trusteesreport/default.asp. Accessed October 6, 2002.

Boufford JI. 1999. Health future: the managerial agenda. Journal of Health Administration Education 17(4):271–295.

Breen N, Wagener DK, Brown ML, Davis WW, Ballard-Barbash R. 2001. Progress in cancer screening over a decade: results of cancer screening from the 1987, 1992, and 1998 National Health Interview Surveys. Journal of the National Cancer Institute 93:1704–1713.

Brewster LR, Rudell LS, Lesser CS. 2001. Emergency room diversions: a symptom of hospitals under stress. Issue Brief No. 38. Washington, DC: Center for Studying Health System Change.

Brodie M, Foehr U, Rideout V, Baer N, Miller C, Flournoy R, Altman D. 2001. Communicating health information through the entertainment media: a study of the television drama ER lends support to the notion that Americans pick up information while being entertained. Health Affairs 20(1):192–199.

Burstin HR, Swartz K, O'Neill AC, Orav EJ, Brennan TA. 1998. The effect of change of health insurance on access to care. Inquiry 35:389–397.

Calleson DC, Seifer SD, Maurana C. 2002. Forces affecting community involvement of AHCs: perspectives of institutional and faculty leaders. Academic Medicine 77(1):72–81.

CDC (Centers for Disease Control and Prevention). 1997. Estimated expenditures for essential public health services-selected states, fiscal year 1995. Morbidity and Mortality Weekly Report 46(7):150–152.

CDC. 1998. Use of clinical preventive services by adults aged <65 years enrolled in health-maintenance organizations—United States, 1996. Morbidity and Mortality Weekly Report 47(29):613–619.

CDC. 1999. Summary of notifiable diseases, United States, 1999. Morbidity and Mortality Weekly Report 48(53):1–104.

CDC. 2002. Emerging Infections Program. CDC, National Center for Infectious Diseases Surveillance Resources. Available online at www.cdc.gov/ncidod/ osr/EIP.htm. Accessed October 21, 2002.

CMS (Centers for Medicare and Medicaid Services). 2002a. CMS program operations. Section II. In Program Information on Medicare Medicaid, SCHIP & Other Programs of the Centers for Medicare & Medicaid Services. Available online at http://cms.hhs.gov/charts/ series/. Accessed October 4, 2002.

CMS. 2002b. Medicare program information, Section III.B.1. In Program Information on Medicare Medicaid, SCHIP & Other Programs of the Centers for Medicare & Medicaid Services. Available online at http://cms.hhs.gov/charts/series/. Accessed October 4, 2002.

CMS. 2002c. State Children's Health Insurance Program: Fiscal year 2001 annual enrollment report. Available online at www.cms.hhs.gov/schip/schip01.pdf. Accessed October 15, 2002.

Coffey RM, Mark T, King E, Harwood H, McKusick D, Genuardi J, Dilonardo J, Chalk M. 2001. National Estimates of I xpenditures for Substance Abuse Treatment, 1997. Rockville, MD: Center for Substance Abuse Treatment, Substance Abuse and Mental Health Services Administration, Department of Health and Human Services.

Connolly C. 2002. Health-care costs jump at CalPERS: big premium increase may signal trend. Washington Post, April 17, p. E01.

Cooper-Patrick L, Gallo JJ, Powe NR, Steinwachs DM, Eaton WW, Ford DE. 1999. Mental health service utilization by African Americans and whites: The Baltimore Epidemiologic Catchment Area Follow-up. Medical Care 37:1034–1045.

Department of Defense. 2002. TRICARE Homepage. Available online at www.tricare.osd.mil. Accessed August 3, 2002.

Department of Veterans Affairs. 1993. Clinical Guidelines for Major Depressive Disorder. Washington, DC: Veterans Health Administration.

Derlet R, Richards J, Kravitz R. 2001. Frequent overcrowding in U.S. emergency departments. Academic Emergency Medicine 8(2):151–155.

DHHS (Department of Health and Human Services). 1999. Mental Health: A Report of the Surgeon General. Rockville, MD: Substance Abuse and Mental Health Administration, National Institute of Mental Health, National Institutes of Health, Department of Health and Human Services.

DHHS. 2000a. Objective 18: mental health and mental disorders. In Healthy People 2010, Vol. II, 2nd ed. Washington, DC: Department of Health and Human Services.

DHHS. 2000b. Oral Health in America: A Report of the Surgeon General. Rockville, MD: National Institute of Dental and Craniofacial Research, National Institutes of Health, Department of Health and Human Services.

DHHS. 2002. 2002 CMS Statistics. CMS Publication 03437. Baltimore, MD: Department of Health and Human Services. Available online at http://cms.hhs.gov/researchers/pubs/CMSStatistics BlueBook2002.pdf. Accessed online October 15, 2002.

Dranove D, Simon CJ, White WD. 2002. Is managed care leading to consolidation in health-care markets? Health Services Research 37(3):573–594.

Draper DA, Hurley RE, Lesser CC, Strunk BC. 2002. The changing face of managed care. Health Affairs 21(1):11–23.

Farley T, Flannery JT. 1989. Late-stage diagnosis of breast cancer in women of lower socioeconomic status: public health implications. American Journal of Public Health 79:1508–1512.

Franks P, Fiscella K. 1998. Primary care physicians and specialists as personal physicians. Health care expenditures and mortality experience. Journal of Family Practice 47:105–109.

Fronstin D. 2002. Trends in health insurance coverage: a look at early 2001 data. Health Affairs 21(1):188–193.

GAO (General Accounting Office). 2000. Oral health: dental disease is a chronic problem among low-income populations. Letter Report GAO/HEHS-00-72, April 12. Washington, DC: General Accounting Office.

GAO. 2001a. Medicaid: Stronger Efforts Needed to Ensure Children's Access to Health Screening Services. Report to Congressional Requesters, GAO-01-749. Washington, DC: General Accounting Office.

GAO. 2001b. Strategic objective: the health needs of an aging and diverse population. In Strategic Plan 2002–2007. Available online at www.gao.gov. Accessed October 6, 2002.

Glick M. 1999. The mouth is a mirror of the body. In Closing the Gap, a newsletter. July. Washington, DC: Office of Minority Health, Department of Health and Human Services.

Haas JS, Adler NE. 2001. The causes of vulnerability: disentangling the effects of race, socioeconomic status and insurance coverage on health. Background paper prepared for the Institute of Medicine Committee on the Consequences of Uninsurance.

Hadley J, Steinberg EP, Feder J. 1991. Comparison of uninsured and privately insured hospital patients: condition on admission, resource use, and outcome. Journal of the American Medical Association 265(3):374–379.

Harris Interactive. 2001. Computing in the physician's practice. A Harris Interactive Study. Available online at www.harrisinteractive.com/. Accessed July 29, 2002.

Hayward RA, Shapiro MF, Freeman HE, Corey CR. 1988. Inequities in health services among insured Americans: do working-age adults have less access to medical care than the elderly? New England Journal of Medicine 318(23):1507–1512.

HCFA (Health Care Financing Administration). 2001. Your Medicare Benefits: Your Health Care Coverage in the Original Medicare Plan for Part A (Hospital Insurance), Part B (Medical Insurance), including Preventive Services. Publication No. HCFA – 10116. Baltimore, MD: Federal Medicare Agency, Health Care Financing Administration, Department of Health and Human Services.

HCFA. 2002. National health expenditures. Available online at www.hcfa.gov/ stats/NHE-OAct/. Accessed April 17, 2002.

Heffler S, Smith S, Won G, Clemens MK, Keehan S, Zezza M. 2002. Trends: health spending projections for 2001–2011: the latest outlook. Health Affairs 21(2):207–218.

HELP (Health & Education Leadership for Providence). 2001. Building the city's future: HELP's impact on the Providence economy. Prepared by Appleseed for HELP. Available online at www.helprov.org/pubs/building.pdf. Accessed October 18, 2002.

Henry J. Kaiser Family Foundation and Health Research and Educational Trust (HRET). 2000. Employer Health Benefits: 2000 Annual Survey. Primary authors: Levitt L, Holve E, Wang J, Gabel JR, Whitmore HH, Pickreign JD, Miller N, Hawkins S. Menlo Park, CA and Chicago: Henry J. Kaiser Family Foundation and HRET.

Hetzel L, Smith A. 2001. The 65 Years and Over Population: 2000. Census 2000. October. U.S. Bureau of the Census, Department of Commerce.

HRSA (Health Resources and Services Administration). 2001. The Registered Nurse Population, March 2000. Rockville, MD: Health Resources and Services Administration, Department of Health and Human Services.

Hsia J, Kemper E, Kiefe C, Zapka J, Sofaer S, Pettinger M, Bowen D, Limacher M, Lillington L, Mason E. 2000. The importance of health insurance as a determinant of cancer screening: evidence from the Women's Health Initiative. Preventive Medicine 31(3):261–270.

IHS (Indian Health Service). 2002a. Year 2002 IHS profile. Available online at http://info.ihs.gov/Infrastructure/Infrastructure6.pdf. Accessed October 1, 2002.

IHS. 2002b. Indian Health Service 10 year expenditure trends. Available online at www.his.gov/nonmedicalprograms/ihdt2/bd/IHS10YR.pdf. Accessed August 5, 2002.

IOM (Institute of Medicine). 1996. In Wunderlich GS, Sloan FA, Davis CK (Eds.). Nurse Staffing in Hospitals and Nursing Homes: Is It Adequate? Washington, DC: National Academy Press.

IOM. 1998. In Edmunds M, Coye MJ (Eds.). America's Children: Health Insurance and Access to Care. Committee on Children, Health Insurance, and Access to Care, Institute of Medicine and National Research Council. Washington, DC: National Academy Press.

IOM. 2000a. America's Health Care Safety Net: Intact but Endangered. Washington, DC: National Academy Press.

IOM. 2000b. To Err Is Human: Building a Safer Health System. Washington, DC: National Academy Press.

IOM. 2001a. Coverage Matters: Insurance and Health Care. Washington, DC: National Academy Press.

IOM. 2001b. Crossing the Quality Chasm: A New Health System for the 21st Century. Washington, DC: National Academy Press.

IOM. 2001c. The Right Thing to Do, The Smart Thing to Do: Enhancing Diversity in Health Professions. Summary of the Symposium on Diversity in Health Professions in Honor of Herbert W. Nickens, M.D. Washington, DC: National Academy Press.

IOM. 2002a. Care Without Coverage: Too Little, Too Late. Washington, DC: The National Academies Press.

IOM. 2002b. Unequal Treatment: Confronting Racial and Ethnic Disparities in Health. Washington, DC: The National Academies Press.

IOM. 2002c. Setting the Course: A Strategic Vision for Immunization Part 1: Summary of the Chicago Workshop. Committee on the Immunization Finance Dissemination Workshops, Division of Health Care Services, Institute of Medicine. Washington, DC: The National Academies Press.

Johnson R, Morris TF (Ed.). 1998. Stabilizing the Rural Health Infrastructure. National Advisory Committee on Rural Health. Health Resources and Services Administration and the North Carolina Rural Health Research and Policy Analysis Program, the Cecil G. Sheps Center for Health Services Research, University of North Carolina at Chapel Hill.

Jones R, McConville J, Mason D, Macpherson L, Naven L, McEwen J. 1999. Attitudes towards, and utility of, an integrated medical-dental patient-held record in primary care. British Journal of General Practice 49(442):368–373.

Kaiser Family Foundation and Health Research and Educational Trust. 2000. 2000 Employer Health Benefits Survey. Menlo Park, CA: The Henry J. Kaiser Family Foundation.

Kasper JD, Giovannini TA, Hoffman C. 2000. Gaining and losing health insurance: strengthening the evidence for effects on access to care and health outcomes. Medical Care Research and Review 57(3):298–318.

Keane C, Marx J, Ricci E. 2001. Local health departments' changing role in provision and assurance of safety-net services. A project funded by the Center for Health Services Financing and Managed Care of the Health Resources and Service Administrative through a cooperative agreement with the Association of Schools of Public Health.

Kessler RC, McGonagle KA, Zhao S, Nelson CB, Hughes M, Eshleman S, Wittchen HU, Kendler KS. 1994. Lifetime and 12-month prevalence of DSM-III-R psychiatric disorders in the United States. Results from the National Comorbidity Survey. Archives of General Psychiatry 51:8–19.

King JS. 2000. Grant results report: assessing insurance coverage of preventive services by private employers. Robert Wood Johnson Foundation. Available online at www.rwjf.org/app/rw_grant_results_reports/rw_grr/029975s.htm. Accessed April 19, 2002.

Krall MA. 1998. Achieving clinician use and acceptance of the electronic medical record. The Permanente Journal 2(10):48–53.

Lasker RD, Committee on Medicine and Public Health. 1997. Medicine and Public Health: The Power of Collaboration. New York: The New York Academy of Medicine.

Lazarus R, Kleinman K, Dashevsky I, Adams C, Kludt P, DeMaria A Jr, Platt R. 2002. Use of automated ambulatory-care encounter records for detection of acute illness clusters, including potential bioterrorism events. Emerging Infectious Diseases 8(8):753–760.

Legnini MW, Anthony SE, Wicks EK, Mayer JA, Rybowski LS, Stepnick LS. 1999. Summary of Findings: Privatization of Public Hospitals. Prepared for the Henry J. Kaiser Family Foundation by the Economic and Social Research Institute. Available online at: www.kff.org/content/archive/1450/private_s.pdf. Accessed September 2, 2002.

Leigh WA, Lillie-Blanton M, Martinez RM, Collins KS. 1999. Managed care in three states: experiences of low-income African Americans and Hispanics. Inquiry 36:318–331.

Levit K, Smith C, Cowan C, Lazenby H, Martin A. 2002. Inflation spurs health spending in 2000. Health Affairs 21(1):172–181.

Lumpkin JR, Landrum LB, Oldfield A, Kimel P, Jones MC, Moody CM, and Turnock BJ. 1998. Impact of Medicaid resources on core public health responsibilities of local health departments in Illinois. Journal of Public Health Management and Practice 4(6):69–78.

Lurie N, Ward NB, Shapiro MF, Brook RH. 1984. Termination from Medi-Cal: does it affect health? New England Journal of Medicine 311:480–484.

Lurie N, Ward NB, Shapiro MF, Gallego C, Vaghaiwalla R, Brook RH. 1986. Termination of Medi-Cal benefits: a follow-up study one year later. New England Journal of Medicine 314:1266–1268.

Macinko JA, Starfield B, Shi L. [in press]. The Contribution of Primary Care Systems to Health Outcomes within Organization for Economic Cooperation and Development (OECD) Countries, 1970–1998. Health Services Research.

Mandelblatt J, Andrews H, Kerner J, Zauber A, Burnett W. 1991. Determinants of late stage diagnosis of breast and cervical cancer. American Journal of Public Health 81:646–649.

Mandelblatt J, Andrews H, Kao R, Wallace R, Kerner J. 1996. The late-stage diagnosis of colorectal cancer: demographic and socioeconomic factors. American Journal of Public Health 86:1794–1797.

Mandelblatt JS, Gold K, O'Malley AS, Taylor K, Cagney K, Hopkins JS, Kerner J. 1999. Breast and cervix cancer screening among multiethnic women: role of age, health and source of care. Preventive Medicine 28(4):418–425.

Mark DH, Gottlieb MS, Zellner BB, Chetty VK, Midtling JE. 1996. Medicare costs in urban areas and the supply of primary care physicians. Journal of Family Practice 43:33–39.

Markus A, Roby D, Rosenbaum S. 2002. A profile of federally funded health centers serving a higher proportion of uninsured patients. Prepared for the Kaiser Commission on Medicaid and the Uninsured. Available online at http://www.kff.org/content/2002/4033/. Accessed October 6, 2002.

Martinez RM, Closter E. 1998. Public Health Departments Adapt to Medicaid Managed Care. Issue Brief No. 16. Washington, DC: Center for Studying Health System Change.

Mays GP, Miller CA, Halverson PK. 2000. Local Public Health Practice: Trends & Models. Washington, DC: American Public Health Association.

McGinnis JM, Foege WH. 1993. Actual causes of death in the United States. Journal of the American Medical Association 270(18):2207–2212.

McManus M. 2001. Emergency department overcrowding in Massachusetts : making room in our hospitals. The Massachusetts Health Policy Forum, Issue Brief No. 12. Discussion moderated by CM McManus.

Meadows M. 1999. Making oral health a priority. In Closing the Gap, a newsletter. July. Washington, DC: Office of Minority Health, Department of Health and Human Services.

Mills RJ. 2000. Health Insurance Coverage: Consumer Income. Current Population Reports P60-211. Washington, DC: U.S. Bureau of the Census.

Mills RJ. 2002. Health Insurance Coverage: 2001. Current Population Reports, P60–220. Washington, DC: U.S. Bureau of the Census, Department of Commerce.

Mitchell JB, McCormack LA. 1997. Time trends in late-stage diagnosis of cervical cancer: differences by race/ethnicity and income. Medical Care 35(12):1220–1224.

Montefiore Medical Center. 2001. Community relations. Available online at www.montefiore. org/about/community/services/. Accessed October 21, 2002.

Moos MK, Miller CA. 1981 Relationships between public and private providers of health care. Public Health Reports 96(5):434–438.

Murray CJL, Lopez AD. 1996. The Global Burden of Disease. A Comprehensive Assessment of Mortality and Disability from Diseases, Injuries, and Risk Factors in 1990 and Projected to 2020. Cambridge, MA: Harvard University Press.

NACCHO (National Association of County and City Health Officials). 2001. Local Public Health Agency Infrastructure: A Chartbook. Washington, DC: NACCHO.

NASBO (National Association of State Budget Officials). 2002a. Medicaid and Other Health Care Issues. 2002. Medicaid and Other State Healthcare Issues: The Current Situation. Washington, DC: NASBO and National Governors' Association.

NASBO. 2002b. NASBO analysis: Medicaid to stress state budgets severely into fiscal 2003. Available online at www.nasbo.org/Publications/PDFs/medicaid2003. pdf. Accessed October 13, 2002.

NCHS (National Center for Health Statistics). 2002. Early release of selected estimates based on data from the January–June 2001 National Health Interview Survey. Available online at www.cdc.gov/nchs/nhis.htm. Accessed March 2, 2002.

NCVHS (National Committee on Vital and Health Statistics). 2002. Information for Health: A Strategy for Building the National Health Information Infrastructure. Report and Recommendations from the National Committee on Vital and Health Statistics. Atlanta, GA: NCVHS, CDC.

Needleman J, Buerhaus PI, Mattke S, Stewart M, Zelevinsky K. 2001. Nurse Staffing and Patient Outcomes in Hospitals. Final Report. Contract No. 230-99-0021. Washington, DC: Health Resources and Services Administration, Department of Health and Human Services.

NRC (National Research Council). 2000. Networking Health: Prescriptions for the Internet. Washington, DC: National Academy Press.

Office of the President of the United States. 2001. The budget for fiscal year 2002. Office of Management and Budget. Available online at www.whitehouse.gov/omb/budget/fy2002/bdg12.htm. Accessed June 14, 2002.

Olson K, Perkins J, Pate T. 1998. Children's Health under Medicaid: A National Review of Early Periodic Screening, Diagnosis and Treatment. Washington, DC: National Health Law Program.

O'Malley AS, Mandelblatt J, Gold K, Cagney KA, Kerner J. 2001. Continuity of care and the use of breast and cervical cancer screening services in a multiethnic community. Archives of Internal Medicine 157:1462–1470.

OPM (Office of Personnel Management). 2001. Fiscal Year 2001 performance and accountability report. Consolidated Financial Statements and Appendix A. Available online at www.opm.gov/gpra/opmgpra/par2002/. Accessed October 18, 2002.

Pacific Business Group on Health. 2002. Driving the market to reduce medical errors through the Leapfrog California Patient Safety Initiative. Available online at www.pbgh.org/programs/leapfrog/default.asp. Accessed September 27, 2002.

Partnership for Prevention. 1999. Why Invest in Disease Prevention? Results from the William M. Mercer/Partnership for Prevention Survey of Employer Sponsored Plans. Washington, DC: Partnership for Prevention.

Partnership for Prevention. 2001. Prevention Priorities: Employers' Guide to the Highest Value Preventive Health Services. Washington, DC: Partnership for Prevention.

Pew Environmental Health Commission. 2001. Transition Report to the New Administration: Strengthening Our Public Health Defense Against Environmental Threats January 17. Baltimore: Pew Environmental Health Commission.

Phillips KA, Mayer ML, Aday LA. 2000. Barriers to care among racial/ethnic groups under managed care. Health Affairs 19:65–75.

Politzer RM, Yoon J, Shi L, Hughes R, Regan J, Gaston M. 2001. Inequality in America: the contribution of health centers in reducing and eliminating disparities in access to care. Medical Care Research and Review 58:234–248.

Providence Public School District. 2002. Community partners in education. Available online at www.providenceschools.org/community_groups.cfm. Accessed September 26, 2002.

Rabinowitz J, Bromet EJ, Lavelle J, Hornak KJ, Rosen B. 2001. Changes in insurance coverage and extent of care during the two years after first hospitalization for a psychotic disorder. Psychiatric Services 52(1):87–91.

Rees T. 1999. Demand for health care information prompts media–institution alliances. Profiles in Healthcare Marketing 15(5):24–28.

Regier DA, Narrow W, Rae DS, Manderscheid RW, Locke BZ, Goodwin FK. 1993. The de facto US mental and addictive disorders service system. Epidemiologic Catchment area prospective 1-year prevalence rates of disorders and services. Archives of General Psychiatry 50:85–94.

Reinhardt UE, Hussey PS, Anderson GF. 2002. Cross-national comparisons of health systems using OECD data, 1999. Health Affairs 21(3):169–181.

Rice DP, Miller LS. 1996. The economic burden of schizophrenia: conceptual and methodological issues, and cost estimates. In Moscarelli M, Rupp A, Sartorious N (Eds.). Handbook of Mental Health Economics and Health Policy: Schizophrenia, Vol. 1. New York: John Wiley & Sons.

Rice T, Pourat N, Levan R, Silbert LJ, Brown ER, Gabel J, Kim J, Hunt KA, Hurst KM. 1998. Trends in job-based health insurance coverage. Los Angeles, CA: UCLA Center for Health Policy Research and KPMG Peat Marwick.

Robert Wood Johnson Foundation (RWJF). 2001. Substance Abuse: The Nation's Number One Health Problem. Key Indicators for Policy. February 2001 update. Waltham, MA: The Schneider Institute for Health Policy, Brandeis University.

Rosenbach ML, Gavin NI. 1998. Early and periodic screening, diagnosis and treatment and managed care. Annual Review of Public Health 19:507–525.

Schiff GD, Aggarwal HC, Kumad S, McNutt RA. 2000. Prescribing potassium despite hyperkalemia: medication errors uncovered by linking laboratory and pharmacy information systems. American Journal of Medicine 109(6):494–497.

Schoen C, DesRoches C. 2000. Uninsured and unstably insured: the importance of continuous insurance coverage. Health Services Research 35(1 Pt 2):187–206.

Schoenbaum M, Unützer J, Sherbourne C, Duan N, Rubinstein LV, Miranda J, Carney MF, Wells K. 2001. Cost-effectiveness of practice-initiated quality improvement for depression. Journal of the American Medical Association 286(11):1325–1330.

Schulberg H, Katon W, Simon G, Rush AJ. 1999. Best clinical practice: guidelines for managing major depression in primary care. Journal of Clinical Psychiatry, 60(Suppl. 7):19–24.

Seedco and the Non-Profit Assistance Corporation (N-PAC). 2002. Case studies: Montefiore Medical Center Loan. Available online at www.seedco.org/ loan/case/montefiore.html. Accessed October 21, 2002.

Sherer RA. 2001. How can a nursing shortage be prevented? Geriatric Times 2(4). Available online at www.geriatrictimes.com/g010704a.html. Accessed March 2, 2002.

Shi L, Starfield B, Kennedy BP, Kawachi I. 1999. Income inequality, primary care, and health indicators. Journal of Family Practice 48:275–284.

Smith V, Ellis E, Gifford K, Ramesh R, Wachino V. 2002. Medicaid spending growth: results from a 2002 Survey. Health Management Associates and Kaiser Commission on Medicaid and the Uninsured. Available online at www.kff.org/content/2002/4064/. Accessed October 6, 2002.

Solanki G, Schauffler HH, Miller LS. 2000. The direct and indirect effects of cost-sharing on the use of preventive services. Health Services Research 34(6):1331–1350.

Solis JM, Marks G, Garcia M, Shelton D. 1990. Acculturation, access to care, and use of preventive services by Hispanics: findings from NHANES, 1982–1984. American Journal of Public Health 80(Suppl.):11–19.

Spratley E, Johnson A, Sochalski J, Fritz M, Spencer W. 2000. The Registered Nurse Population. Findings from the National Sample Survey of Registered Nurses. Rockville, MD: Division of Nursing, Bureau of Health Professions, Health Resources and Services Administration.

Stagg Elliott V. 2002. Public health reporting flaws spell trouble: doctors complain about requirements that appear to lack follow-through. American Medical News, April 22/29, 2002. Available online at http://www.ama-assn.org/sci-pubs/amnews/pick_02/hll20422.htm. Accessed March 14, 2003.

Starfield B. 1998. Primary Care: Balancing Health Needs, Services and Technology. New York: Oxford University Press.

Starfield B. 2002. The role of primary care in improving population health and equity in the distribution of health: an unappreciated phenomenon. Presented at the Macy-Morehouse Conference on Primary Care, Atlanta, GA, September 17–19, 2002.

Starfield B, Shi L. 2002. Policy-relevant determinants of health: an international perspective. Health Policy 60:210–218.

Strasz M, Allen DJ, Paterson Sandie AK. 2002. EPSDT: Early Periodic Screening Detection and Treatment: a snapshot of service utilization. The Michigan Council for Maternal and Child Health. Available online at www.mcmch.com/docs/EPSDT.pdf. Accessed September 29, 2002.

Sturm R, Wells K. 2000. Health insurance may be improving—but not for individuals with mental illness. Health Services Research 35(1 Pt. 2):253–262.

Sturm R, Jackson CA, Meredith LS, Yip W, Manning WG, Rogers WH, Wells KB. 1995. Mental health care utilization in prepaid and fee-for-service plans among depressed patients in the medical outcomes study. Health Services Research 30(2):319–340.

Substance Abuse and Mental Health Services Administration. 2001. SAMHSA fact sheet: analysis of alcohol and drug abuse expenditures in 1997. SAMHSA News Release. Available online at www.health.org/newsroom/releases/ 2001/april01/12.htm. Accessed April 16, 2002.

Teutsch SM, Churchill RE (Eds.). 1994. Principles and Practices of Public Health Surveillance. New York: Oxford University Press.

Thacker SB, Stroup DF. 1994. Future directions for comprehensive public health surveillance and health information systems in the United States. American Journal of Epidemiology 140:383–397.

Trude S, Christianson JB, Lesser CS, Watts C, Benoit AM. 2002. Employer-sponsored health insurance: pressing problems, incremental changes. Health Affairs 21(1):66–75.

University of Illinois at Chicago. 1999. Linking affordable housing to community development. University of Illinois at Chicago City Design Center, Community Design Excellence. Available online at www.uic.edu/aa/cdc/files/LinkingAffordableHousing.html. Accessed September 26, 2002.

U.S. Department of Housing and Urban Development. 2002. Building Higher Education—Community Development Corporation Partnerships. Washington, DC: Department of Housing and Urban Development.

U.S. House of Representatives. 2001. National Preparedness: Ambulance Diversions Impede Access to Emergency Rooms. Washington, DC: Special Investigative Division, Minority Staff for Representative Henry A. Waxman, Committee on Government Reform, U.S. House of Representatives.

U.S. Office of Management and Budget (OMB). 2001. Budget of the United States Government. Fiscal year 2002. Washington, DC: Government Printing Office. Available online at www.whitehouse.gov/omb/budget. Accessed March 2, 2002.

VHA Health Foundation and the AHA Health Research and Educational Trust (HRET). 2000. Sustaining community health: the experience of health care system leaders. White paper. Irving, TX: VHA Health Foundation

Viccellio P. 2001. Emergency department overcrowding: an action plan. Academic Emergency Medicine 8(2):185–187.

Wagner EH, Austin BT, Von Korff M. 1996. Improving outcomes in chronic illness. Managed Care Quarterly 4(2):12–25.

Wagner EH, Austin BT, Davis C, Hindmarsh M, Schaefer J, Bonomi A. 2001. Improving chronic illness care: translating evidence into action. Health Affairs 20(6):64–78.

Wagner TH, Guendelman S. 2000. Health care utilization among Hispanics: findings from the 1994 Minority Health Survey. American Journal of Managed Care 6:355–364.

Wang PS, Berglund P, Kessler RC. 2000. Recent care of common mental disorders in the United States. Journal of General Internal Medicine 15(5):284–292.

Welch WP, Miller ME, Welch HG, Fisher ES, Wennberg JE. 1993. Geographic variation in expenditures for physician' services in the United States. New England Journal of Medicine 328:621–627.

Wells BL, Horm JW. 1992. Stage at diagnosis in breast cancer: race and socioeconomic factors. American Journal of Public Health 82(10):1383–1385.

Wells KB, Sherbourne C, Schoenbaum M, Duan N, Meredith L, Unützer J, Miranda J, Carney MF, Rubinstein LV. 2000. Impact of disseminating quality improvement programs for depression in managed primary care: a randomized controlled trial. Journal of the American Medical Association 283(2):212–220.

Woolhandler S, Himmelstein DU. 1988. Free care: a quantitative analysis of health and cost effects of a national health program for the United States. International Journal of Health Services 18(3):393–399.

Young AS, Grusky O, Jordan D, Belin TR. 2000. Routine outcome monitoring in a public mental health system: the impact of patients who leave care. Psychiatric Services 51(1):85–91.

Young AS, Klap R, Sherbourne CD, Wells KB. 2001. The quality of care for depressive and anxiety disorders in the United States. Archives of General Psychiatry 58:55–61.

Zambrana RE, Breen N, Fox SA, Gutierrez-Mohamed ML. 1999. Use of cancer screening practices by Hispanic women: analyses by subgroup. Preventive Medicine 29:466–477.

Zuvekas SH, Banthin JS, Selden TM. 1998. Mental health parity: what are the gaps in coverage? Journal of Mental Health Policy and Economics 1(3):135–146.

Zuvekas SH. 2001. Trends in mental health services use and spending, 1987–1996. Health Affairs 20(2):214–224.

6

Employers and Business

The main function of American employers is the production and sale or direct provision of goods and services. Through these economic activities, employers provide jobs and incomes to America's families. As noted in Chapter 2, employment and the workplace are important determinants of health that can generate protective health effects through income and social ties as well as adverse health effects (i.e., poor work conditions and job strain). This chapter provides information regarding the ways in which employers (both public and private), as actors in the public health system, can make important contributions to the health of the population through activities that are specifically directed toward health concerns.

The chapter begins with a discussion of how American employers, as providers of health care benefits to their employees, contribute significantly to supporting the conditions for health of a large proportion of American workers and their dependents. The discussion then addresses the important role that employers play in ensuring quality and accountability for the health care services purchased by and for their employees. The chapter then discusses the rationale for employer investment in the health of employees and how sponsoring health promotion and disease prevention activities in the workplace and improving workplace conditions promote employee health. Finally, the chapter ends with a discussion of a range of health-promoting activities—lessening environmental pollution and involvement in civic activities in the community, for example—in which employers and the business sector at large can engage to help promote the health of the population.

EMPLOYERS' ROLE IN HEALTH INSURANCE COVERAGE

Employers make a major contribution to population health and health security because of the important role they play in providing health insurance. Employers are primarily motivated to offer health insurance benefits to recruit and retain employees and to be competitive in the marketplace. Employees value health insurance and benefits and the opportunity to extend such coverage to their dependents.

For a number of historical reasons, employment is the foundation of the private health insurance system in the United States. Ninety percent of persons under the age of 65 who are privately insured obtain their health insurance through employers. Voluntary employer-sponsored health insurance is offered to employees and their dependents as part of a typical compensation package. In 2002, 62 percent of all firms (including both public and private employers) offered health benefits to their employees, a decline from a high of 67 percent in 2000 (Kaiser Family Foundation, 2002).

The percentage of firms offering health benefits varies by the size of the firm. For example, in 2002, 99 percent of firms with more than 200 workers offered health benefits to their employees, whereas less than 61 percent of small firms (those with 3 to 199 employees) offered such benefits (see Figure 6–1) (Kaiser Family Foundation, 2002).

Small firms are less likely to offer health insurance for a number of reasons, including the increased cost of a comparable insurance package because of higher administrative costs, lower employee wages, and more part-time workers (Custer and Ketsche, 2000).

Employees place a high value on health insurance. According to the Employee Benefit Research Institute and Mathew Greenwald & Associates, Inc.'s Value of Benefits Survey, 60 percent of employees rank health insurance as the most important benefit. Employees also report that benefits (e.g., health insurance and retirement plans) continue to be a very important factor in job selection (EBRI, 2002; Lave et al., 1999; Peele et al., 2000).

Most employers (both private and public) believe that they play an important role in providing health insurance coverage and that they can provide better coverage than employees could buy on their own. However, changing economic pressures are causing employers, particularly private firms, to reconsider the nature of their health insurance offerings. Pressures resulting from the slowing of the U.S. economy, rising health care costs associated in part with increasingly looser forms of managed care, rising prescription drug prices, and employee demands are making it more difficult for small employers to offer insurance coverage and for large employers to maintain premiums at affordable levels (Custer and Ketsche, 2000; Lambrew, 2001; Kaiser Family Foundation, 2002). Data indicate that pre-

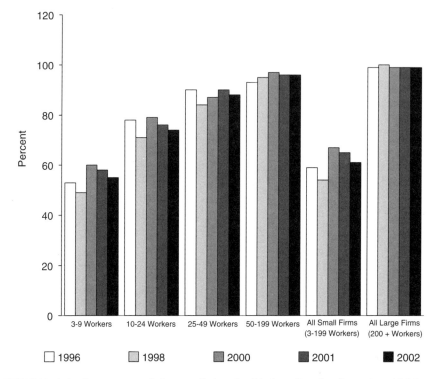

FIGURE 6–1   Percentage of firms offering health benefits, by firm size, 1996–2001.
NOTE: Nationwide, there are an estimated 5,355,412 firms with 3 to 199 workers and 86,957 with 200 plus workers. Firms include both public and private employers.
SOURCES: Kaiser Family Foundation (2000, 2001, 2002); KPMG (1996, 1998).

miums have already begun to rise. Premiums for employer-based health insurance increased an average of 11 percent in 2001, the largest increase since 1992. Large employers faced, on average, a 10.2 percent increase in health insurance costs, whereas the smallest employers (those with three to nine employees) experienced an average increase in premiums of 16.5 percent (Kaiser Family Foundation, 2002). As their costs rise, many employers expect to ask employees to pay more for insurance in the years to come and to pay for a higher proportion of the costs of care in terms of higher deductibles or copayments when they actually use services.

Increasing health insurance premiums influence whether an employee (as well as dependents) has coverage or joins the ranks of the uninsured. Employees typically pay between one-quarter and one-third of the total cost of the insurance premium, in addition to deductibles, copayments, and the costs of health services that are not covered or that are covered only in part. The proportion of employees who choose to participate in employer-sponsored health insurance is inversely related to the employee's contribution to the cost. The expense and competing demands on family income are the main reasons individuals report for declining an offer of employment-based coverage (Cooper and Schone, 1997; Rowland et al., 1998; Hoffman and Schlobohm, 2000). Individuals who decline employer-based health insurance are typically covered through a spouse or some other type of coverage, and about 4 percent remain uninsured. The consequences of being uninsured are described in Chapter 5 and in past reports of the Institute of Medicine (IOM, 2001a, 2002).

EMPLOYERS' ROLE IN ASSURING HEALTH CARE QUALITY

As purchasers for the health services of a large proportion of American families, the employer sector has an important role to play in ensuring the availability of high-quality health care services. Recent Institute of Medicine (IOM) reports have noted that the American health care delivery system is in need of fundamental change and that purchasers (employers and governmental agencies such as the Centers for Medicare and Medicaid Services) can play an important role in demanding health care services that are safe, effective, patient centered, timely, efficient, and equitable (IOM, 2001a).

Over the years, many employers (both private and public) have been strong partners of health plans and other health care organizations in efforts to improve health care quality. They were active participants in the National Committee for Quality Assurance initiative to develop the Health Plan Employer Data and Information Set in the early 1990s. The data set attempts to standardize a process for assessing and comparing health plan performance so that purchasers and consumers have a better sense of the quality of services provided. Another partnership, the Washington Business Group on Health, has worked over the past 27 years with approximately 170 employer members to improve employee health and productivity through attention to employee mental health issues and clinical preventive service guidelines, among others.

More recently, the Leapfrog Group, founded in 1999 and composed of growing numbers of Fortune 500 companies and other large health care purchasers, has joined forces to "trigger a giant leap forward in quality, customer service and affordability of health care." The two-pronged strategy to achieve this goal involves educating the public about patient safety and defining a set of purchasing principles designed to promote safety and increase the value of health care. Other employer-based initiatives include the National Business Coalition on Health, a membership organization of nearly 85 employer-led coalitions representing more than 11,000 mid- and large-sized employers and approximately 21 million employees and their dependents. These coalitions have joined together to collectively purchase health care, to proactively challenge high costs and the inefficient delivery of health care, and to share information on quality. Through these efforts and others across the country, the business community can be proactive in shaping the health care delivery system and promoting quality.

Illustrations of other employment-based efforts to improve health care quality include specific activities of the California Public Employees Retirement System (CalPERS) and the Minnesota Health Plan Initiative to Improve Health Care. Many employer groups are also involved in prevention activities sponsored by the Partnership for Prevention, a national nonprofit organization dedicated to increasing the resources for and knowledge about effective disease prevention and health promotion policies and practices.

CalPERS is one of the oldest purchasing coalitions in the country, representing one-third of public agencies in California; it holds the purchasing power of more than 1 million people and $1.7 billion a year in premiums. CalPERS pioneered the use of patient satisfaction and medical quality reports to encourage the provision of high-quality medical care from its participating plans (CalPERS, 2002). The combination of consumerism and strong purchasing influence is working to help improve the quality of health care for CalPERS members.

In another pioneering move to improve health care quality, five health plans (HealthPartners, Blue Cross and Blue Shield of Minnesota, Medica, PreferredOne, and UCare Minnesota) covering the majority of Minnesota residents came together to endorse evidence-based standard treatments and prevention procedures. This was the first time that the majority of health plans in a state have collaborated around setting and adopting evidence-based standards. Under the auspices of the Institute for Clinical System Improvements, a not-for-profit corporation, physicians and other health care professionals reviewed the scientific evidence and recommended the best course of action for 50 health problems such as urinary tract infection, hypertension, diabetes, and lower back pain. The health plans believe that use of the treatment guidelines is responsive to the health care quality concerns raised by IOM (2001b) and will lead to improved and more consistent care across the state (Freudenheim, 2001).

Recognizing that employers often have a difficult time balancing decisions about which benefits to purchase for their employees, the Partnership for Prevention convened a 25-member advisory panel to provide guidance on the clinical and preventive services that provide the "best bang for the buck." To begin, the panel—composed of public- and private-sector purchasers of care, health plan medical directors, state and local public health officials, clinicians, and consumer advocates—identified 30 clinical and preventive services and groups of services recommended by the U.S. Preventive Services Task Force (USPSTF)[1] for average-risk patients (AHRQ, 2002). The relative value of these services was then assessed on the basis of two dimensions: health impact and value. Health impact refers to the portion of disease, injury, and premature death that would be prevented if the service was delivered—that is, the clinical preventive burden. The value of the service refers to cost-effectiveness, in which the net cost of the service is compared to its health impact. Cost-effectiveness provides a standard measure for comparing services' return on investment (ROI). The results of the assessment identified 14 services that employers may want to purchase to improve the delivery of clinical preventive services (see Box 6–1). The Partnership for Prevention has disseminated its results to employers through its publication *Prevention Priorities: Employers' Guide to the Highest Value Preventive Health Services* (Partnership for Prevention, 2001b).

The committee acknowledges the crucial role that employers, particularly large employers, play in creating health security for millions of Americans as providers of employer-based health insurance coverage and purchasers of health care services. It also notes that, to the extent that the quality improvement activities lead to improvements in the processes of care, these improvements should benefit not only the employees of specific companies but all people who use the health care system.

In recent years, however, the current role of employer-sponsored health has been challenged. Some of the criticism points out that employers are under no legal mandate to offer health insurance and that the employer is an unstable source of insurance for some employees, particularly those who work for small firms or firms that hire a disproportionate number of low-income employees (Long and Marquis, 2001). Other criticism is directed at the employer's "role" per se (Reinhardt, 1999). A number of critics have argued that the employer should be removed from these decisions and that the employee, not the employer, should make decisions about what type of insurance to hold (Gavora, 1997; American Medical Association, 1999; Health Policy Consensus Group, 1999). In addition, critics point out that although employees ultimately bear the cost of insurance through lower wages, they are not aware of the trade-offs that are being made between wages and benefits and are demanding more benefits (or resisting cost containment) because such benefits are viewed as being "free" (Pauly, 1986,

---

[1] The USPSTF is a panel of independent experts in prevention and primary care tasked with identifying a core set of clinical preventive services known to improve health. The USPSTF recommendations are published in the *Guide to Clinical Preventive Services*, 2nd edition (U.S. Preventive Services Task Force, 1996), and most recent updated recommendations are available at www.ahrq.gov/clinic/uspstfix.htm.

BOX 6–1
Priorities for Employers: Recommended Clinical Preventive Services with High Health Impact and Value

- Vaccinate children: DTP/DTaP, MMR, oral polio/IPV, Hib, Hep B, varicella.
- Assess adults for tobacco use and provide tobacco cessation counseling.
- Screen adults aged ≥65 years for vision impairment.
- Assess adolescents for drinking and drug use and counsel them on abstinence from alcohol and drug use.
- Assess adolescents for tobacco use and provide an antitobacco message or advice to quit.
- Screen sexually active women aged ≥18 years for cervical cancer.
- Screen all persons aged ≥50 years for colon cancer (FOBT or sigmoidoscopy).
- Screen newborns for hemoglobinopathies, PKU, and congenital hypothyroidism.
- Screen all persons for hypertension.
- Vaccinate adults aged ≥65 years against influenza.
- Screen sexually active women aged 15 to 24 for chlamydia.
- Screen men aged 35 to 65 and women aged 45 to 65 for high blood cholesterol levels.
- Screen for problem drinking among adults and provide brief counseling.
- Vaccinate adults aged ≥65 against pneumococcal disease.

NOTE: DTP/DtaP = diphtheria, tetanus, pertussis/diphtheria, tetanus, acellular pertussis; FOBT = fecal occult blood testing; Hep B = hepatitis B; Hib =*Haemophilus influenzae* type b; IPV = poliovirus vaccine, inactivated; MMR = measles, mumps, rubella; PKU = phenylketonuria.
SOURCE: Partnership for Prevention (2001a).

1997). Furthermore, critics point out that employer-sponsored health insurance distorts the labor market by favoring large businesses over small ones, encourages employers to outsource certain workers, and affects workers' decisions about work and retirement (Congressional Budget Office, 1994; Gruber and Madrian, 1996). These critics recommend changes in tax policy so that tax incentives for the purchase of health insurance would not favor employer-sponsored coverage (Pauly, 1986; Congressional Budget Office, 1994; Gruber and Madrian, 1996; Gavora, 1997; American Medical Association, 1999; Health Policy Consensus Group, 1999).

Until reforms are enacted to assure access to affordable health insurance for all Americans, the committee urges employers to continue to provide and improve health insurance coverage for their employees. Employers should endorse the purchase of evidence-based benefits and work diligently to ensure the quality of the services that they purchase. **The committee recommends that the federal government develop programs to assist small employers and employers with low-wage workers to purchase health insurance at reasonable rates.**

EMPLOYER INTEREST IN PROMOTING
THE HEALTH OF EMPLOYEES:
A RATIONALE FOR CORPORATE INVESTMENT IN HEALTH

Employers should be concerned about the health and well-being of their employees for a number of reasons. Healthy employees consume fewer benefits in the form of benefit payments for medical care, short- and long-term disability, and workers' compensation. Furthermore, healthy employees are more productive than their nonhealthy counterparts because they are absent less often and are more focused on their tasks while at work.

Through health insurance premiums and self-insured plans, employers pay large sums of money for the treatment of diseases and disorders, many of which are lifestyle related and often preventable. The leading causes of death in the United States are heart disease, followed by cancer, stroke, chronic lower respiratory disease, accidents, diabetes, pneumonia/influenza, Alzheimer's disease, nephritis, nephritic syndrome and nephrosis, and septicemia (NCHS, 2002). A significant proportion of some of these diseases and disorders can be attributed to lifestyle habits and behaviors. For example, one study suggests that about 57 percent of heart disease deaths, 37 percent of cancer cases, 50 percent of strokes, 60 percent of accidents, 23 percent of pneumonias, 34 percent of diabetes cases, 60 percent of suicides, and 70 percent of chronic liver disease and cirrhosis cases are related to habits and behavior (NCHS, 1999). In the case of cancer and cardiovascular disease, seven modifiable risk factors account for 23 and 65 percent of the cases of morbidity, respectively (Amler and Dull, 1987).

More than 10,000 peer-reviewed articles in scientific journals show a clear causal relationship between specific modifiable risk factors and adverse health consequences. The following modifiable risk factors increase rates of mortality, morbidity, disability, and, in many cases, productivity loss: tobacco use, alcohol and drug use, sedentary behavior, poor nutrition, being overweight, having elevated serum cholesterol levels and high blood pressure, exhibiting high levels of stress and hostility, a lack of social support networks, and having unsafe sex. About half of all deaths in the United States are attributable to nine modifiable risk factors, including tobacco use (Box 6–2), diet and activity patterns, alcohol use (Box 6–3), firearm use, sexual behavior, motor vehicle accidents, and illicit drug use (McGinnis and Foege, 1993). Tobacco use alone caused approximately 440,000 premature deaths annually from 1995 to 1999 (CDC, 2002).

A number of studies have presented information on the distribution of illnesses in different companies. In a comprehensive study of Fortune 500 companies, coronary artery disease was the most costly disease for employers and represented 6.72 percent of total payments (Goetzel et al., 2000). The annual mean payment for claims related to coronary artery disease was $4,639 per patient and more than double the average payment of $2,230

BOX 6-2
Smoke-Free Policies in the Workplace

Tobacco use is the number one cause of preventable disease and death in the United States (DHHS, 2000). Private-sector restrictions on smoking in the workplace are effective strategies that can make a difference for a significant number of employees. A comprehensive review of workplace smoking policies from the National Cancer Institute's tobacco use supplement to the Current Population Survey found that slightly more than 80 percent of workers are covered by an official workplace smoking policy; however, less than half are protected by smoking policies that prohibit smoking in both the work area and the public or common areas of the workplace (smoke-free policy). Furthermore, the study found that those workers who work indoors—an estimated 58 million Americans, 40 million of whom are nonsmokers—are not protected by a smoke-free workplace policy. These data suggest that access to smoke-free workplace environments could be improved (Gerlach et al., 1997).

BOX 6-3
Creating Work Environments That Discourage Alcohol Misuse

Drinking while at work and heavy drinking outside of work are a real headache for employers. Alcohol-related performance problems include absenteeism, tardiness, feeling ill at work, and sleeping. Alcohol misuse can undercut productivity (quality and quantity) and can aggravate problems between coworkers (Bernstein and Mahoney, 1989; Ames et al., 1997; Mangione et al., 1999).

Health care costs for employees with alcohol problems are typically double those for other employees (Schneider Institute for Health Policy, 2001). Moreover, workers who drink even relatively small amounts of alcohol can raise the risk of alcohol-related death and injury in occupational accidents, especially if they drink before operating a vehicle (Partnership for Prevention, 2001a).

In 1994, more than 8 percent of full-time workers (more than 6.5 million employees) engaged in heavy drinking, defined as five or more drinks on 5 or more days in the past 30 days.

To stem the cost of lost productivity, work-site accidents, and excess health care because of alcohol and drug use, employers can do the following:

- Offer health plans that cover the cost of screening, counseling, and treatment for substance misuse;
- Participate in community programs to prevent alcohol and drug misuse;
- Establish work-site alcohol and drug policies;
- Integrate alcohol prevention into existing work-site health promotion programs;
- Educate supervisors about alcohol and drugs so they are better equipped to make caring and effective interventions and referrals;

BOX 6–3 Continued

- Sponsor confidential employee assistance programs with on-site external counselors to help workers resolve substance abuse problems and link them with treatment services (especially those in safety-sensitive positions); and
- Educate employees about health problems associated with drinking and stress (National Institute on Alcohol Abuse and Alcoholism, 1999; Partnership for Prevention, 2001a).

The U.S. Department of Labor's Working Partners program offers resources to help employers develop drug and alcohol-free workplaces (Partnership for Prevention, 2001a).

Promoting Mental Health in the Workplace

The employer community can take active steps to ensure that employees with depression remain productive. Estimates show that the annual cost of depression in the United States due to work loss and work cutback reaches $33 billion (Greenberg et al., 1995). Evidence suggests that the gains in productivity from effective treatment for depression could far exceed the direct costs of treatment (Simon et al., 2001). Employers who cut back on mental health benefits face increased costs for non-mental health services and more sick days (Rosenheck et al., 1999). Therefore, the business community has an economic incentive to ensure the timely, high-quality treatment of depression in employees.

One option is for businesses to become more active in improving employee awareness of the importance of the detection and treatment of depression. Another option is to require quality care for depression through private health insurance. Businesses increasingly finance mental health care for their employees through contracts with managed care organizations (OPEN MINDS, 1999). These contracts can be used as a means to require managed care organizations to improve the quality of care for depression via quality improvement programs.

for all conditions examined. These very large payments are for the treatment of heart disease and not its prevention.

Other high-cost health conditions highlighted in the study of Fortune 500 companies either were caused by or were the consequence of lifestyle factors. Some were highly prevalent but the cost of treatment was relatively low, such as diseases of the gastrointestinal tract (2.49 percent of total payments), essential hypertension (2.23 percent of total payments), and back disorders (2.07 percent of total payments) (Goetzel et al., 2000). Other conditions had lower prevalence rates but high average treatment costs and high total payments, such as cerebrovascular disease (1.65 percent of total payments) and cholecystitis and cholelithiasis (1.58 percent of total payments).

The analysis of Fortune 500 companies also uncovered costly mental health and substance abuse disorders that may be initiated or exacerbated by stress. Bipolar disorders with major depressive episodes were the most costly (1.25 percent of total payments), followed by neurotic, personality, and nonpsychotic disorders (1.11 percent of total payments) and depression (0.77 percent of total payments). Alcoholism, with an average cost of $3,012 per patient, is the most costly substance abuse disorder on a per patient basis, although it accounts for less than 1 percent of total payments (Goetzel et al., 2000).

A clear relationship exists between modifiable risk factors in a typical employed population and the employers' health care expenditures for the treatment of the diseases and disorders caused by these risk factors. For example, in a study of 10,000 employees of the Control Data Corporation, researchers documented lower health care costs for employees who exercised regularly, ate nutritious foods, abstained from smoking cigarettes, and had low blood pressure (Brink, 1987). A 5-year study of Steelcase Corporation employees showed that as modifiable health risks increased for employees, so did their medical expenditures (Yen et al., 1992). Another study examined the effects of 10 risk factors (obesity, high serum cholesterol levels, high blood pressure, stress, depression, smoking, inappropriate diet, excessive alcohol consumption, physical fitness and lack of exercise, and high blood glucose levels) on employer health care costs (Goetzel et al., 1998a; Anderson et al., 2000).

The study examined medical claims for more than 46,000 employees from both private- and public-sector organizations for 6 years. These 10 modifiable risk factors accounted for about 25 percent of all health care expenditures for the six employers in the study (Anderson et al., 2000). Interestingly, the two risk factors with the greatest effect on health care expenditures within 3 years were psychosocial: depression and stress. Health care expenditures for employees who reported depression were 70 percent greater than those for employees not reporting depression. Health care expenditures for employees with high levels of stress were 46 percent greater than those for employees who did not have high levels of stress, after controlling for demographics and other risk factors. When risk factors were combined, as they normally are for individuals at risk in multiple categories, health care expenditures increased to a far greater extent. For example, when health care expenditures for individuals with multiple risks for heart disease (i.e., smoking, hypertension, hypercholesterolemia, high stress, sedentary lifestyle, and obesity [Box 6–4], high blood glucose) were examined, they were found to be more than 200 percent greater than the expenditures for those without these risk factors. Similarly, health care expenditures for individuals at high risk for the two psychosocial risks, depression and stress, were nearly 150 percent greater than those for individuals lacking these risks.

BOX 6–4
Obesity and Employers

Employers represent another group of stakeholders adversely affected by the growing epidemic of obesity in America, but they also have ample opportunities to reverse this trend. As the problem of obesity in America grows, businesses are confronted with escalating health care costs, missed days of work, lost productivity, and much more. Because more than 134 million Americans (BLS, 2001) spend a majority of their day at work, businesses can help promote healthy lifestyles through work-site policies, changes in the physical and social work environment, educational programs, and connections with resources and programs in the surrounding community. Employers must first understand the direct and indirect costs of obesity and the return on investment that can be realized when obesity prevention and treatment strategies are implemented. Then, employers can communicate their commitment to helping employees be healthy by creating flexible work schedules that permit regular physical activity; providing healthy, accessible, and affordable food options at or near work; establishing on-site exercise facilities or creating incentives for employees to join or participate in other fitness-oriented activities; working with health insurers to provide healthy eating and physical activity counseling for all employees and their families; and offering incentives (e.g., time off and decreased insurance rates) to employees who participate in exercise or weight maintenance programs.

Furthermore, there is growing evidence that these modifiable risk factors not only increase health care costs but also increase worker absenteeism and decrease on-the-job productivity (Golaszewski et al., 1989; Bertera, 1991; Yen et al., 1994; Burton et al., 1999; Pronk et al., 1999; Edington, 2001). One of these studies found a consistent relationship between obesity, stress, multiple risk factors, and subsequent health care expenditures (Aldana, 2001). A similar relationship existed between modifiable risk factors and illness-related employee absenteeism.

For an employer, the implications of this research are enormous. When all else is held constant, the risk profile for the population covered by the employer's medical plan and human resource policies can significantly affect labor costs. What options does an employer have for managing the risk of its labor pool? It cannot fire employees, for self-evident legal and ethical reasons. However, the employer can institute risk reduction programs that, if successful, will significantly reduce the employer's costs.

One company undertook a study of the implications of undertaking a risk reduction program. In a study of 56,000 employees of Union Pacific Railroad, investigators estimated that the company would save $20.7 million over 10 years compared with the amount that it would spend in a "do-nothing" scenario if it were able to reduce each of 10 modifiable risk factors by 0.1 percent during those 10 years (Leutzinger et al., 2000). If risk reduction programs were even more successful and the risk factors were reduced by 1 percent per year, economic models predicted that the company would save $77.4 million over 10 years. As a result of this study, senior management at Union Pacific Railroad decided that improving the health and productivity of its employees was a priority for the railroad and elevated this initiative to the status of a "big financial deal" in 2001 (Leutzinger, 2001).

Changing the Health Risk Profiles of Employees

In many ways, the workplace should be an ideal setting for the introduction and maintenance of health promotion and disease prevention programs. Employees are concentrated in a finite number of geographic sites, they share a common purpose and a common culture, and communication and information exchanges are relatively straightforward. Individual goals and organizational goals are generally aligned with one another. Social support is available when changes are tried, and organizational norms can encourage certain behaviors and discourage others. Financial or other incentives can be introduced to encourage participation in programs, and the consequences of the programs can be measured by using existing administrative systems for data collection and analysis. Employers can also create a set of programs to encourage employees to participate in risk reduction activities. It is important, however, that employers conduct health promotion activities and implement incentives programs in ways that assure nondiscrimination and privacy for persons with disabilities. Nondiscrimination and privacy are required under the Americans with Disabilities Act of 1990 and represent good practices for any employer.

If the work site represents an ideal setting for changing people's behaviors and improving their risk profiles, do workplace health promotion and disease prevention programs actually work? Can the workplace serve as a catalyst for health improvement and risk reduction? Certainly, a number of companies have introduced workplace health promotion and disease prevention programs. Twenty years ago, less than 10 percent of U.S. businesses with 50 or more employees offered some kind of health promotion or disease prevention programs to their workforces. Today, many more companies are offering such programs. Twenty years ago there was little credible evidence that such programs were effective. Companies invested in them because they believed it was the right thing to do. Today's employers are seeking information that these programs work to retain or enhance them.

There is increasing evidence that health promotion and disease prevention programs based in the workplace can change the behavior, psychosocial risk factors, and biometric values for individual employees and the overall risk profile of the employed population (Bly et al., 1986; Bertera, 1990, 1993; Fries et al., 1993, 1994; Breslow et al., 1994; Goetzel et al., 1994, 1996; Wilson et al., 1996; Heaney and Goetzel, 1997; Pelletier, 1999; Gold et al., 2000; Ozminkowski et al., 2000).

Overall Cost Savings and Returns on Investment

Employers are concerned not only whether health promotion and disease prevention programs work in the sense that they can change the behavior, psychosocial risk factors, and biometric values for individuals employees but also whether these programs save money overall. They are concerned about whether investment in these activities has a positive rate of return.

Growing evidence shows that well-designed and well-resourced health promotion and disease prevention programs can produce savings in medical costs and possibly a positive rate of ROI in the program. The return on investment for health programs and for demand and disease management programs has been reported to range from $1.40 to $13 in benefits per dollar spent on the program, depending on the type of program (Goetzel et al., 1999). Traditional health promotion programs had a median return on investment of $3.14 per dollar spent; demand management programs had a median return on investment of $4.50 per dollar spent; and disease management programs achieved a median return on investment of $8.88 per dollar spent. Multiple-category programs that combined the elements of health programs and demand and disease management programs achieved returns on investment ranging from $5.50 to $6.50 per dollar spent, with a median value of about $6 (Goetzel et al., 1999). Other studies report an average benefit–cost ratio of $3.48 for every dollar spent. For example, in one of the programs studied, Citibank invested $1.9 million in a health promotion program. It saved $8.9 million in medical expenditures as a result of the program and realized a return on investment of $4.56 to $4.73 per dollar spent (Ozminkowski et al., 1999, 2000). Additionally, the health care costs of participating employees with preexisting chronic medical conditions (heart disease, diabetes, back problems, and hypertension) were less than those of employees who did not participate.

Need for More Information on the
Effectiveness of Health Promotion Programs

Although evidence indicates that workplace programs can work to reduce risk factors and that programs that are well designed can lead to cost savings, much still remains to be determined about such programs.

Much more needs to be known about which interventions are the best for facilitating behavioral change and risk reduction. For example, although individualized risk reduction counseling is effective in creating behavioral change, there are many ways of providing risk reduction counseling. However, the most effective way of providing this service is not known. Does this intervention work best when delivered in person, by telephone, or through tailored print communication? Which messages work best for which people? What social factors can be brought into play? What is the ideal balance between individual and group change processes? Should employers use social marketing techniques to influence employee behavior?

In addition to learning more about the effectiveness of specific intervention strategies, more needs to be known about how to structure these programs. Health promotion and disease prevention programs vary considerably in intensity, comprehensiveness, content, the communications media used, the staff involved, and other characteristics. Such programs include the following components:

• **Program awareness.** Health promotion and disease prevention must be "sold" to eligible employees in the same way that Band-Aids, Tylenol, and detergents are sold. Eligible employees need to be aware, at an individual level, of the importance of health promotion and disease prevention and the availability of programs to address health risk factors. This is accomplished through successful implementation of communications, public relations, and marketing programs.

• **Participation.** A large proportion of eligible employees must be engaged in the program and participate in its activities. Program participation rates significantly affect program savings and estimates of return on investment because program expenses are typically spread across an entire eligible population, whereas program savings apply only to participants.

• **Employee attitudes.** Attitudes, health beliefs, feelings of being in control, readiness to change behaviors, stress management, and other psychosocial factors significantly influence an individual's health and well-being (see also Chapter 2). Changing employee attitudes and altering behavior are critical because a change in behavior cannot be maintained unless individuals believe intrinsic psychological or social value is associated with the change.

• **Behavioral change and risk reduction.** The extent to which corporate programs achieve significant and long-lasting changes in employee health and well-being will influence the likely economic benefits that follow.

Finally, more needs to be known about how to measure the effectiveness of such programs. The benefits of these programs should be measured in terms of health care cost savings, decreases in absenteeism, and improvements in productivity. Absenteeism can be used to measure employee productivity. As discussed earlier, health promotion and disease prevention activities have been shown to improve health and decrease costs, and one indication of improved health may be a decrease in absenteeism.

Employee health and productivity are apparently closely related, and effective management of one will positively affect the other (Goetzel et al., 1998b; Burton et al., 1999; Claxton et al., 1999; Cockburn et al., 1999). However, of the three benefits of these programs, measuring on-the-job productivity is the most difficult. On-the-job productivity losses are harder to measure than absenteeism because traditional ways of measuring productivity (i.e., counting the number of widgets produced per unit of time) are quickly becoming outdated as the U.S. economy changes from a manufacturing economy to a service economy, in which quality is more important than quantity. Nonetheless, several tools and systems are under development to assess gains or losses in on-the-job productivity. These include self-assessment tools, simulation studies, and sophisticated tracking and monitoring systems (Reilly et al., 1993; Van Roijen et al., 1996; Endicott and Nee, 1997; Berger et al., 2001; Burton et al., 2001; Goetzel et al., 2001; Kessler et al., 2001; Lerner et al., 2001). Once these tools and systems are perfected, the potential impact of health promotion and disease prevention programs on employee productivity and overall business performance should be easier to document. Results from these studies are expected to overshadow any savings realized from cost-cutting and expense management initiatives.

Workplace Safety Programs Promoting the Health of Employees

Promoting the health of the workforce requires a safe workplace and a healthy workforce. At the turn of the century, premature death often resulted from diseases, injuries, and unhealthy work conditions. The Department of Labor's Bureau of Labor Statistics documented that 23,000 workers died from work-related injuries in 1913; this is equivalent to a rate of 61 deaths per 100,000 workers (CDC, 1999). However, with the identification of the etiologic factors that contribute to occupational health hazards and the implementation of federal legislation to assure safe and healthy working conditions, data from multiple sources indicate that work-related deaths, injuries, and illnesses have declined dramatically over time.

In 1970, the Occupational Safety and Health Act was specifically framed "to assure so far as possible every working man and woman in the nation safe and healthful working conditions." That act established, in 1971, both the Occupational Safety and Health Administration (OSHA), which is part of the Department of Labor, and the National Institute for Occupational Safety and Health (NIOSH) (2000a), which is part of the Centers for Disease Control and Prevention.

BOX 6–5
Federal Legislation to Promote Occupational Safety and Health

The first federal legislation pertaining to occupational health and safety granted limited compensation benefits to civilian service workers for injuries sustained during employment (1908, Federal Workers' Compensation Act). Subsequent legislation established occupational health and safety standards for employees of federal contractors (1936, Walsh-Healey Public Contracts Act) and regulations to protect mine workers (1969, Federal Coal Mine Health and Safety Act).

The Occupational Safety and Health Act of 1970 authorized the federal government to develop and set mandatory occupational safety and health standards and to establish the National Institute for Occupational Safety and Health to conduct research on workplace standards. The Toxic Substances Control Act of 1976 requires industry to provide data on the production, use, and health and environmental effects of chemicals. The act also led to the development of "right-to-know" laws, which provide employees with information on the nature of potential occupational exposures.

The Federal Mine Safety and Health Act of 1977 (Mine Act) strengthened and expanded the rights of miners and enhanced the protection of miners from retaliation for exercising such rights.

The Pollution Prevention Act of 1990 established policy to ensure that pollution is prevented or reduced at the source, recycled or treated and disposed of, or released only as a last resort. The act also led to the substitution of less toxic substances in a wide range of industrial processes, with significant reductions in worker exposure to toxic substances.

OSHA was created to assure safe and healthy workplaces in America by enforcing workplace safety and health regulations (see Box 6–5). Since 1971, workplace fatalities have been halved and occupational injury and illness rates have declined 40 percent. Over the same period, U.S. employment nearly doubled from 56 million workers at 3.5 million work sites to 105 million workers at nearly 6.9 million sites. OSHA forms cooperative relationships with labor and management through Voluntary Protection Programs, which "recognize and promote effective safety and health management" at numerous sites around the United States and in more than 180 industries (OSHA, 2002b). These programs have resulted in millions of dollars in savings each year because injury and illness rates have declined below the averages for the industries at the participating sites. In addition, OSHA's Strategic Partnership Program focuses on safety and health programs and includes outreach and training components along with enforcement (OSHA, 2002a).

Although the reductions in workforce injuries and the improvements in working conditions have been impressive, an average of 137 individuals die each day from work-related diseases; an additional 16 die from injuries received while on the job. Every 5 seconds a worker is injured; every 10 seconds a worker is temporarily or permanently disabled (NIOSH, 1996).

NIOSH is the only federal agency responsible for conducting research and making evidence-based recommendations on the prevention of work-related diseases and injuries. NIOSH is responsible for conducting research on the full scope of occupational diseases and injuries, ranging from lung disease in miners to carpal tunnel syndrome in computer users. In addition, NIOSH investigates potentially hazardous working conditions; makes recommendations and disseminates information on preventing work-related diseases, injuries, and disabilities; and trains occupational safety and health professionals.

NIOSH data show that the direct and indirect costs of occupational injuries and illnesses are $171 billion annually for all businesses, compared to "$33 billion for AIDS, $67.3 billion for Alzheimer's disease, $164.3 billion for circulatory diseases, and $170.7 billion for cancer" (NIOSH, 2000b).

NIOSH has brought together numerous organizations and individuals to focus on the creation of a research agenda. NIOSH and its public and private sponsors have developed the National Occupational Research Agenda (NORA) to provide a framework to guide the entire occupational safety and health community to help reduce the high toll of occupational injuries and illnesses. NORA priorities reflect a significant degree of concurrence among the large number of stakeholders. The priority research areas have been grouped into three broad categories: disease and injury, work environment and workforce, and research tools and approaches (see Table 6–1). NIOSH and its partners, through NORA, will guide and coordinate research for the entire occupational safety and health community. Fiscal constraints on occupational safety and health research are increasing, however, making it important for NIOSH to focus on the topics that will benefit workers and the nation and to ensure a coordinated research agenda.

In addition to implementing NORA, NIOSH operates programs in every state to improve the health and safety of workers. NIOSH evaluates workplace hazards, builds state worker safety and health capacity through grants and cooperative agreements, funds occupational safety and health research, and supports occupational safety and health training programs.

Occupational safety and health programs are specific to the work site and operations. Programs usually focus on basic principles of control technology that include engineering controls, work practices, personal protective equipment, and monitoring of the workplace for emerging hazards. Work site safety and health training and a long-term commitment to such programs are also critical to achieving occupational safety and health goals. However, the majority of safety and health regulations and enforcement

TABLE 6-1   NORA Priority Research Areas

Category	Illness or Injury
Disease and injury	Allergy and irritant dermatitis
	Asthma and chronic obstructive pulmonary disease
	Fertility and pregnancy abnormalities
	Hearing loss
	Infectious diseases
	Lower back disorders
	Musculoskeletal disorders of the upper extremities
	Traumatic injuries
Work environment and workforce	Emerging technologies
	Indoor environment
	Mixed exposures
	Organization of work
	Special populations at risk
Research tools and approaches	Cancer research methods
	Control technology and personal protective equipment
	Exposure assessment research
	Risk assessment methods
	Social and economic consequences of workplace illness and injury
	Surveillance research methods

SOURCE: NIOSH (1996).

efforts have been designed to focus on large employers. Therefore, small businesses face specific challenges in ensuring a safe and healthy workplace.

Small employers employ more than half of the employees in private industry, and they experience higher levels of work-related hazards. Data from a survey of businesses in 1994–1995 found that about one-third of all work-related deaths occur at workplaces with 10 or fewer employees, although they employ only 15 percent of all workers in private industry. The challenges to ensuring safe workplaces and healthy workers include a lack of onsite occupational safety and health professionals, difficulties in recognizing the magnitudes of specific hazards, and a lack of strategies for dealing with hazards in a small-business environment (NIOSH, 2002c).

The importance of occupational hazard assessment and worker protection is exemplified by the recovery, demolition, and site-clearing operations at the World Trade Center (WTC) in the aftermath of September 11, 2001, when occupational hazard assessment and worker protection were critical. First-response workers—firefighters, police, rescue workers, and volunteers—faced numerous occupational exposures, including fire and smoke, falling debris, and air contaminants such as asbestos, lead, silica, and volatile organic compounds, to name a few. OSHA became an integral part of response efforts at WTC. Box 6–6 provides a summary of OSHA activities performed to identify and abate serious hazards and to protect the workers in WTC site operations.

The committee acknowledges the progress that has been made in reduc-

---

BOX 6–6
OSHA's Role at the World Trade Center Emergency Project

After the September 11, 2001, terrorist attack, the Occupational Safety and Health Administration (OSHA) worked at the World Trade Center site 24 hours a day, 7 days a week, to help protect rescue and recovery workers involved in recovery, demolition, and site-clearing operations. By September 21, 2002, about 800 federal and state OSHA staffers and several private-sector Voluntary Protection Program volunteers from throughout the United States assisted in the following roles:

Risk Assessment and Monitoring
- Taking more than 6,642 air and bulk samples to test for asbestos, silica, lead and other heavy metals, carbon monoxide, and numerous organic and inorganic compounds. Noise testing was also conducted.
- Providing 24-hour laboratory support at the Salt Lake Technical Center to analyze air and bulk samples taken at the site.
- Distributing sampling results directly to the workers as well as to contractors, unions, and other safety and health representatives at the site and posting the sampling results on the agency website (www.osha.gov).

Respiratory Distribution and Fit Checking
- Distributing about 121,000 respirators—some 4,000 daily during the first weeks after the attack but now down to about 500 daily.
- Conducting quantitative fit testing of negative-pressure respirators for the New York Fire Department and assisting in quantitative fit testing of this type of respirator for other rescue workers at the World Trade Center site.

Safety Monitoring
- Conducting an initial assessment of the site within 24 hours of the attack to identify hazards and potential health and safety risks to workers involved in the recovery.
- Providing around-the-clock monitoring of the site to identify and alert workers to safety and health hazards.

Site Safety and Health Support
- Helping to develop the World Trade Center Emergency Project Environmental, Safety, and Health Plan to ensure the highest level of worker safety and health protections at the site.
- Assisting in the development and coordination of a site orientation training program to familiarize workers with potential hazards, personal protective equipment requirements, and overall safety rules at the site.

continued

BOX 6–6 Continued

- Participating with contractors at the site to conduct job hazard analyses of unique operations to identify hazardous operations at the site and recommend ways to abate or reduce the hazards involved.

Site Safety and Health Coordination
- Initiating the World Trade Center Emergency Project Partnership to promote cooperation and unified support for safety and health at the site among contractors, employees, employee representatives, and federal, state, and city agency representatives participating in the recovery operation.
- Providing full-time staffing at the New York City Office of Emergency Management Emergency Operation Center to exert leadership on safety and health issues and maximize coordination and information sharing among the federal, state, and city agencies involved in the effort.

SOURCE: OSHA (2002c).

---

ing work-related mortality, injuries, and diseases, especially among large employers. The committee also acknowledges that employers and employees must continue to be vigilant and proactive in recognizing hazards in the workplace. The committee encourages a greater sharing between large and small employers of the best practices and strategies that can reduce work-related mortality, injuries, and diseases and protect workers' health.

Other Workplace Policies That Promote Health

Employers implement a number of policies related to family leave, flexible work practices, and other benefits and organize work (e.g., through the creation of teams and the assignment of multiple tasks) in ways that may have important health consequences. Employers implement some of these policies voluntarily; they implement others to comply with the law. For example, the federal Family and Medical Leave Act of 1993 requires employers with 50 or more employees to provide up to 12 weeks of unpaid leave for the birth or adoption of a child; to take care of a seriously ill child, parent, or spouse; and to recover from a serious illness. The business and public health sectors rarely consider these policies and practices as influential determinants of health. Chapter 2 presents evidence that job characteristics, such as job demands and control, job insecurity, and issues related to part-time, shift work, and current practices on outsourcing have important effects on health. A range of policies related to work organization, the interface between work and family, and long-term employment practices have often been evaluated for their effects on employee productivity and satisfaction. The committee believes that these same work practices, along with the more traditional concerns about occupational health and safety practices, have important consequences for health. These types of private-sector policies may be among the most important determinants of population health. Evaluation of the effects of these policies and practices on health is a high priority.

ROLE OF BUSINESSES AND INDUSTRIES IN PROMOTING A HEALTHY ENVIRONMENT

The private and public sectors significantly influence health when their goals are incompatible with conditions that promote healthy behaviors or physical environments. When such goals are in conflict and significant health hazards arise, governmental agencies have a responsibility to act. Over the past 30 years, the U.S. government has passed numerous environmental laws and regulations to protect the health of the public (see Table 6–2). These laws have often been passed in response to industrial contami-

TABLE 6–2   Selected Environmental Legislation

Legislation	Purpose
Safe Drinking Water Act, 1974	Passed to protect the public from waterborne diseases, chemicals, and heavy metals in drinking water
Clean Air Act Amendments, 1977	Established the regulatory structure and an enforceable timetable for reducing urban air pollution
Clean Water Act, 1977	Sought to make rivers and lakes safe for fishing and swimming
Comprehensive Environmental Response, Compensation, and Liability Act (Superfund statute), 1980	Passed in response to the contamination at Love Canal, New York and Times Beach, Missouri to protect communities from health dangers at hazardous waste disposal sites
Federal Insecticide, Fungicide, and Rodenticide Act, 1972, and Toxic Substances Control Act, 1976	Enacted to require analysis of chemicals to which the public might be exposed through food and other pathways
Toxics Release Inventory, 1987, mandated by the Emergency Planning and Community Right-to-Know Act of 1986	Enacted to inform citizens about toxic chemicals in the environment; it is also known as Title III of the Superfund amendments and is based on the premise that citizens have a right to know

nation. In recent years, however, the roles of private-sector businesses and industry and of the public sector have become important in improving the environments of the communities in which they operate. Additionally, the private sector has formed partnerships with governmental agencies to help promote the health of the public.

One example is the Environmental Protection Agency's (EPA's) Design for the Environment (DfE) program. Through voluntary partnerships with businesses, industries, and others (e.g., public interest groups, universities, and research institutions), EPA provides businesses and industry with information to make environmentally informed choices regarding their products, processes, and practices (EPA, 1998). According to EPA, the DfE program strives to promote the incorporation of environmental considerations into the traditional parameters of cost and performance on which businesses base their decisions.

Businesses and industries have come to realize that responsible entrepreneurship can play a major role in protecting human health by improving the environmental quality of the community through the efficient use of resources and the minimization of waste. Businesses and industries are developing techniques that reduce harmful environmental impacts. Some business and industry leaders are also fostering openness and dialogue with employees and the public and carry out environmental audits and assessments of their compliance with environmental laws and regulations. An example of a company initiative to improve community health is described in Box 6–7.

Thus, investing in community and environmental health not only is an example of corporate responsibility but also can provide economic returns to the business or industry. These programs succeed when there is a commitment from the leadership of the organization and, in many cases, when they are part of the business's mission and vision statements. Another example is provided in Box 6–8.

The food and beverage industry generates products that may contribute to disease and disability if consumers make choices potentially incompatible with good health. In light of the intensifying obesity epidemic in the United States, the industry has been asked to work in partnership with other sectors to help consumers in their efforts to make healthier lifestyle decisions that will promote health by reducing obesity. In October 2002, the Health and Human Services Secretary, Tommy Thompson, and the Agriculture Secretary, Anne Veneman, met with officials from the National Restaurant Association and the National Council of Chain Restaurants to begin a dialogue about how the food and beverage industries can help to reduce obesity. Potential strategies to be considered are delivering healthy food choices, providing easy-to-understand nutritional information, integrating healthiness into mass-marketing strategies, and offering an increased

BOX 6–7
Dow Chemical Company: Improving Environmental Health

The Dow Chemical Company has 40 global manufacturing sites. The third largest is in Midland, Michigan, with 550 buildings and 40 chemical production plants on a 1,900-acre facility. Air emissions were such that, in the late 1990s, the attitude and belief inside the company were that no further gains could be made in emission control at the facility. However, Dow set two important goals: (1) to accrue by April 30, 1999, capital that could be used to cut waste and emissions by 35 percent and (2) to begin to foster institutional changes within Dow to shift the corporation's thinking from compliance to pollution prevention and to further integrate health and environmental concerns into core business practices.

Working with the community, activists, and pollution control consultants, Dow engineers identified pollution prevention opportunities. The result of this activity reduced waste and emissions by 12 million pounds per year, a 37 percent reduction. Yet, the common belief in this facility had been that there were no cost-effective pollution prevention projects left to pursue. Ultimately, 17 projects were identified with a combined return on investment of 180 percent, or a savings of $5.4 million per year.

BOX 6–8
Intel: Improving Environmental Health Through Corporate Vision and Mission

Intel, a manufacturer of microprocessors, changes it manufacturing processes every 2 years as it miniaturizes the next generation of microprocessors. Intel considers this an opportunity for environmental improvement, for example, through chemical selection, facility design, waste management, ergonomics, and manufacturing equipment selection. Other aspects of planning include projecting environmental health and safety impacts over 10 years, or five generations of manufacturing. It sets goals that must be integrated into the design and development processes. For example, Intel reduced water use by 40 percent in one process that uses hydrofluoric acid to etch wafers and achieved better management of the exhaust, which reduced energy use. In another process, it recycled hazardous wastes and reduced emissions of volatile organic compounds.

A key to Intel's success in improving the environmental health of the community has been the company's vision to develop a "green" plan that integrates design for the environment while aiming for sustainable activities as part of its operations.

variety of healthy meals. The secretaries will also engage other organizations in the attempt to help combat the obesity epidemic, including fruit and vegetable growers, grocery manufacturers, public health groups, and state leaders through the National Governors' Association and the National Conference of State Legislatures, as well as physical fitness groups (DHHS, 2002). This example shows how federal leadership can be used to encourage voluntary change. Other voluntary efforts, such as those made to develop standards to protect children on the Internet, demonstrate that industries can be mobilized to deal with problems of social significance. In the absence of voluntary agreements, potential legislative and regulatory strategies could be developed; for example, federal school lunch grants could be contingent upon schools' removal of soft drinks and other fast-food sources from junior high schools and high schools.

A CASE FOR IMPROVING THE
HEALTH AND WELL-BEING OF COMMUNITIES

Although the primary contribution of businesses to creating the conditions for health is the provision of jobs and creation of economic wealth, major employers as leaders of the business sector can also consider investing in community health as an example of corporate social responsibility. The investment, in turn, can provide social and economic returns to the company. These programs succeed only if senior and middle managers view them as directly aligned with the company's mission and vision. Company mission and vision statements, such as "becoming the preferred employer in the community," "attracting and retaining the best and brightest," and "emphasizing worker safety above all else," can be leveraged by champions of health promotion and disease prevention programs to, very simply, "help the company achieve its mission and vision."

Beyond the theoretical, philosophical, or even emotional reasons for supporting investments in employee and community health, there are practical reasons for these investments. A company, especially one that is large and dominant, that assumes a leadership position in improving community health and emphasizing disease prevention, health promotion, and accountability is likely to stand out in that community and is likely to affect the norms and practice patterns of health care practitioners for the better.

Another rationale for increased employer leadership and corporate investment in community health is the scarcity of mentally and physically capable employees able to take the place of employees who retire or voluntarily leave the organization. This scarcity is most pronounced in the service and high-technology sectors, where "knowledge workers" are in high demand. Many companies have begun to invest in the educational infrastructures of their communities to produce a large pool of well-educated and technologically advanced workers from which the company can recruit new employees with the skills that the companies need (see Box 6–9). A similar philosophy could be applied to health. Corporate investment in an improved community health infrastructure can create a larger pool of healthy and productive employees who are better able to face the physical and mental challenges of today's work environment.

Many corporate leaders seek to present an image of their companies as caring and responsible employers, and many companies try to distinguish themselves by being the preferred place to work (Johnson & Johnson, 1989; Levering and Moskowitz, 1994; Goetzel et al., 1998b; Mercer, 2000; Fortune Magazine, 2002). Investing in health promotion and disease prevention can also expand a corporation's social connections with the community. Organizations that are actively engaged in their communities and that act in socially responsible ways can also achieve a sense of purpose, relevance, social connectedness, and leadership in the community. They can do this by, for example, implementing no-smoking rules in buildings, in company vehicles, in front of company premises, and at client meetings; instituting work–life balance policies such as flexible working hours and telecommuting; allowing employees to take time off to participate in health promotion programs; offering healthy food choices in workplace eating facilities; and limiting air and water pollution in the community. Some businesses have begun to offer employees computers and access to e-health programs (i.e., that use the Internet) to help them better manage their own health (Box 6–9).

Organizations that are socially responsible and that exhibit a sense of caring for employees and the community can realize significant business gains as well, even when the gains are measured in traditional accounting terms. Across every financial outcome measured, socially responsible businesses perform no worse and, perhaps, perform better than non-socially responsible firms (Stalling, 1998). Furthermore, consumers are more likely to purchase products from companies, such as Ben & Jerry's Ice Cream, that they believe are more socially responsible (Stalling, 1998) (see Box 6–10).

The reasons and incentives for companies to enhance their cooperation with the community described in this section have also been summarized by Helperin (2000). The author notes that the public perception that "your company is a good corporate citizen isn't just for nice guys anymore; it's for everyone." The involvement of corporations in aligning or branding themselves with a social cause (i.e., a strategic, stakeholder-based approach to integrating social issues into business strategy, brand equity, and an organization's identity) affects employee recruitment and retention, employee morale, community and supplier relationships, public affairs, and the company's overall operating philosophy. A recent example of corpo-

---

BOX 6–9
Ford Motor Company: Model E Program

In February 2000, the Ford Motor Company, together with United Auto Workers leadership, launched the Model E Program for its employees. This program, the first of its kind, provides computer and Internet access to 350,000 Ford employees and their families in their homes for a nominal fee. The program is intended to help employees enhance their computer skills and comfort with the Internet environment, as well as their access to Internet learning opportunities. Ford management also envisions benefits for the company: employees will gain a deeper understanding of customer needs, communications with plant workers who do not have desktop computers will improve, and the costs of some human resource and other corporate services will be lower. By February 2002, 93 percent of employees had accepted the offer (Denise Clement, personal communication, February 4, 2002). Other companies have followed Ford's lead in sponsoring employees to become computer savvy (e.g., Fleet Bank-Boston, General Motors and Daimler-Chrysler, Intel Corp., Ollin Corporation, and the U.S. Army) (www.hconline.org/industry.php).

With large numbers of employees participating in the Model E Program, in July 2001 Ford moved to provide access to online tools that help empower employees in the management of their health. Through a licensing agreement, Ford provides access to the WellMed Personal Health Manager, a product of WellMed Inc., for 170,000 U.S.-based Ford employees and their families. According to WellMed:

> The product allows employees and their families to assess, record and improve their health on a daily basis. It includes general and gender-specific health risk assessment tools that cover past health issues, family history, and lifestyle habits; a secure location for individuals to create, gather, and store health records; a source of education information on conventional and alternative treatment options for important health topics such as allergies, asthma, depression, diabetes, cancer, and stress; and interactive, self-paced programs designed to assist individuals in achieving positive, healthful change such as quitting smoking, improving nutrition and fitness, or preparing for a healthy pregnancy. (www.wellmed.com/wellmed/c/c0802pr.asp?prID=62)

---

rate alignment with a significant social issue involves Viacom, a global media company. It has embraced its role as a participant in the public health system by strategically aligning itself with the Kaiser Family Foundation to launch a major media campaign to foster HIV awareness and prevention domestically and internationally (www.kff.org). This campaign is described more fully in Chapter 7.

Engaging Corporate Partnership in the Public Health System

As discussed above, the arguments for corporate investment in promoting the health of workers and their communities are compelling. However, more must be done to encourage American business leaders to view them-

BOX 6-10
Vignettes of Business Involvement in Community Activities

Mellon Bank, Pittsburgh, Pennsylvania

The Mellon Bank Chief Executive Officer, Martin McQuinn, serves as the Chair of the Community Health Committee for the University of Pittsburgh Medical Center and is a member of the Healthy Communities Business Advisory Panel for the Institute for Healthy Communities. One of Mellon's projects is the Community Bridge Project, a model designed to show how local businesses can partner with other agencies to address critical social and economic issues in their communities.

Community Bridge Project

The program model calls for the formation of community advisory committees consisting of business managers, educators, human services professionals, and local residents. The committees will assess their communities' business climates and recruit a pool of local residents willing to volunteer as mentors for welfare clients. A Penn State Cooperative Extension Program facilitator will be hired to coordinate existing extension resources and to work with volunteer mentors. Mentors will be trained to offer support and guidance for clients, helping them to identify workable strategies for improving their circumstances.

Participants will also undergo employment skills assessments and take part in appropriate job skills training. In addition, clients will receive help in matching their current skills to available training opportunities in the community, and they will be coached to match employment goals with realistic employment opportunities.

Mellon Financial Corporation Foundation

The Mellon Financial Corporation Foundation provides support for initiatives in economic development, health and human services, culture, and education. Mellon is a leader in workforce development and job readiness initiatives. In addition to the Community Bridge Project, Mellon has partnerships with the National Council on Aging as well as welfare-to-work programs in Pittsburgh, Philadelphia, and Boston. In 1999, Mellon was awarded the Goodwill Industries of Pittsburgh's Power of Work award (Stefani McAullife, Director of Community Planning at the Institute for Healthy Communities, personal communication, 2001).

Manufacturer's Association of Mideastern Pennsylvania

Darlene Robbins of the Manufacturer's Association of Mideastern Pennsylvania has seen a return on the investment that her organization made when it began focusing on the wellness of employees. Having programs such as Wellness in the Workplace decreased turnover, decreased absenteeism, and improved employee retention and morale. Through this program, the association invites small-, mid-, and large-sized organizations to attend a breakfast to discuss wellness in the workplace and the important role that it plays in production. The breakfasts are attended by several dozen business representatives who exchange a variety of useful information. The Manufacturer's Association wants to attract high-quality employees to Schuylkill County and realizes that a community with a high quality of life attracts the type of potential employees who will bring revenue to the business community. In addition, the association aims to attract new businesses into the

continued

BOX 6-10 Continued

area and recognizes that executives look at the quality of the community when deciding whether to move their families and businesses there. Representatives from potential new businesses explore factors such as competition, wages, cost of living, and the employee base, as well as the educational system, economic development potential, and the attitude of the community. The association and other Schuylkill County partners recognize that collaborative efforts are needed to bring new resources to the communities but note that a community does not have to be big to be successful (McAullife, personal communication, 2001).

GTE

GTE, which has recently merged with Bell Atlantic to form Verizon, is a founding member of the Georgia Healthcare Leadership Council. The council is an organization of managed care plans and local employers such as Delta Air Lines, Georgia Pacific, Lockheed, GTE, UPS, and pharmaceutical companies. Its goal is to improve the medical care provided to Atlanta residents. The primary focus of the council, formed in the fall of 1999, has been the development of preventive care standards based on evidence-based medicine. The council distributed posters to 3,500 metropolitan Atlanta doctors outlining standard prevention measures for children and adults. Upcoming initiatives include issuing guidelines for women's health and standardizing treatments for asthma and allergies.

GTE also has provided funding to support a Washington Business Group on Health project, Community Partnerships to Prevent Violence. The project will create a forum consisting of Texas-based employers; community organizations; school, mental health, and public health organizations; and parents. Its objective is to jointly develop strategies for businesses to assist parents (including their own employees) and schools in working to prevent school and youth violence. Forum participants will assess the community's inherent ability to work cooperatively on these issues and identify their roles and responsibilities in meeting this challenge. The participants will develop a set of goals and recommendations. They will also identify resources to share, such as information to be provided to parents on identifying risk behavior, working with school personnel on children's emotional and behavioral issues, and identifying community resources for children who need educational, mental health, and other services (WBGH, 2000).

3M

A core value at 3M is to embrace a commitment to strengthening the communities that are home to 3M locations. Through the 3M Foundation and the 3M Community Affairs Department, 3M links resources to community needs. 3M employees volunteer in multiple activities, such as tutoring programs and visiting scientist programs in local schools. Employees who participate are given paid time off from work to provide these services (WBGH, 2000).

selves as engaged partners in the public health system. Groups such as the Washington Business Group on Health are leading efforts to identify strategies to build greater collaboration between corporate leaders and governmental public health agencies.

In 1999, the Washington Business Group on Health hosted a public health forum for employers that brought together large employers and governmental public health leaders to discuss maternal and child health. A summary of the findings from the forum highlights the difficulties that employers and public health agencies must overcome if collaborative actions toward common health goals are to be achieved (WBGH, 2000). These findings include:

1. Employers and governmental public health agencies have had little interaction; this situation needs to change, and both will benefit from such a change.
2. There is a need for a common language and for dialogue among public health employers about issues related to health care costs.
3. Employers need data on pressing community health problems, but the data gathered need to be interpreted in ways that are meaningful to corporate health leaders.
4. There are significant limits to both the extent and the efficacy of employee health education.
5. There is a need to improve employee utilization of preventive health services that are covered but not being accessed by employees.

The findings from the forum also noted that partnership and collaboration could bring needed public health expertise to employers and business expertise to public health agencies (WBGH, 2000).

Governmental public health officials and business leaders would benefit from a formal dialogue on the health issues facing communities and the workforce. For example, corporate leaders should be invited to participate in community assessments and health planning and promotion activities (see Chapter 4). Such communication with corporate leaders and the participation of corporate leaders would allow the exchange of data on employee health as well as population-based health data from the community that are interpreted in ways that are meaningful to both public health officials and corporate health leaders. Such a dialogue would also provide the public health community with a better understanding of the processes that business leaders use to diagnose problems, review options, make decisions, and implement actions. Business leaders would gain a better understanding of the reasoning behind public health statutes, regulations, and other requirements that may affect businesses. Moreover, such a dialogue would help businesses leaders better understand their critical role as partners in the public health system.

The scientific basis of the health promotion and disease prevention programs needs to be better explained so that employers can better determine the most effective and efficient strategies to promote and sustain employee health, lower costs, and increase worker productivity. The public health community, the business community, and philanthropies may all play a role in such an effort. Public health researchers and philanthropies could be active partners in helping employers who want to develop, manage, and evaluate these types of programs.

Strong communications strategies must be developed to disseminate information on the costs (to employers and businesses) of modifiable health risk factors and the evidence-based interventions available to reduce these risk factors. This is especially critical if employees (as noted in the forum of the Washington Business Group on Health) are not taking advantage of covered preventive services. The corporate world is already steeped in marketing techniques but could benefit from the social marketing and media advocacy strategies described in Chapter 7 to motivate behavioral change among individuals (e.g., to increase the levels of use of preventive services) or to change public policies that would contribute to a healthier community and workforce (e.g., support educational programs in the community).

In addition to contributing to the health of employees and communities, greater corporate engagement in the public health system can improve public opinion about companies. A 2000 *Business Week*/Harris Poll explored Americans' views of corporate America. Two findings are of particular relevance to this discussion. When asked to rate large U.S. employers on "really caring about what is good for America," 25 percent of respondents answered "pretty good" and 7 percent answered "excellent." The remaining 66 percent answered only "fair" or "poor." Respondents were also asked to show their agreement with one of the following two statements: (1) "U.S. corporations should have only one purpose—to make the most profit for their stakeholders—and the pursuit of that goal will be best for America in the long run" and (2) "U.S. corporations should have more than one purpose. They also owe something to their workers and the communities in which they operate, and they should sometimes sacrifice some profit for the sake of making things better for their workers and communities" (Business Week, 2000). The respondents were almost unanimous (95 percent) in agreeing with the second statement.

Recognition of exemplary corporate responsibility can affect the public's view of a company's social responsibility and corporate reputation. A number of programs recognize corporations for their investments, and several partnerships between governmental and nongovernmental bodies recognize corporate efforts. For example, EPA, the Department of Energy, and the Center for Resource Solutions sponsor the Green Power Leadership Award, which recognizes the actions of organizations that advance the development and use of renewable energy sources. The Ron Brown Award for Corporate Leadership is a presidential award that rewards corporate leadership for promoting employees' development and well-being and for enhancing the communities where the employers work and live. For the past 10 years, the C. Everett Koop National Health Award, sponsored by the Health Project,[2] has been presented to U.S. companies that have documented improved employee health and cost savings from the health promotion and disease prevention programs at their work sites (Tully, 1995; Ziegler, 1998, 1999).

The committee recommends that the corporate community and public health agencies initiate and enhance joint efforts to strengthen health promotion and disease and injury prevention programs for employees and their communities. As an early step, the corporate and governmental public health community should:

a. Strengthen partnership and collaboration by

- Developing direct linkages between local public health agencies and business leaders to forge a common language and understanding of employee and community health problems and to participate in setting community health goals and strategies for achieving them, and
- Developing innovative ways for the corporate and governmental public health communities to gather, interpret, and exchange mutually meaningful data and information, such as the translation of health information to support corporate health promotion and health care purchasing activities.

b. Enhance communication by

- Developing effective employer and community communication and education programs focused on the benefits of and options for health promotion and disease and injury prevention, and
- Using proven marketing and social marketing techniques to promote individual behavioral and community change.

---

[2] The Health Project is a White House-initiated public–private partnership of health care leaders dedicated to improving family, individual, and community health through programs that are also proven to reduce overall costs.

c. Develop the evidence base for workplace and community interventions through greater public, private, and philanthropic investments in research to extend the science and improve the effectiveness of workplace and community interventions to promote health and prevent disease and injury.

d. Recognize business leadership in employee and community health by elevating the level of recognition given to corporate investments in employee and community health. The Secretaries of DHHS and the Department of Commerce, along with business leaders (e.g., chambers of commerce and business roundtables), should jointly sponsor a Corporate Investment in Health Award. The award would recognize private-sector entities that have demonstrated exemplary civic and social responsibility for improving the health of their workers and the community.

CONCLUDING OBSERVATIONS

Strong partnerships among governments, communities, philanthropies, and the corporate community to facilitate actions to improve the health of employees and their communities are critical for the public health system to achieve its goals. These partnerships could stimulate national debate and commentary to draw more attention to the importance of health promotion and disease and injury prevention in improving the health of the nation. Such partnerships could also serve to identify the incentives that can be used as tools to further engage the corporate community in providing high-quality programs that promote employee and community health and to develop shared actionable strategies to achieve the vision of healthy people living in healthy communities.

REFERENCES

AHRQ (Agency for Healthcare Research and Quality). 2002. Guide to Clinical Preventive Services, 3rd Edition (2000–2003). Available online at http://www.ahrq.gov/clinic/prevnew.htm. Accessed March 18, 2003.

Aldana SG. 2001. Financial impact of health promotion programs: a comprehensive review of the literature. American Journal of Health Promotion 15:(5):296–320.

AMA (American Medical Association). July 1999. Rethinking health insurance: the AMA's proposal for reforming the private health insurance system. Available online at www.ama.assn.org/ad.com. Accessed September 18, 2002.

Ames GM, Grube JW, Moore RS. 1997. The relationship of drinking and hangovers to workplace problems; an empirical study. Journal of Studies on Alcohol 58(1):37–47.

Amler RW, Dull HB (Eds.). 1987. Closing the Gap: The Burden of Unnecessary Illness. New York: Oxford University Press.

Anderson DR, Whitmer RW, Goetzel RZ, Ozminkowski RJ, Dunn RL, Wasserman J, Serxner S, HERO Research Committee. 2000. The relationship between modifiable health risks and health care expenditures: a group-level analysis of the HERO database. American Journal of Health Promotion 15(1):45–52.

Berger ML, Murray JF, Xu J, Pauly M. 2001. Alternative valuations of work loss and productivity. Journal of Occupational Environmental Medicine 43:18–24.

Bernstein M, Mahoney JJ. 1989. Management perspectives on alcoholism: the employer's stake in alcoholism treatment. Occupational Medicine 4(2):223–232.

Bertera R. 1990. Planning and implementing health promotion in the workplace: a case study of the Dupont company experience. Health Education Quarterly 17:307–327.

Bertera R. 1991. The effects of behavior risks on absenteeism and health-care costs in the workplace. Journal of Occupational Medicine 33(11):1119–1124.

Bertera R. 1993. Behavioral risk factor and illness day changes with workplace health promotion: two-year results. American Journal of Health Promotion 7:365–373.

BLS (Bureau of Labor Statistics). 2002. The Employment Situation, June 2002. Bureau of Labor Statistics news release. Available online at HtmlResAnchor http://www.bls.gov/schedule/archives/empsit_nr.htm#2002. Accessed September 23, 2002.

Bly J, Jones R, Richardson J. 1986. Impact of worksite health promotion on health care costs and utilization: evaluation of the Johnson and Johnson Live for Life program. Journal of the American Medical Association 256:3236–3240.

Breslow L, Fielding J, Herrman A, Wilbur CS. 1994. Worksite health promotion: its evolution and the Johnson & Johnson experience. Preventive Medicine 19:13–21.

Brink SD. 1987. Health Risks and Behavior: The Impact on Medical Costs. Seattle: Milliman & Robertson, Inc..

Burton WN, Conti DJ, Chin-Yu C, Schultz AB, Edington DW. 1999. The role of health risk factors and disease on worker productivity. Journal of Occupational and Environmental Medicine 41(10):863–877.

Burton WN, Conti DJ, Chen CY, Schultz AB, Edington DW. 2001. The impact of allergies and allergy treatment on worker productivity. Journal of Occupational and Environmental Medicine 43:64–71.

Business Week Online. 2000. Business Week/Harris Poll: how business rates: by the numbers. Available at www.businessweek.com. Accessed September 18, 2002.

CalPERS. 2002. The CalPERS Record: How CalPERS Functions as a Health Care "Purchasing Coalition." Web Page. Available online at: http://www.calpers.ca.gov/about/record/record02.htm. Accessed July 21, 2002.

CBO (Congressional Budget Office). 1994. An Analysis of the President's Health Proposal. Washington, DC: Government Printing Office.

CDC (Centers for Disease Control and Prevention). 1999. Achievements in Public Health, 1990-1999. Improvements in Workplace Safety—United States, 1900-1999. Mortality and Morbidity Weekly Report 48(22):461–469.

CDC. 2002. Annual smoking; attributable mortality, years of potential life lost, and economic costs—United States 1995–1999. Morbidity and Mortality Weekly Report 51(14):300–303.

Claxton AJ, Chawla AJ, Kennedy S. 1999. Absenteeism among employees treated for depression. Journal of Occupational and Environmental Medicine 41:605–611.

Cockburn IM, Bailit HI, Berndt ER, Finkelstein SN. 1999. Loss of work productivity due to illness and medical treatment. Journal of Occupational and Environmental Medicine 41(11):948–953.

Cooper P, Schone S. 1997. More offers, fewer takers for employment based health insurance: 1987 and 1996. Health Affairs 16(6):142–149.

Custer W, Ketsche P. 2000. Employment-Based Health Insurance Coverage. Washington, DC: Health Insurance Association of America.

DHHS (Department of Health and Human Services). 1990. Healthy People 2000: National Health Promotion and Disease Prevention Objectives. PHS Publication 91–50213. Washington, DC: DHHS.

DHHS. 2000. Reducing Tobacco Use: A Report of the Surgeon General. Atlanta, Georgia: U.S. Department of Health and Human Services, Centers for Disease Control and Prevention, National Center for Chronic Disease Prevention and Health Promotion, Office on Smoking and Health.

DHHS. 2002. HHS, USDA take next step in obesity fight, Secretaries Thompson and Veneman meet with leaders from food industry. DHHS News Release, October 15, 2002. Available online at http://www.hhs.gov/news/press/2002pres/20021015c.html. Accessed October 18, 2002.

EBRI (Employee Benefit Research Institute). 2002. EBRI General Benefits Research: 2002 Findings. Available online at http://www.ebri.org/ findings/gb_findings.htm. Accessed March 14, 2003.

Edington DW. 2001. Emerging research: a view from one research center. American Journal of Health Promotion 15(5):341–349.

Endicott J, Nee J. 1997. Endicott Work Productivity Scale (EWPS): a new measure to assess treatment effects. Psychopharmacology Bulletin 33:13–16

EPA (Environmental Protection Agency). 1997. Partners for the Environment: A Catalogue of the Agency's Partnership Program. EPA Report 100-B-97-003. Washington, DC: EPA.

EPA. 1998. Partnerships for a cleaner future. Available online at http://www.epa.gov/dfe/. Accessed November 1, 2002.

Fortune Magazine. 2002. Best companies to work for: America's top employers. Available online http://www.fortune.com. Accessed November 1, 2002.

Freudenheim M. 2001. Minnesota health insurers to standardize treatments. The New York Times, March 13. Available online at http://www.nytimes.com. Accessed March 13, 2002.

Fries J, Bloch D, Harrington H, Richardson N, Beck R. 1993. Two-year results of a randomized controlled trial of a health promotion program in a retiree population: the Bank of America Study. American Journal of Medicine 94:455–462.

Fries J, Harrington H, Edwards R, Kent L, Richardson N. 1994. Randomized controlled trial of cost-reductions from a health education program: the California Public Employees Retirement System (PERS) study. American Journal of Health Promotion 8:216–223.

Gavora C. 1997. How Health Insurance Mandates Misdiagnose the Disease. Backgrounder No. 1108. April 10. Washington, DC: Heritage Foundation.

Gerlach KK, Shopland DR, Hartman AM, Gibson JT, Pechacek TF. 1997. Workplace smoking policies in the United States: results of a national survey of more than 100,000 workers. Tobacco Control 6:199–206.

Goetzel RZ, Ozminkowski RJ. 2000. Disease management as a part of total health and productivity management. Disease Management and Health Outcomes 8:121–128.

Goetzel RZ, Sepulveda M, Knight K, Eisen M, Wade S, Wong J, Fielding J. 1994. Association of IBM's "A Plan for Life" health promotion program with changes in employees' health risk status. Journal of Occupational Medicine 36:1005–1009.

Goetzel RZ, Kahr TY, Aldana SG, Kenny GM. 1996. An evaluation of Duke University's Live for Life health promotion program and its impact on employee health. American Journal of Health Promotion 10(5):340–342.

Goetzel RZ, Anderson DR, Whitmer RW, Ozminkowski RJ, Dunn RL, Wasserman J, HERO Research Committee. 1998a. The relationship between modifiable health risks and health care expenditures: an analysis of the multi-employer HERO health risk and cost database. Journal of Occupational and Environmental Medicine 40(10):843–854.

Goetzel RZ, Guindon A, Humphries L, Newton P, Turshen J, Webb R. 1998b. Health and productivity management: consortium benchmarking study best practice report. Houston, TX: American Productivity and Quality Center International Benchmarking Clearinghouse. Available online at http://www.apqc.org. Accessed September 18, 2002.

Goetzel RZ, Juday TR, Ozminkowski RJ. 1999. What's the ROI? A systematic review of return on investment (ROI) studies of corporate health and productivity management initiatives. Association for Worksite Health Promotion's Worksite Health (Summer, 1999).

Goetzel RZ, Ozminkowski RJ, Meneades L, Stewart M, Schutt DC. 2000. Pharmaceuticals—cost or investment? An employer's perspective. Journal of Occupational and Environmental Medicine 42(4):338–351.

Goetzel RZ, Guindon AM, Turshen J, Ozminkowski RJ. 2001. Health and productivity management: establishing key performance measures, benchmarks, and best practices. Journal of Occupational and Environmental Medicine 43:10–17.

Golaszewski T, Lynch W, Clearie A, Vickery DM. 1989. The relationship between retrospective health insurance claims and a health risk appraisal-generated measure of health status. Journal of Occupational Medicine 31:262–264.

Gold DB, Anderson DR, Serxner SA. 2000. Impact of a telephone-based intervention in the reduction of health risks. American Journal of Health Promotion 15(2):97–106.

Greenberg PE, Finkelstein SN, Berndt ER. 1995. Economic consequences of illness in the workplace. Sloan Management Review 36(Summer):4–26.

Greenberg PE, Kessler RC, Nells TL, Finkelstein SN, Berndt ER. 1996. Depression in the workplace: an economic perspective, pp. 327–363. In Feighner JP, Boyer WF (Eds.). Selective Serotonin Re-Uptake Inhibitors: Advances in Basic Research and Clinical Practice. New York: John Wiley and Sons.

Gruber J, Madrian B. 1996. Health insurance and early retirement: evidence from the availability of continuation coverage, pp. 115–143. In Wise D (Ed.). Advances in the Economics of Aging. Chicago: University of Chicago Press.

Harris JS, Fries JF. 2001. The health effects of health promotion. In O'Donnell M (Ed.). Health Promotion in the Workplace, 3rd ed. Albany, NY: Delmar Press.

Health Policy Consensus Group. 1999. A Vision for Reform: Consumer-Driven Health Care Reform. Washington, DC: Galen Institute.

Heaney CA, Goetzel, RZ. 1997. A review of health-related outcomes of multicomponent worksite health promotion programs. American Journal of Health Promotion 11(3):290–308.

Helperin, J. 2000. All for the Cause: Cause marketing is helping dot-coms profit through philanthropy. Business2.0, October 2000. Available online at www.business2.0.com. Accessed March 18, 2003.

Hoffman C, Schlobohm A. 2000. Uninsured in America: A Chart Book. Washington, DC: The Kaiser Commission on Medicaid and the Uninsured.

IOM (Institute of Medicine). 2000. America's Health Care Safety Net: Intact but Endangered. Washington, DC: National Academy Press.

IOM. 2001a. Coverage Matters: Insurance and Health Care. Washington, DC: National Academy Press.

IOM. 2001b. Crossing the Quality Chasm: A New Health System for the 21st Century. Washington, DC: National Academy Press.

IOM. 2002. Care Without Coverage: Too Little, Too Late. Washington, DC: National Academy Press.

Johnson & Johnson. 1989. Customer advisory board survey results. Unpublished manuscript. Santa Monica, CA: Johnson & Johnson Health Management, Inc.

Kaiser Family Foundation. 2000. Kaiser Family Foundation/Health Research and Educational Trust (HRET) 2000 Annual Employer Benefits Survey. Available online at http://www.kff.org/docs/ehbs/. Accessed October 1, 2002.

Kaiser Family Foundation. 2001. Kaiser Family Foundation/Health Research and Educational Trust (HRET) 2001 Annual Employer Benefits Survey. Available online at http://www.kff.org/docs/ehbs/. Accessed October 1, 2002.

Kaiser Family Foundation. 2002. Kaiser Family Foundation/Health Research and Educational Trust (HRET) 2002 Annual Employer Benefits Survey. Available online at http://www.kff.org/docs/ehbs/. Accessed October 1, 2002.

Kessler RC, Greenberg PE, Mickelson KD, Meneades LM, Wang PS. 2001. The effects of chronic medical conditions on work loss and work cutback. Journal of Occupational and Environmental Medicine 43:218–225.

KPMG Peat Marwick. 1996. Health benefits in 1996. KPMG survey of employer sponsored health benefits.

KPMG Peat Marwick. 1998. Health benefits in 1998. KPMG survey of employer sponsored health benefits.

Lambrew JM. 2001. How the Slowing Economy Threatens Employer-Based Health Insurance. New York: The Commonwealth Fund.

Lave JR, Peele PB, Black JT, Evans JH, Amderbach G. 1999. Changing the employer sponsored health plan system: the views of employees in large firms. Health Affairs 18(4):112–117.

Leapfrog Group. 2002. Web Page. Available online at www.leapfroggroup.org. Accessed March 14, 2002.

Lerner D, Amick BC, Rogers WH, Malspeis S, Bungay K, Cynn D. 2001. The Work Limitations Questionnaire. Medical Care 39:72–85.

Leutzinger, JA 2001. The Health Project Application for the 2001 C. Everett Koop National Health Awards, May 14(1).

Leutzinger JA, Ozminkowski RJ, Dunn RL, Goetzel RZ, Richling DE, Stewart M, Whitmer RW, Anderson DR. 2000. Projecting health care costs using the HERO database and prevalence rates of lifestyle risks at Union Pacific Railroad. American Journal of Health Promotion 15(1):35–44.

Levering R, Moskowitz M. 1994. The 100 Best Companies to Work for in America. New York: Plume.

Long SH, Marquis MS. 2001. Low wage and health insurance coverage: can policymakers target them through their employees? Inquiry 38:331–337.

Mangione TW, Howland J, Amick B, Cote J, Lee M, Bell N, Levine S. 1999. Employee drinking practices and work performance. Journal of Studies on Alcohol 60(2):261–270.

McGinnis JM, Foege W. 1993. Actual causes of death in the United States. Journal of the American Medical Association 270:2207–2212.

Mercer WM. 2000. National Worksite Health Promotion Survey. Prepared in collaboration with the Association for Worksite Health Promotion and DHHS, Office of Disease Prevention and Health Promotion. Northbrook, IL: Association for Worksite Health Promotion.

Mosser G. 2001, July. Continuous improvement: a Minnesota model. Minnesota Physician 15(4):1–10.

National Institute on Alcohol Abuse and Alcoholism. 1999. Alcohol Alert No. 44. Available online at http://www.niaaa.nih.gov/publications/aa44.htm. Accessed March 14, 2002.

NCHS (National Center for Health Statistics). 1999. Advance Report of Final Mortality Statistics, 1997. Hyattsville, MD: Department of Health and Human Services.

NCHS. 2002. Deaths: Leading Causes for 2002. National Vital Statistics Report, Vol. 50 (16). Hyattsville, MD: Department of Health and Human Services.

NIOSH (National Institute for Occupational Safety and Health). 1996. National occupational research agenda. Available online at http://www.cdc.gov/niosh/nora.html. Accessed September 19, 2002

NIOSH. 2000a. Safety and health resource guide for small business. Publication 2000–148. Available online at http://www.cdc.gov/niosh/00-148pd.html. Accessed September 18, 2002.

NIOSH. 2000b. National Occupational Research Agenda. Update 2000. Available online at http://www.cdc.gov/niosh/pdfs/nora2000.pdf. Accessed September 19, 2002.

NIOSH. 2000c. Safety and Health Resource Guide for Small Businesses. NIOSH Publication No. 2000-148. Available online at http://www.cdc.gov/niosh/00-148pd.html. Accessed March 14, 2002.

OPEN MINDS. 1999. Over 72% of insured Americans are enrolled in MBHOs: Magellan Behavioral Health continues to dominate the market. OPEN MINDS Behavioral Health and Social Service Industry Analyst 11(9).

OSHA (Occupational Safety and Health Administration). 2002a. Strategic partnership overview. OSHA, Department of Labor. Available online at http://www.osha.gov/fso/vpp/partnership/what_is.html. Accessed September 18, 2002.

OSHA. 2002b. An overview of Voluntary Protection Programs. Available online at http://www.osha.gov/oshprogs/vpp/overview.html. Acessed March 14, 2002.

OSHA. 2002c. OSHA's Role at the World Trade Center Emergency Project. Available online at http://www.osha.gov/nyc-disaster/ny7summaries.html. Accessed January 14, 2003.

Ozminkowski RJ, Dunn RL, Goetzel RZ, Cantor RI, Murnane J, Harrison M. 1999. A return on investment evaluation of the Citibank, N.A. health management program. American Journal of Health Promotion 14(1):31–43.

Ozminkowski RJ, Goetzel RZ, Smith MW, Cantor RI, Shaughnessy A, Harrison M. 2000. The impact of the Citibank, N.A. health management program on changes in employee health risks over time. Journal of Occupational and Environmental Medicine 42(5):502–511.

Partnership for Prevention. 2001a. Health Workforce 2010: An Essential Health Promotion Sourcebook for Employers, Large and Small. Washington, DC: Partnership for Prevention.

Partnership for Prevention. 2001b. Prevention Priorities: Employers' guide to the highest value preventive health services. Available online at http://www.prevent.org/publications/PrevPriorities-Sm-Employers.pdf. Accessed March 18, 2003.

Pauly MV. 1986. Taxation, health insurance and market failure in the medical economy. Journal of Economic Literature 24:629–675.

Pauly MV. 1997. Health Benefits at Work: An Economic and Political Analysis of Employment-Based Health Insurance. Ann Arbor: University of Michigan Press.

Peele PB, Lave JR, Black JH. 2000. Employer sponsored health insurance: employers' choice and employee preferences. Milbank Quarterly: 78:5–21.

Pelletier K. 1999. A review and analysis of the clinical and cost-effectiveness studies of comprehensive health promotion and disease management programs at the worksite: 1995–1998 update (IV). American Journal of Health Promotion 13:333–345.

Pronk NP, Goodman MJ, O'Connor PJ, Martinson, BC. 1999. Relationship between modifiable health risks and short-term health care charges. Journal of the American Medical Association 282(23):2235–2239.

Reilly MC, Zbrozek AS, Dukes EM. 1993. The validity and reproducibility of a work productivity and activity impairment instrument. PharmacoEcon 4:353–365.

Reinhardt, UE. 1999. Employer-based health insurance: a balance sheet. Health Affairs 18(6):124–132.

Rosenheck RA, Druss B, Stolar M, Leslie D, Sledge W. 1999. Effect of declining mental health service use on employees of a large corporation. Health Affairs 18(5):193–203.

Rowland D, Feder J, Keenan P. 1998. Uninsured in America: the causes and consequences, pp. 25–44. In Haltman SH, Reinhart UE, Shields AE (Eds.). The Future U.S. Healthcare System: Who Will Care for the Poor and Uninsured? Chicago: Health Administration Press.

Schneider Institute for Health Policy. 2001. Substance Abuse: The Nation's Number One Health Problem. Princeton, NJ: Schneider Institute for Health Policy, Brandeis University, for the Robert Wood Johnson Foundation.

Simon GE, Barber C, Birnbaum HG, Frank RG, Greenberg PE, Rose RM, Wang PS, Kessler RC. 2001. Depression and work productivity: the comparative costs of treatment versus non-treatment. Journal of Occupational Environmental Medicine 43:2–9.

Stalling, B. 1998. Volunteerism and corporate America. U.S. Society and Values September:23–26.

Tully S. 1995. America's healthiest companies. Fortune 131(11):98–106.

U.S. Preventive Services Task Force. 1996. Guide to Clinical Preventive Services, 2nd edition. Washington, DC: Public Health Service. Available online at http://php.osophs.dhhs.gov/pubs/guideps.

Van Roijen L, Essink-Bot ML, Koopmanschap MA, Bonsel G, Rutten FF. 1996. Labor and health status in economic evaluation of health care. The Health and Labor Questionnaire. International Journal of Technology Assessment and Health Care 12:405–415.

WBGH (Washington Business Group on Health). 2000. The business interest in a community's health. Washington, DC: Washington Business Group on Health.

WBGH. 2002. Mental Health. Available online at http://www.wbgh.com/programs/mentalhealth/mental. Accessed September 18, 2002.

Wilson M, Holman P, Hammock A. 1996. A comprehensive review of the effects of worksite health promotion on health related outcomes. American Journal of Health Promotion 10(6):429–435.

Yen LT, Edington DW, Witting P. 1992. Prediction of prospective medical claims and absenteeism costs for 1,284 hourly workers from a manufacturing company. Journal of Occupational Medicine 34(4):428–435.

Yen LT, Eddington DW, Witting P. 1994. Corporate medical claim cost distributions and factors associated with high-cost status. Journal of Occupational Medicine 36(5):505–515.

Ziegler J. 1998. America's healthiest companies. Business and Health 16(12):29–31.

Ziegler J. 1999. High honors for encouraging health. Fitness, productivity and fresh thinking featured prominently in this year's Koop Awards. Business and Health 17(11):37–38.

7

Media

Mass media plays a central role in people's lives. Its importance is evident in the amount of time people spend watching television, surfing the World Wide Web, listening to music, and reading newspapers and magazines. The delivery of information through mass media is instant and available around the clock. The proliferation of communication technologies— miniature TVs, handheld radios, and personal computer companions such as Blackberry and Palm Pilot—contribute to the omnipresence of the media in daily life. More and more, a growing proportion of "life experience" is mediated through communication technologies instead of being directly experienced or witnessed. The public health community and policy makers often do not appreciate the importance and power of the media in shaping the health of the public. More importantly, media outlets or organizations do not see themselves as a part of, or contributing to the public health system. As this chapter discusses, however, the media plays a number of roles in educating the public about health issues and has a responsibility to report accurate health and science information to the public.

In this chapter, the committee examines the potential role of the media as an actor in the public health system, that is, how it can use its presence and power to lead to the mobilization of societal action that creates the conditions for health. The chapter specifically discusses how the news media can place health issues on the national public agenda and can catalyze action at the national and local levels. The chapter also addresses how advertising media, entertainment media, and the Internet provide health-related information that can reinforce or alter norms and attitudes that influence individual behavioral and societal changes. The chapter concludes with a brief discussion of the theories that help us understand the impact of the media on behavioral change and on evaluation and research issues, including the difficulties in predicting the outcomes of media campaigns. The committee recommends a number of steps that can be taken to further enhance the role of the media in improving the population's health.

NEWS MEDIA AND THE NATIONAL PUBLIC AGENDA

The ubiquitous nature of the news media, in particular, makes it a powerful tool for directing attention to specific issues. Generally, Americans look to the news media for coverage of events and to help us understand the world around us. Although the news media does not specifically tell us what to think, it plays an important role in identifying what issues we should think about (McCombs and Shaw, 1972). The more coverage a topic receives in the news, the more likely it is to be a concern of the public. Conversely, issues not mentioned by the media are likely to be ignored or to receive little attention.

The unfolding news coverage of HIV/AIDS provides a good example of how an important health issue may be invisible to the public eye until the media bring it to light. The first publicly documented cases of AIDS were reported in the June 5, 1981, issue of *Morbidity and Mortality Weekly Report* (*MMWR*) (CDC, 1981a). The publication provided five case histories of previously healthy, young (ages 29 to 36) homosexual men from the Los Angeles area who developed *Pneumocystis carinii* pneumonia (PCP), an affliction usually seen in severely immunodepressed patients, and a myriad of other opportunistic infections. A July issue of *MMWR* (CDC, 1981a) reported Kaposi's sarcoma in 26 homosexual men and additional cases of PCP in Los Angeles and San Francisco. Physicians were alerted about Kaposi's sarcoma, PCP, and other opportunistic infections associated with immunosuppression in homosexual men. A subsequent issue of *MMWR* (CDC, 1982c) reported 70 additional cases of Kaposi's sarcoma and PCP, and by December 1981, the Centers for Disease Control and Prevention (CDC) had reported more than 150 deaths.

During this time, news media coverage of the illnesses that appeared to be affecting homosexual men was limited. According to an analysis conducted by the Kaiser Family Foundation (1996), it was only in August 1982 that the *New York Times* brought readers up to date on an emerging and puzzling health crisis in the homosexual community. The article, "A Disease's Spread Provokes Anxiety," used the term *acquired immune deficiency syndrome*, or AIDS, for the first time. Later that year, the *Washington Post* reported on the death of an infant who had received a transfusion of blood from a donor with AIDS (CDC, 1982b). By 1983, a *Newsweek*

TABLE 7–1   Media Coverage of AIDS

Year	News Story
October 1985	Death of Rock Hudson, a well-known public figure
August 1987	Florida family burned out of home; a dramatic case of public anxiety concerning AIDS leading to violence. Arsonists were seeking to keep the family's AIDS-afflicted hemophiliac sons out of the local school system
April 1990	Ryan White's death at age 18. White contracted HIV at age 13 through blood products used to treat his hemophilia. He was the country's best-known victim of AIDS as a result of nonsexual transmission
June 1991	Public request by Kimberly Bergalis to test health professionals for AIDS. Kimberly contracted HIV from her dentist. Her dramatic case raised the controversial issue of AIDS testing for health care professionals
November 1991	Magic Johnson reveals his HIV-positive status. Johnson was the first major public figure not in a higher-risk group to announce his HIV-positive status and to attribute it to heterosexual activity and was the first major professional athlete (he was the National Basketball Association's most valuable player three times) to leave his sport because of HIV infection
February 1993	Arthur Ashe dies of AIDS. Ashe, a renowned tennis star, political activist, and social commentator, contracted HIV through a blood transfusion during a surgical procedure

SOURCE: Kaiser Family Foundation (1996).

poll found that 9 in 10 Americans over 18 years of age had heard about AIDS but were generally uninformed or misinformed. Subsequent coverage of AIDS included several newsmaker and public interest stories that further increased the public's concern about AIDS.

News media coverage during the mid- to late 1980s may have contributed to improved public awareness and knowledge of AIDS. By 1989, Gallup surveys indicated that nearly all adults were aware that HIV, the virus that causes AIDS, can be transmitted by shared needles (98 percent), homosexual intercourse (96 percent), and heterosexual intercourse (95 percent) (Kaiser Family Foundation, 1996). Table 7–1 gives examples of the media coverage of AIDS from 1985 to 1993.

The media also play an important role in gaining the attention of specific opinion leaders, including politicians, governmental regulators, community leaders, and corporate executives, among others. Between 1982 and 1987, several members of the U.S. Congress placed AIDS on the political agenda by holding hearings on the growing numbers of people afflicted by it and research into its causes and prevention. Celebrity activists and spokespersons covered by the media also increased the visibility of AIDS on the political agenda. However, it was not until 1987 that President Ronald Reagan gave his first public speech about AIDS. During that year the Congress also passed legislation that took into account the larger societal implications of the epidemic and that went beyond funding for AIDS prevention, research, and treatment efforts. The AIDS Federal Policy Act of 1987 prevented discrimination against individuals with disabilities—including those with HIV/AIDS.

In 1988, as public recognition of the burgeoning AIDS epidemic increased, the growing need for information was addressed by a booklet sent to all 107 million U.S. households by then-Surgeon General C. Everett Koop. *Understanding AIDS: A Message from the Surgeon General* was one of the largest educational public health mailings in U.S. history (Koop, 2002).

Political attention to AIDS continued to grow from the late 1980s through 1990. Advocacy groups and celebrities used news media coverage to bring attention to the case of Ryan White, an Indiana teenager who acquired AIDS through blood products used to treat his hemophilia, and to AIDS issues in general (AIDS Project Los Angeles, 2001). In August 1990, the Ryan White Comprehensive AIDS Resources (CARE) Act was enacted, a few months after Ryan's death. This landmark legislation authorized funds in emergency relief to cities devastated by the AIDS epidemic (P.L. 101–381).

As noted earlier, a high level of media coverage about a topic elicits public attention and concern. In the case of HIV/AIDS, the news media engaged public attention and stimulated policy response. Shuchman (2002) provides several examples of journalism as a catalyst of health care system change.

> A *New York Times* probe of fraudulent practices at the Columbia/HCA Healthcare Corp. chain of hospitals in March of 1997 led to a federal criminal investigation of the company (Gottlieb et al., 1997). A *Los Angeles Times* series on the U.S. Food and Drug Administration's system of drug approval in 2000 strengthened the claims of those advocating tighter controls at the agency (Willman, 2000). Extensive coverage by the *Washington Post* and others of the death of a young patient in a university-based gene therapy experiment resulted in stronger federal protections for patients enrolled in clinical trials (Nelson, 2000). A *Boston Globe* series on the hazards of placebo-control trials in psychiatry was one of several journalistic investigations that resulted in changes in the way psychiatric patients are enrolled in research protocols (Whitaker and Kong, 1998) (quoted in Shuchman, 2002).

News attention to specific issues, however, may also distort public perceptions and change behavior in adverse ways. Gilliam and colleagues (1995) found that the public's concern regarding crime increased, despite little actual change in the frequency of criminal activity and national survey statistics indicating a declining population-adjusted rate of crime over the previous two decades. The authors note that although Americans do not experience crime directly, they receive large doses of crime coverage from the media. The authors suggest that such coverage drives Americans to name crime as the most important problem facing the country and shapes public attitudes toward criminals, the death penalty, mandatory jail sentences, and "three strikes" laws. In response to public concerns, policy makers endorse strategies to strengthen law enforcement and the criminal justice system. Dorfman and Thorson (1998) also note that one by-product of media reporting on crime and violence is that readers receive a distorted picture of the world and that people react to reading and hearing news about crime and violence by fearing their world. Dorfman and colleagues (2001) have developed techniques to enable journalists to report on highly unusual crimes without misrepresenting the patterns of violence in their communities and creating misguided fears. Such techniques for reporting on violence integrate a public health perspective and offer readers information to understand the determinants of violence and to develop strategies for reducing violence in the community (Stevens, 1998).

NEWS MEDIA AS A CATALYST TO PROMOTE HEALTH AT THE COMMUNITY LEVEL

The AIDS example illustrates the role of the news media in placing the AIDS epidemic in the public light and on the national political and legislative agendas. The news media can also function as a catalyst for action at the local or community level. The story of "motel families" living across the street from Disneyland in Orange County, California, demonstrates the power of the news media to highlight social issues and stimulate action by local government and community members.

Over a period of 6 months in 1998, Laura Saari, a writer for the *Orange County Register*, brought to light the sharp social and economic contrast that exists in one of California's more affluent counties, where one in five children lives in poverty. The article on motel children uses the voices of children to poignantly communicate the impact of poverty on their lives (see Box 7–1).

The story had a significant influence on the community; more that 1,100 people contacted the paper to offer $200,000 in donations, 50 tons of food, 8,000 toys, and thousands of volunteer hours. The media coverage also activated a response by the local government. The Orange County

BOX 7–1
Growing Up in "Toxic Communities"
Sunday, August 2, 1998
Copyright © *The Orange County Register*
By Laura Saari

Five children sit on the lip of the Dumpster and spear cans to get the money for a McDonald's.

A broken fan, onion peels, a gravy-stained box from a Salisbury steak TV dinner, a can of Hype Morning Rush Energy.

"A toy bucket," shouts Jeffrey Littlefield, 6. He wiggles a stick to get to the bucket before the other kids. He pulls up a fast-food chicken pail and smiles. Two black teeth.

"I'm fishin'," he says. "It's a contest, whoever gets the most cans."

"Can I help?" asks Anthony Chavez, 3, trying to climb up.

"I see French fries!" says a girl. She jumps in.

The children live at a motel across from Disneyland.

There was a time when tourists checked into motels such as this one, drawn to the U-Dial telephones and color TVs and a balcony view of the Happiest Place on Earth.

Today, the vacancy signs are still up, but their neon tubes have lost their gas. Newer high-rise hotels lure the vacationers.

And so the old rooms-by-the-day have become $140 rooms-by-the-week that soon become rooms-by-the-year, even though everyone always says they're moving out tomorrow.

For families who can't find a way into the county's rental market, the motels are the last stop before the homeless shelter or the street. And it's not just here. A healthy economy and rising home prices have driven families across the nation into motels.

Often, the buildings are in decay. The ceilings fall, the locks don't latch, and the roaches don't wait until dark. Some families live six or more people to a room.

For the hundreds of children living in Orange County motels, violence often is a thin wall away, if that. Drug deals, prostitution, stabbings, assaults, theft, an occasional murder, a fugitive in hiding.

The children are transient. Because of new occupancy limits in some cities, families must move on after 28 days. Social workers who are trying to protect the children often have difficulties just finding them, says Michael Riley, director of Orange County Children and Family Services.

At some schools near motels, a third of the kids who sign up in the fall aren't there at the end of the year. Head lice are chronic. Nurses have found roaches lodged deep inside children's ears. "These children are consumed, 24 hours a day, with poverty—and it's not just financial," says Linda Dunlap, a nurse whose volunteer group, Project Dignity, works with families in motels. "It's spiritual and emotional. They didn't just decide one day they were going to surrender their spirits. They did it to survive."

The little ones seem too wise for their years, and too angry. Yet they share their last piece of bread with a neighbor. They protect each other fiercely. They try to create order where there is none.

BOX 7–1 Continued

In grade school, many children are still hanging onto their dreams of what their lives could be. By the time they are teenagers, anger often has hardened into resentment, hopelessness, defiance. "I think the general population doesn't understand what kind of lifestyle is being led in these places," says Sgt. Joe Vargas of the Anaheim Police Department.

"These are toxic communities. The kids are really starving for stability, and they don't get it. We're breeding criminals. We're breeding kids who are growing up without the life skills necessary to function to their full potential."

That is the way grown-ups see life in motels. But things look different when you're a kid.

SOURCE: Saari (1998). Excerpted with permission of the *Orange County Register*.

Board of Supervisors ordered an audit of services for motel children and directed $1 million in funds to create a housing program to help families move out of motels (Leaman, 1998). A nonprofit agency launched a $5 million capital campaign for a shelter to help motel families with drug abuse problems. The city of Anaheim, where the motels are located, also moved services into the motels so that families would have easier access to parenting classes, job training, and food programs.

Many public health issues are not considered newsworthy. In contrast to the coverage of a frightening infectious disease epidemic such as AIDS or, more recently, the anthrax attacks, the story on motel children illustrates the everyday work of public health that involves struggles with endemic conditions and risk factors that are not considered news. The journalist was able to capture interest in an endemic situation by presenting the story in a novel way, and subsequent advocacy helped to keep the story and the public interest alive.

NEWS MEDIA COVERAGE AND HEALTH INFORMATION

Although news media coverage can help place a specific health issue on the national agenda, tensions exist among news reporters, scientists, and public health professionals as they seek to convey health news and information to the public, especially during a crisis. It is important to understand these tensions if the news media is to be involved in the public health system.

The results of a survey of scientists and journalists are particularly helpful in understanding the attitudes of each toward the other and their views on transmitting and translating scientific information through the media to the public. Hartz and Chappell (1997) found that scientists complained that reporters do not understand many of the basics of their methods, including the proper interpretation of statistics, probabilities, and risk. Journalists viewed scientists as being too immersed in esoteric jargon and unable to explain their work simply and cogently, whereas scientists said the news media oversimplify complex issues. Reporters also noted that scientists do not understand that "news" is a perishable commodity that must be made relevant to the reader and viewer (see Table 7–2).

These findings allude to many of the tensions between the scientific community (including the public health community) and the journalism community that arise because of differences in defining what is newsworthy, differences in styles of communication (Nelkin, 1996, 1998; Hartz and Chappell, 1997), and differences in perceptions about the role of the media (Nelkin, 1996, 1998).

In identifying newsworthy topics, journalists often seek out stories that are potential attention grabbers. The tenets of newsworthiness include controversy, broad interest, injustice, irony, local "peg," personal angle, breakthrough, anniversary peg, seasonal peg, celebrity peg, and visuals that can make the story interesting (Wallack et al., 1999).

Scientists and public health professionals believe that journalists, in writing attention-grabbing stories, often violate the traditional norms that guide scientific communication. Nelkin (1996, 1998) notes that media con-

TABLE 7–2 Scientists' and Journalists' Agreement with Various Negative Statements About the News Media

Statement	Scientists' Agreement (%)	Journalists' Agreement (%)
Few members of the news media understand the nature of science	91	77
News media reporters are ignorant of the process of science	69	46
News media reporters cannot interpret results	66	48
News media reporters overblow risks	61	45
News media reporters rarely get details right	56	62
Member of the media seek the sensational	76	69
Members of the news media focus on the trendy	79	67
News media reporters focus on personalities, not on findings	49	70
News media reporters want instant answers	75	52

SOURCE: Hartz and Chappell (1997).

straints of time, brevity, and simplicity, for example, impede the careful documentation, nuanced positions, and caveats that scientists believe are necessary to discuss and present their work. Journalists, on the other hand, often see the use of caveats or qualifications as information that can be dismissed to improve the readability of a story. Furthermore, journalistic efforts to enhance audience interest may violate other traditional scientific norms. For example, to create a human interest angle, journalists may look for personal stories and individual cases, although this may distort research findings that have meaning only in a broader statistical context.

Scientific journals may also contribute to the distortion of research findings. Scientific journals often prepare press releases for the news media to assist them in getting the story right. These attempts to translate research into news can be misleading. Woloshin and Schwartz (2002) reviewed the content of journal press releases and interviewed press officers at nine prominent medical journals. The study found that press releases do not routinely highlight study limitations or the role of industry funding. Formats for presenting data were also found to exaggerate the perceived importance of findings.

Fueling these tensions is the fact that scientists, health care professionals, and policy experts rarely receive training in public communication, and reporters are not well trained in science, medicine, and statistics. Both groups are generally untrained in risk communication.

A recent study (Voss, 2002) highlights reporters' self-perceptions about their own ability to report health news. The study surveyed reporters and newspapers in five Midwestern states. In response to questions about reporting ability, 49.7 percent of respondents reported it was sometimes easy and sometimes difficult to understand key health issues, and 31 percent found it often or nearly always (2.7 percent) difficult to do. Also, 51.3 percent of respondents reported that it was sometimes easy or sometimes difficult to interpret statistical data, whereas 27.4 percent found it often or nearly always (6.2 percent) difficult. More than three-quarters of respondents (83 percent) reported that they had no training to cover health topics. Similarly, a national survey of journalists and news executives found that only 12 percent of reporters covering health care are viewed as "extremely prepared" and 43 percent are viewed as "prepared" to cover health care issues (Foundation for American Communications, 2002).

To help ease these tensions and to improve the quality of the information delivered to the public, scientists and public health officials as well as journalists and editors should seek opportunities for training. The need for media training is acknowledged in the statement of Al Cross, President of the Society of Professional Journalists, who notes that "training is a good way to meet your public responsibilities" (quoted in Kees, 2002) and in the words of Melinda Voss, executive director of the Association of Health Care Journalists:

> It seems to me that it is more important than ever that we as journalists really know how to do our jobs right, because so many critical policy decisions are being made that affect everyone. The ability to properly report medical studies and survey research and the ability to interpret statistics are all a part of doing the job right. We owe it to our audiences. (quoted in Kees, 2002)

In response to the need for better health and science reporting, governmental agencies and foundations have developed programs for journalists that seek to provide them with experiences that will deepen their subject matter knowledge and strengthen their reporting. With funding from the John S. and James L. Knight Foundation, the CDC Foundation sponsors the Knight Journalism Fellowship at CDC (CDC Foundation, 2002). The fellowship provides classroom instruction in epidemiology and biostatistics, public health intervention, public health structure, and health reporting. Fellows are also provided with opportunities to observe investigations of disease outbreaks and participate in research and field practice (http://www.cdcfoundation.org/fellowships/knight/fellowship.html).

The Kaiser Family Foundation (2002b) sponsors three fellowship programs for journalists. The Kaiser Media Fellowships in Health provide print or broadcast journalists and editors interested in health issues with an annual stipend that allows them to pursue individual projects on a wide range of health and social policy issues. The Kaiser Media Internships in Urban Health provide minority journalists interested in urban public health reporting with practical experiences in reporting on the health beat. The Kaiser Media Mini-Fellowships provide travel and research grants to journalists to research and report on health policy and public health issues. Both the Kaiser Family Foundation and the CDC-Knight fellowships, as well as others,[1] facilitate a healthy dialogue between health officials and reporters and contribute to the development of a well-trained cadre of health journalists.

Journalist associations also have begun to take a lead in providing opportunities for journalists to improve the quality of information they provide to the public. The Association of Health Care Journalists (AHCJ), for example, is an independent, nonprofit organization dedicated to advancing public understanding of health care issues. Its mission is to improve the quality, accuracy, and visibility of health care reporting, writing, and editing. One of the ways the association works to enhance the understand-

---

[1] Although not dedicated specifically to health issues, the Pew Charitable Trusts sponsors the Fellowships in International Journalism (www.pewfellowships.org), which may cover health issues in other countries.

ing between journalists and health care experts is by offering workshops and training resources on current and emerging issues in health care and reporting skills. With support from the Robert Wood Johnson Foundation, the association recently published *Covering the Quality of Health Care—A Resource Guide for Journalists* (AHCJ, 2002b).

The importance of effective communication among public health officials, the media, and the public is particularly critical during crises. During such times, the news media play an important role in amplifying or attenuating the public's perception of risk and serve as a key link in the risk communication process. The media played a key role in reporting the anthrax attacks following the terrorist attacks on September 11, 2001. The events emphasized the need to communicate scientific and medical information in a way that the public can understand and to provide clear information about the concepts of risk and how to apply them.

In November 2001, Dr. Kenneth Shine, president of the Institute of Medicine, advised Congress that communication to the public and to health professionals about the anthrax terrorist attack were found to be insufficient and needed improvement to deal more effectively with future situations that may compromise public health or national security. He stated:

> Within the Department of Health and Human Services, there must be a single credible medical/public health expert spokesperson that reports regularly, most likely daily, to the American people in regard to an outbreak with national significance. This is analogous to the situation in local communities where there is a need for such an individual to communicate on behalf of the local health department. Several months before the anthrax outbreak, uninformed statements on local television in a community with two cases of meningococcal meningitis resulted in thousands of individuals taking antibiotics or seeking immunizations that were not indicated. Local stores of antibiotics were depleted and many people were subjected to risk from unnecessary treatment. This episode emphasizes the need for credible medical/public health information during natural events, as well as during those that are produced by terrorism.

> In the case of the anthrax episodes, the media responded by interviewing countless number of individuals. Among them was a self-professed pundit who announced he was an expert on the "anthrax virus." Anthrax is a bacterium, not a virus. In many cases, well-intentioned infectious disease specialists who knew a good deal about the literature on anthrax could provide accurate retrospective information, but when pressed about the current events, they were not privy to the information about the cases that had occurred. They were then forced to either acknowledge their limitations, which the responsible experts did, or in the case of others less responsible, to speculate based on news reports, rumors, and a variety of other kinds of incomplete or false information.

In the case of anthrax, less than 20 cases resulted in thousands of people taking antibiotics that were not indicated. Perhaps 20 percent of these individuals experienced some side effects from these drugs. These antibiotics changed the bacteriological environment and may have rendered some organisms resistant to the antibiotics employed. (Shine, 2001).

In response to Department of Health and Human Services plans to reorganize communication, legislative, and public affairs offices, the Association of Health Care Journalists and the National Association of Science Writers warned that tight control of information by top department managers may be efficient, but it can also increase the risk of communication bottlenecks that can deprive the public of timely and vital health information, and raises questions about how the public's access to objective information will be protected (AHCJ, 2002a).

Analyzing the communication response to the anthrax attacks may present potentially critical lessons, and a rigorous review of the handling of the incident by the media and public health officials is needed to improve communication strategies for the future. The summary proceedings of a recent conference of media and public health representatives highlighted a number of lessons learned from coverage of public health crises (Joseph, 2002). First, the primary goal of both the press and public health professionals is to serve the public, and the communication of accurate information is a crucial factor in this service. Second, a credible spokesperson or expert must be available to the press to help ensure that information is accurate. This is especially critical during a crisis when there is pressure for both health and nonhealth reporters to cover an incident. Ideally, the spokesperson(s) should have an ongoing dialogue and relationship with reporters as well as editors. Third, public health professionals need to acknowledge the independence of the news media. The press attempts to provide a balanced story for its audience and must be careful not to serve just as a "vehicle" for a specific group's message. For the press, there is a fine line between cooperation and the risk of losing independence, or cooptation. Furthermore, the audience or public is not a single entity; it can be segmented into different groups with different experiences, social determinants, cultures, and languages. Thus, it is essential to consider different ways of presenting information, especially when dealing with "risks." Fourth, both public health officials and journalists share a concern that the U.S. public is unaccustomed to uncertainty and that public levels of literacy are low. The continuation of this dialogue is essential; there is much that media and public health professionals can learn from each other that will help both improve their service to the public.

Understanding and appreciating the perspectives and needs of all parties will create a better climate for accurately informing the public. **The committee recommends that an ongoing dialogue be maintained between medical and public health officials and editors and journalists at the local** level and their representative associations nationally. Furthermore, foundations and governmental health agencies should provide opportunities to develop and evaluate educational and training programs that provide journalists with experiences that will deepen their knowledge of public health subject matter and provide public health workers with a foundation in communication theory, messaging, and application. Results from these activities would contribute knowledge on how best to structure training and other educational opportunities for health and media specialists so that they are better prepared to bring accurate health information to the public.

MEDIA AND HEALTH COMMUNICATION

Health communication campaigns are interventions intended to generate specific outcomes for a relatively large number of individuals within a specified period of time and through an organized set of communication activities (Rogers and Storey, 1987). Large-scale health communication campaigns seeking to change behaviors were first seen in the United States in the eighteenth century in the form of efforts to educate the public about infectious diseases and the benefits of immunization. In 1721, Reverend Cotton Mather used pamphlets and personal appeals to promote immunization during a smallpox epidemic in Boston (Paisley, 2001). Another illustrative example of a public health campaign was associated with the newly found knowledge that the *Mycobacterium tuberculosis* bacillus caused tuberculosis (TB) and that TB was communicable and could be prevented. In 1896, the New York City Department of Health, responding to a report on TB developed by D. Hermann Biggs, issued an ordinance that prohibited spitting on sidewalks. The public and civil sectors helped to drive behavioral change at the individual level by placing notices in public areas warning that spitting on the floor spread disease. Hospitals joined the effort by posting signs proclaiming "spit is poison" (Ruggiero, 2000). More recently, health communication campaigns have used a variety of ways to present health messages.

This section discusses the use of specific media to promote health messages. It first addresses public service announcements (PSAs) and then discusses the role of emerging media channels—the entertainment media and the Internet—in conveying health messages. The section concludes with an examination of social marketing and media advocacy, strategies that use media as part of a broader approach to changing individual behavior or promoting social change.

Advertising Media: Public Service Announcements

Broadcasters can help create conditions for improved population health by choosing to donate time for PSAs that convey health-promoting messages. PSAs became a possible conduit for disseminating health-related messages when the Federal Communications Commission (FCC) required that stations donate a certain amount of airtime to serve the public and the community in exchange for the use of public airways.

The FCC defines PSAs as "any announcement (including network) for which no charge is made and which promotes programs, activities, or services of federal, state, or local governments or the programs, activities, or services of nonprofit organizations and other announcements regarded as serving community interests" (FCC Rules, Section 73.1810 [d][4]). The requirement, however, does not specify the length of time or the time of day that broadcasters should make PSAs available. In fact, PSAs are only one option for fulfilling the FCC requirement; broadcasters can meet their public interest obligations without running any PSAs at all. Furthermore, new broadcasting venues such as cable networks have no statutory obligation to serve the public interest (Kaiser Family Foundation, 2002a).

The Kaiser Family Foundation recently conducted a study to examine the amount of airtime that television broadcasters donate for PSAs.[2] They found that broadcast and cable television networks donate an average of 15 seconds an hour to air PSAs. This represents just under one-half of 1 percent (0.4 percent) of all airtime. Much of this donated airtime (43 percent) is made available between midnight and 6 a.m., and only 9 percent is available during prime time. The major broadcast networks (ABC, CBS, Fox, and NBC) donate an average of 5 seconds an hour to PSAs during prime time. The study also found that health issues are the top priority of PSAs at some networks: 52 percent of all donated airtime on MTV, 35 percent of all donated airtime on Fox, and 33 percent on CBS are devoted to health issues (Kaiser Family Foundation, 2002a).

In addition to donated airtime for PSAs, paid PSAs have become another mode to deliver public service messages. According to the Kaiser Family Foundation study, of all PSAs aired, 36 percent are paid for by sponsors (e.g., governmental agencies such as the Office of National Drug Control Policy and community-based organizations). Sponsors buy an average of 9 seconds an hour of advertising time for paid PSAs per network. Paid PSAs are not only longer (on average, 9 seconds compared to 5 seconds for donated PSAs), but they are better placed. Only 18 percent of paid PSAs are run between midnight and 6 a.m., whereas 43 percent of donated spots run between those hours. Health issues are also a primary focus of paid PSAs—39 percent convey health messages.

The growing use of paid PSAs has raised concerns about the degree to

---

[2] The study examined a week's worth of television programming for 10 channels: the major broadcast networks ABC, CBS, Fox, and NBC and the cable channels CNN, ESPN, MTV, Nickelodeon, TNT, and the Spanish-language network Univision.

which networks are meeting their public service obligations. Paid PSAs are regarded by some as an indication that the traditional public service model—relying on donated airtime from broadcasters seeking to fulfill their public service obligations—is no longer working (LaMay, 2002). Some paid PSA sponsors report that before turning to paying for PSAs, they encountered significant difficulties getting messages on the air, especially during prime time (Berger, 2002).

Struggles to get PSAs with health messages on the air can significantly challenge efforts to educate and persuade the public to adopt healthy practices or to avoid behaviors that pose a risk to health. Reviews of the impacts of PSAs have found them to increase public recognition or awareness of a problem and in some cases to motivate action or change behavior. Hu and colleagues (1995), for example, found that California's paid antismoking media campaign accounted for a 2 to 3 percent lower level of cigarette sales, or an estimated reduction of 232 million packs of cigarettes during the 2-year study period. The $1 million investment in media messages reduced per capita cigarette sales by 7.7 packs. Part of the success of this campaign was that the paid nature of the PSAs allowed greater freedom in their design, which was considered controversial and attracted news media attention (Dorfman and Wallack, 1993). Antismoking media campaigns in Massachusetts and Florida also report significant reductions in smoking behavior. Siegel and Biener (2000) report that among a panel of Massachusetts adolescents (aged 12 to 13 years at the baseline), those who were exposed to television antismoking advertisements were significantly less likely to progress to established smoking 4 years later (odds ratio = 0.49; 95 percent confidence interval = 0.26, 0.93). Similarly, Zucker and colleagues (2001) report a 19 percent decline in smoking among Florida middle school students and an 8 percent decline among Florida high school students exposed to antismoking media campaigns.

The outcomes noted above are well documented. Atkin (2001) notes, however, that "effects may unfold indirectly and gradually as messages increase knowledge, stimulate information seeking, and interpersonal discussion and move individuals through early stages of decision making."

In addition to specific behavioral change, Balbach and Glantz (1998) emphasize that public service advertising can also have an effect on public discourse and can create pressure for changes in policy and regulations:

> The media, both paid advertising and free media, are important vehicles for putting pressure on public agencies. By running their own advertisements, program advocates can create a forum in which they are able to frame issues publicly in a way that reflects their viewpoint. This is a particularly powerful strategy if other forums, such as legislatures or oversight bodies, have not been responsive. Such advertisements reach deci-

sion makers, the public, and reporters, and call attention to the fact that there are problems with the program. (Balbach and Glantz, 1998: 407)

The results noted are compelling; however, researchers and health communicators increasingly understand that PSAs play a significant but limited role in promoting health messages and should be considered part of a broader health communication strategy.

A question often debated when discussing PSAs is: Why should broadcasters be motivated to donate public service announcements, especially if there are monetary implications for them? There are at least three responses to the question; first, the FCC, through its licensing agreements, imposes on broadcasters a commitment to serve the public interest. Second, when broadcasters do so, it creates good will among their audiences, and as evidenced earlier, studies demonstrate that PSAs contribute to improving the health of the public who consume the broadcasters' media. Third, when broadcasters comply freely, calls for tighter and more specific regulatory actions to ensure broadcasters' commitment to the public interest are less likely to be made.

As noted earlier, not all broadcasters are averse to donating time for PSAs, and some have made significant contributions of time and effort to promote the health of the public. Viacom, a global media company with leading positions in broadcast and cable television, radio, outdoor advertising, and online, recently announced (October 2002) that it has partnered with the Kaiser Family Foundation to create an unprecedented, public information campaign to eradicate ignorance about HIV/AIDS. The campaign capitalizes on Viacom's global brand power and strong audience relationships to reach the public at large and those most affected by the disease. The Kaiser Family Foundation brings to the partnership its expertise in HIV/AIDS and public education. The campaign includes domestic and international public messaging, television and radio programming, and outdoor, print, and online content and employee education. The $120 million campaign will be launched in January 2003 (www.viacom.com; www.kff.org). This partnership demonstrates strong corporate responsibility and the role that the public health sector can play to engage media gatekeepers in the task of promoting the public's health.

In light of the important opportunity that PSAs provide as a vehicle for the dissemination of messages to educate and persuade the public to adopt healthy practices or avoid behaviors that pose a risk to health and of the limited amount of time donated to PSAs throughout the broadcasting schedule, **the committee recommends that television networks, television stations, and cable providers increase the amount of time they donate to PSAs as a partial fulfillment of the public service requirement in their FCC licensing agreements.** In doing so, the public would benefit from more opportunities to obtain health messages, the media would be seen as demonstrating greater corporate and civic responsibility, and the need for tighter regulation to ensure that licensing agreement requirements are being met would be diminished.

Historically, as mentioned above, the FCC has required that broadcast networks allot a certain amount of time to "the public interest." Networks complied but often aired PSAs late at night, when few viewers were watching. This was, of course, the least valuable time that the networks had, and because the networks competed with one another, using late night television for nonpaid advertisements was sensible. A critical opportunity, however, was missed as corporations advertised their products, and the public interest was not served. The FCC should review the regulations governing broadcast and broadband media with an eye toward finding ways in which media institutions can serve the public's interest in accurate health information without being unfairly burdened in the process.

Better placement of PSAs would benefit the public as well as the media, which will be seen as fully contributing to the public good. **The committee recommends that the FCC review its regulations for PSA broadcasting on television and radio to ensure a more balanced broadcasting schedule that will reach a greater proportion of the viewing and listening audiences.** This will benefit the public as well as the media's image as a vital contributor to the public good.

Policy makers may ask if PSAs are more effective in reducing cigarette consumption than other measures, such as tobacco taxation. Hu and colleagues (1995) examined the relative effects of taxation versus an antismoking media campaign in California, as noted earlier. The study results indicate that both taxation and antismoking media campaigns are effective means of reducing cigarette consumption. The authors note, however, that the strength of the effects is related to the magnitude of the taxes and the amount of resources expended on the media campaign.

Corporations spend billions of dollars on paid advertising to promote their products. In 2001 (Ad Age, 2001), the 100 leading national advertisers spent well over $40 billion on advertising. The federal government is among these advertisers, with just over $1 billion spent on advertising-related activities. Competition between state government spending on health promotion and prevention activities (which may include advertising) and corporate marketing activities for products that undermine health is also in tremendous imbalance. The public is negatively influenced by corporate advertisers of unhealthy behaviors and products, with little counteradvertising that promotes positive health behaviors. For example, in 2000, state spending on tobacco use prevention was $768.4 million, whereas tobacco companies spent $9.7 billion on marketing across the states (National Center for Tobacco Free Kids, 2002). To deal with such an imbalance in

advertising, researchers have proposed that a federal tax be levied on tobacco advertising and promotion (Bayer et al., 2002). The impact of a 10-
cent tax would generate about $2.1 billion a year, which would substan-
tially increase the funds currently available for antitobacco advertising. The
U.S. Supreme Court has not yet tested the constitutionality of a content-
based tax on commercial speech. More discussion and research are needed
to identify and develop support for strategies that can improve the balance
between advertising that promotes health and advertising for products that
harm the health of the public.

Entertainment Media: Television

Television is one of society's most common and constant learning environments. Television entertainment programs and commercials, with potential positive and negative health messages embedded in them, reach tens
of millions of viewers each day. Often, these messages reach viewers who
may not otherwise expose themselves to such information and do not fully
realize that these messages may influence their thoughts and actions
(Signorielli, 1990). However, concerted efforts to develop strong partnerships between the entertainment media and health communicators are increasingly contributing to more accurate and timely health information in
entertainment programming.

American television producers have a history of working with health
promotion experts to address public health issues. A few examples are
alcoholism on *Hill Street Blues* and *Cagney and Lacey*; AIDS on *St. Elsewhere*, *Designing Women*, and *LA Law*; birth control on *Valerie* (Wallack,
1990); and the Jeanie Boulet storyline on AIDS on *ER*.

A more concerted effort to partner with entertainment media to disseminate health messages was undertaken by researchers at the Harvard
School of Public Health Center for Health Communication. In 1988, the
Harvard Alcohol Project partnered with the three largest television networks—ABC, CBS, and NBC—to demonstrate that a new social concept,
the "designated driver" for avoiding driving after drinking, could be dif-
fused rapidly through American society via mass communication techniques.
As part of the project, television writers agreed to insert drunk driving
prevention messages and references to designated drivers into the scripts of
top-rated television programs. The networks also aired frequent PSAs during prime time that encouraged the use of designated drivers (www.hsph.
harvard.edu/chc/alcohol). Evaluations of the campaign's impact documented a rapid, widespread acceptance and the strong popularity of the
designated driver concept. Before the campaign, 62 percent of Gallup poll
respondents said that they and their families used a designated driver all or
most of the time. By mid-1989, the percentage had risen to 72 percent, a

statistically significant increase in the numbers of individuals using designated drivers. Surveys sponsored by the National Highway Traffic Safety Administration in 1993 and 1995 found that about three-quarters of those surveyed responded that people should not be allowed to drive if they have been drinking any alcohol at all. These results indicate a wide acceptance of the social norm that the driver should not drink (Winsten and DeJong, 2001).

The designated driver concept and the strategy to emphasize it, however, were extremely controversial. Some alcohol control advocates argued that they may have done more harm than good by encouraging excessive drinking by passengers and deflecting attention away from the social determinants that influence alcohol consumption (DeJong and Wallack, 1992).

In a more recent partnership, researchers at the Kaiser Family Foundation, together with a writer and producer of ER, NBC's medical drama, collaborated to test the effect of health information communicated through an ongoing television drama. They learned that a short mention of an important health issue in an entertainment television show can make millions of Americans aware of that issue. The experiment included preshow, postshow, and follow-up surveys of ER viewers. The surveys assessed viewers' knowledge gain, their retention of health information, and their interest in health-related stories and actions taken based on the storylines.

Study results indicate that viewer knowledge increased as a result of the ER episodes. For example, after an episode with a 1-minute story line on emergency contraception, the percentage of viewers who were aware of emergency contraception increased from 50 to 67 percent, and 20 percent of viewers noted that they had learned about the issue from ER. This effect, however, decreased to baseline levels 2 months later. Similar knowledge gains occurred after a short vignette focused on a sexually transmitted disease (STD) caused by human papilloma virus (HPV). HPV is the most common cause of STDs in the country, and it has been linked to more than 95 percent of all cases of cervical cancer. The proportion of ER viewers who had heard of HPV increased from 24 to 47 percent, and 32 percent who had heard of HPV noted that they had learned about it from ER. One month later this effect had decreased but remained above preshow levels; 38 percent of those surveyed reported having heard of HPV, and 16 percent could give a correct description of HPV. Furthermore, the study found that slightly more than half (51 percent) of the regular viewers surveyed were prompted to discuss health issues presented on the show with friends and family, and one in five viewers reported turning to other sources for more information about a health issue presented on ER (Brodie et al., 2001).

Among their conclusions, the researchers noted that although entertainment television is a powerful medium for reaching a diverse and large audience on a regular basis, fictional depiction for the sake of dramatic effect could give viewers inaccurate information or lead them to misperceptions about health issues. This observation confirms the need for a present and competent public health partner to ensure that health information is accurate or to counteract misleading storylines.

As noted above, the increase in knowledge of emergency contraception and HPV decreased over time. This suggests that media initiatives that introduce health messages into entertainment programming should be conceived as ongoing projects because the effects may be short-lived. The example described in the next section shows how *ER* storylines are leveraged to continue health information dissemination and discussion at the local level.

Following ER: The Audience Is Still Watching

Another unique effort to disseminate health messages using television leveraged health-related storylines on *ER* and linked them to health segments that were broadcast on local news stations after *ER*. The *Following ER* health news series initiative aimed to educate and motivate viewers to take action on health issues. The series was sponsored by the Kaiser Family Foundation and implemented by the Johns Hopkins Health Institutions. News staff from NBC affiliate WBAL in Baltimore provided the news reporting. News segments included a 90-second news broadcast that instructed viewers on how to prevent the type of disease or injury depicted in *ER*'s weekly episode. The segments also provided viewers with information about the resources of national organizations or health experts in the form of toll-free numbers or Internet addresses. *Following ER* ran for 4 years and reached an average weekly viewership of 1.7 million.

The use of entertainment media as a strategy for providing health information is well founded. In 1999, the case for presenting health information through entertainment was strengthened by a CDC study of the Healthstyles Survey Database. Healthstyles is a proprietary database developed by Porter Novelli, a social marketing and public relations firm. The database contains responses to the Healthstyles survey. The sample for the survey is drawn from the DDB Needham Lifestyles Survey, which bases its sampling on seven characteristics of the Bureau of the Census, considered by most market research experts to create a sample that best represents the U.S. population (CDC, 2000).

Results of the CDC analysis indicate that viewers of soap operas report that television is a major source of health information. Viewers report that they learn about health topics from soap operas and take positive action as a result. Women and African Americans, who are among the groups with the largest representation among regular soap opera viewers, report the highest rates of learning and action as a result of soap opera viewing (see

---

BOX 7–2
Selected Findings from the 1999 Healthstyles Survey

Regular viewers report that they learned something about a disease or how to prevent it from the following television entertainment shows in the past year:
- Soap operas (48 percent)
- Prime-time television shows (41 percent)
- Television talk shows (38 percent)

More than one-third (34 percent) of regular viewers took one or more actions after hearing something about a health issue or disease on a soap opera in the past year:
- Told someone about it (25 percent)
- Told someone to do something to prevent the health problem (13 percent)
- Visited a clinic or a doctor (7 percent)
- Did something to prevent the problem (6 percent)

Regular viewers seek out and attend to health information more than nonviewers. They:
- Bring up something with their doctor that they read or hear is relevant to their health (63 percent versus 52 percent)
- Make a point to read and watch stories about health (46 percent versus 38 percent)
- Call a toll-free number or hotline for health information (19 percent versus 13 percent)
- Find out more about a health problem for someone else (57 percent versus 48 percent)

SOURCE: CDC (2000).

Box 7–2). Many people report that the information that they receive in the media has an important influence, often indirectly or directly affecting their behavior. Public health officials, however, are typically trained primarily in the sciences and not in using media channels to promote health or convey health information. This disconnect can give rise to confusion and less than optimal utilization of the media to promote public health goals. Consequently, **the committee recommends that public health officials and local and national entertainment media work together to facilitate the communication of accurate information about disease and about medical and health issues in the entertainment media.**

Recognizing the powerful impact of the entertainment media in conveying health information and messages, a number of health agencies and other groups are working to acknowledge the efforts of the Hollywood community. CDC, for example, established the Sentinel for Health Award for Daytime Drama (CDC, 2002b) to recognize exemplary achievements of daytime dramas that inform, educate, and motivate viewers to make choices for healthier and safer lives. CDC also funds the Hollywood, Health, and Society program at the University of Southern California Annenberg Norman Lear Center (University of Southern California, 2002). The program seeks to combine public health expertise with entertainment industry knowledge and outreach. Similarly, The Media Project, operated jointly by the Kaiser Family Foundation and Advocates for Youth, has worked for years to promote accurate descriptions of reproductive health issues in television shows and also administers an awards program. The SHINE Awards (Sexual Health IN Entertainment) honor those in the entertainment industry who do an exemplary job of incorporating accurate and honest portrayals of sexuality into their television, film, and music video programming (The Media Project, 2002). The Entertainment Industries Council, Inc., in partnership with the Robert Wood Johnson Foundation and the National Institute on Drug Abuse of the National Institutes of Health, sponsors the PRISM Awards (www.eiconline.org). These awards honor the correct depiction of drug, alcohol, and tobacco use in television and feature films, music, and comic books. The committee applauds efforts to recognize and highlight the contributions of the entertainment media in conveying accurate health information and messages as part of their programming activities.

Strong partnerships between the health community and the entertainment media are also important because they provide not only an opportunity to promote positive health messages but also an opportunity to educate the entertainment media about the impact of negative health messages on viewers, especially children. According to a 1998 Nielsen report on television viewing, the average child or adolescent watches an average of nearly 3 hours of television per day. Coupled with children's general vulnerability, this makes them especially susceptible to the messages conveyed through television.

A growing body of evidence associating the portrayal of violence in the entertainment media with increased aggression in young people, for example, has led a number of governmental and nongovernmental bodies to express concern regarding the amount of violence in the entertainment media. Those voicing concerns include the U.S. Surgeon General (1972), the National Institute of Mental Health (1982), the American Psychological Association (1993), and the American Academy of Pediatrics (2001). Concerns have also been expressed about the entertainment media's depictions of cigarettes, alcohol, and illicit drug use, sexual behavior, and body concepts because of their potentially negative impacts on children (Roberts, 2000).

Given the important influence of the entertainment media on children and adults, the committee joins the voices of concern raised by other governmental and nongovernmental bodies and encourages entertainment television writers to refrain from glamorizing tobacco, alcohol, and drug use or violence and to incorporate appropriate contextual elements in such programming whenever possible.

The Internet

The Internet is rapidly and radically transforming many aspects of society, including reshaping how information is accessed and shared (NRC, 2000). In the health arena, interactive health communication, or the interaction of an individual—consumer, patient, caregiver, or professional—with an electronic device or communication technology to access or transmit health information or receive guidance and support on a health-related issue, is growing at a rapid pace (Robinson et al., 1998). Consumer health in particular is one area that is being reshaped by interactive health communication. Consumer health refers to a set of activities aimed at empowering consumers in their own health and health care. Activities in this area include the provision of health information, the development of tools for self-assessment of health risks and management of chronic diseases, and home-based monitoring of health status and delivery of care (NRC, 2000).

A recent study of interactive health communication applications conducted by the Science Panel on Interactive Communication and Health, convened by the Office of Disease Prevention and Health Promotion of the Department of Health and Human Services, examined the current status of interactive health communication and its potential to promote health. In its consensus statement, the panel identified 12 potential advantages of using the Internet for health communication (Robinson et al., 1998). These potential advantages are listed in Box 7–3.

The panel also identified six specific functions of interactive health communication, which are listed in Box 7–4. These functions of interactive health communication have been noted by consumers as well as public- and private-sector organizations. According to a recent Harris Poll, an estimated 101 million U.S. web users have sought health care information online in the past year, up from 97 million in 2001 (Harris Poll, 2002). Web users also turn to the Internet to find social support (Bly, 1999). Foote and Etheredge (2002), in a study conducted to identify strategies to improve consumer health information services, found that insurers, provider organizations, consumer groups, foundations, and public-sector agencies are now sponsoring initiatives to strengthen these services. They note as an example that some insurers and provider organizations offer consumer-focused websites, preventive care and disease management outreach programs, and peer support programs for patients and caregivers. Some of the new peer support programs include meetings in person or online, introducing pa-

---

BOX 7–3
Benefits of Interactive Health Communication

1. Improved opportunity to find information tailored to the specific needs or characteristics of individuals or groups of users (Harris, 1995).
2. Improved capabilities of various media to be combined with text, audio, and visuals and of matching specific media to the particular purposes of the intervention or the learning styles of users (Harris, 1995).
3. Increased possibility for users to remain anonymous by providing access to sensitive information that people may be uncomfortable acquiring in a public forum or during a face-to-face discussion. Computer-based interfaces also can increase a participant's willingness to engage in frank discussions about health status, behavioral risks, fears, and uncertainties (Robinson, 1989; Locke et al., 1992; Gustafson et al., 1993; General Accounting Office, 1996).
4. Increased access to information and support on demand because these resources often can be used at any time and from numerous locations (Harris, 1995; General Accounting Office, 1996).
5. Increased opportunity for users to interact with health professionals or to find support from others similarly situated through the use of networking technologies such as e-mail, which enables direct communication between individuals, despite distance or structural barriers (Robinson, 1989; Harris, 1995; General Accounting Office, 1996; Pingree et al., 1996).
6. Enhanced ability for widespread dissemination and for expanding an audience at a limited incremental cost once the necessary hardware infrastructure is in place (General Accounting Office, 1996; Eng et al., 1998).

SOURCE: Robinson et al. (1998).

BOX 7–4
Functions of Interactive Health Communication

- Relay health information in a generalized or individualized way
- Enable informed decision making
- Promote healthful behaviors
- Promote peer information exchange and emotional support
- Promote self-care
- Manage demand for health services

---

tients to "buddies" who have similar medical experiences, chat rooms, bulletin boards, customized websites with online tutorials, links to other relevant websites, referral information to local resources, e-mail access to experts and peers, and computerized management support tools.

Although the potential benefits of interactive health communication applications are many, the growing volume and use of these applications also raise several concerns. This section briefly highlights three areas of concern: (1) the quality of information, (2) the digital divide, and (3) the privacy and confidentiality of personal health information.

A recent National Research Council (NRC) committee charged with studying the Internet and health applications noted the need for tools to help consumers find information of interest and evaluate its quality (NRC, 2000). The sheer volume of health information on the Internet, the NRC committee noted, can be overwhelming. For example, a simple web search for "diabetes mellitus" returned more than 40,000 web pages, and some 61,000 websites contain information on breast cancer (Boodman, 1999). The committee emphasized that consumers need effective searching and filtering tools that can help identify and rank information according to their needs and capabilities and present it in a form they can understand, regardless of educational or cultural background. Consumers also need a way to judge the quality, authoritativeness, and origin of the information. Because the Internet allows anyone to publish information, filtering and credentialing become extremely important. The Scientific Panel on Interactive Health Communication, for example, has called for disclosure statements on websites to make it easier for consumers to evaluate the source and authority of information resources. Other efforts to help consumers evaluate health-related websites focus on systems for classifying information according to characteristics such as accuracy, timeliness, completeness, and clarity (NRC, 2000). Mitretek Systems' Information Quality Tool, a tool that helps educate consumers by evaluating a website's strengths and weaknesses, is an example of such an effort (Mitretek Systems, 2002).

The digital divide is another area of concern that must be addressed if disparities in access to interactive health communication are to be overcome. The digital divide refers to the experiences of two groups of people: one group has access to information technology and relevant training to use that technology; the other group, for a variety of reasons, does not have access to such technology and is not trained to use it. The difference between these two groups of people is what has been called the "digital divide" (NTIA, 2002). A recent Pew Internet Project study reported that the digital divide is narrowing. Internet use is becoming more available to women and minorities. The African-American population online grew 8 percent during the first half of 2000. A large portion of the increase came from African-American women: 45 percent of African-American women had Internet access in November and December, whereas 34 percent had Internet access at midyear (May to June). Access to the Internet also increased for African-American men and access by the Hispanic population increased by 7 percentage points (Fox, 2001).

Even if access to information services were to improve for all groups, disparities could continue to exist because many individuals have low levels of literacy or problems with the English language. Developers of web-based information sites and interactive health applications need to consider that approximately one of five Americans is functionally illiterate and unable to comprehend written materials. One study (Berland et al., 2001) found that the average reading level of English-language websites was collegiate and ranged from 10th grade to graduate school level. Similarly, website developers and those using the Internet to provide health information and applications should consider the growing diversity of the U.S. population and globalization. In response to this problem, federal efforts are under way to develop agency-related non-English-language websites that are accessible to all persons who, as a result of national origin, are not proficient in English or are limited in their ability to communicate in the English language (White House, 2000). Illustrative of the response to the Executive Order is the Department of Health and Human Services' Spanish-language Healthfinder, a guide to health information, and the Food and Drug Administration's efforts to provide food and cosmetic information in 17 languages.

Protection of the privacy and confidentiality of personal health information is a challenge for Internet health communication activities. According to consumer surveys, individuals feel very strongly about keeping their health concerns private. They must have confidence that information that is collected, stored, and made available online is protected. If the information is shared, it should be shared only with a health professional with the capacity and commitment to maintain complete confidentiality (Patrick et al., 1999). Policy making at the federal and other levels is under way to develop steps that will ensure the secure, private, and confidential transmission of information.

This section has focused primarily on the Internet as a medium for personal health care information. The Internet also provides access to a number of data resources that focus on population health. CDC WONDER serves as a single point of access to a variety of CDC public health information that can be valuable in public health research, decision making, priority setting, program evaluation, and resource allocation and for informing the public at large (http://wonder.cdc.gov). Similarly, the Department of Health and Human Services, in collaboration with the Association of State and Territorial Health Officials, National Association of County and City Health Officials, and the Public Health Foundation, manages a website that provides access to community health status indicators (NACCHO, 2002). The Community Health Status Indicators Project was developed in response to community-based requests for data to assess health, plan programs, and develop data-based health policy. Individuals and community groups can access the site for health-related and other data for each of the 3,082 U.S. counties.

More recently, the Internet has become an important tool for providing real-time access to critical information. CDC, for example, webcasts critical briefings on bioterrorism through the site www.bt.cdc.gov. In late September 2002, the site provided a full copy of the revised *Smallpox Response Plan and Guidelines* (CDC, 2002a), an online telebriefing that discusses the plan and that provides a transcript of the briefing and a press release. Another Internet-based initiative is the University of North Carolina School of Public Health's Public Health Grand Rounds, sponsored by CDC (University of North Carolina, 2002) . Grand Rounds covers a variety of public health topics including bioterrorism preparedness. Webcasts are available for simultaneous downlink to a personal computer anywhere in the world. Part of the show allows viewers to call in or e-mail questions. Moreover, webcasts are followed up for 3 weeks with a postshow web forum so that viewers can continue to ask questions and receive answers, share best practices, and network with other participants. These activities can be conducted individually or in groups.

Strategies That Use Media Tools to Promote Population Health

Thus far, this chapter has discussed the use of specific media channels to promote health and has shown how certain media programs have influenced health-related behaviors. Given the prominence of media communication in people's lives, some scholars have argued that the public's health is best served by focusing public health resources on media strategies. These strategies place at the center of their activities the use of media communication to shape public opinion and promote health. By using media communication, the health of the public can be promoted in cost-effective and sustainable ways. Two of the most prominent of these strategies are social marketing and media advocacy.

Social Marketing

Social marketing is an approach that attempts to apply advertising and marketing principles to "sell" positive health behaviors (Kotler and Zaltman, 1971; Kotler and Roberto, 1989; Kotler et al., 2002). Social marketing combines marketing concepts with social influence theories to motivate individuals to change their behavior. Drawing from variables used to plan traditional marketing strategies, social marketing has reinterpreted them for use in planning how to "sell" health objectives (Wallack, 1990). In commercial business, marketing is about getting the right product (what you sell), at the right price (what the consumer pays), in the right place (where it is sold), at the right time, and in such a way as to successfully satisfy the needs of the consumer (what you do to attract the buyer) (Cannon, 1986; Hastings and Haywood, 1991; NCI, 2002). Marketing techniques use the consumer or target audience as the central focus to plan and conduct a marketing program. In social marketing for improved health outcomes, these marketing variables (the "four P's") take on the following definitions:

- "Product" might be defined as the behavior that the program is trying to change within the target audience; more specifically, it could be safer sex or nonsmoking.
- "Price" represents what the consumer must give up to accept the health promoter's offering. Price might include the monetary, time, psychological, or physical costs to the consumer.
- "Place" concerns the distribution channels used to reach the consumer; these could be the mass media, the community, or interpersonal channels of communication.
- "Promotion" is the means (e.g., media outreach and testimonials) by which the health promoter communicates the product to the consumer (Leathar et al., 1986; NCI, 2002) and the benefits of adopting this new product (e.g., practicing safe sex or not smoking).

These variables in an AIDS initiative, for example, could translate into condoms as the product, a free price, health centers, clinics, or schools as the place, and advertising and personal selling for promotion (Leathar et al., 1986).

Key to the social marketing approach is rigorous up-front planning and research, with engineering-style decision making found in traditional marketing processes. At a minimum, the problem and objectives must be clearly defined and stated, the consumer must be heard, and the product must be responsive to consumer needs (Walsh et al., 1993).

Formative research is an important tool used throughout the social marketing process to ensure that consumers are heard and that the product is responsive to their needs. Formative research, for example, can provide consumer input early in the design of a program to better define the nature of the problem to be tackled and to specify the goals. It can also be used to conduct an analysis of the audience for segmentation—the process of partitioning a heterogeneous population into groups or segments of people with similar needs, experiences, or other characteristics. Formative research can also be used to measure the media-viewing habits of the target population so that messages can be placed in the right media, to assess preexisting knowledge and attitudes for specific segments of the population, and to test possible campaign slogans for cultural sensitivity. Lastly, formative research can provide feedback throughout the entire process through surveys, interviews, and focus groups that lead to improvements in the marketing of positive health behaviors or objectives. Evaluation is a critical component of social marketing that assesses whether the product was successfully marketed to the target audience at the right price and place and through the most effective promotion strategies to result in improved health outcomes. As a result, formative research allows the consumer to guide the entire social marketing process (Leathar et al., 1986; Wallack, 1990; Walsh et al., 1993).

In addition to the four P's described above, social marketing adds three more "P's" to influence health behaviors that benefit the target audience and the public at large. These include partnership, policy, and politics:

- "Partnership" involves the identification and interaction of multiple organizations and agencies that share similar goals and that can work together to reach the target audience more effectively. Promoting and sustaining healthy behaviors, such as physical activity among children, requires the participation of all interested parties, including health care providers and clinics, schools, communities, faith-based organizations, and others.
- "Policy" recognizes the need for social and environmental changes to support individual behavioral change. Without supportive policies, social marketing campaigns cannot be sustained. Making convenience stores accountable to the laws regarding the selling of cigarettes to minors is an example of how policy supports a campaign to decrease underage smoking in a particular community.
- "Politics" involves the recognition and strategies incorporated to gain political support for a campaign or ensure political diplomacy within the targeted community and across interested parties. Social marketing programs often target complex and controversial issues, such as gun safety initiatives, that require understanding, involvement, and support from outside organizations or parties who may limit or hinder the program's reach if they are not identified and approached early (Weinreich, 1999).

When a social marketing campaign is being developed, the planning process follows the same steps identified above for general health communication strategies. The needs and perceptions of the consumer remain the primary focus in developing a campaign or program. The process starts with (1) planning and strategy selection, followed by (2) the selection of channels and materials, (3) the development of materials and pretesting, (4) implementation, (5) assessment of effectiveness, and (6) feedback to refine the program. The process is circular, with the last stage feeding back into the first one so that the campaign or program is constantly learning and improving on the basis of past experiences, successes, and failures (Valente and Schuster, 2002).

One example of a social marketing approach is the ABC Immunization Calendar program developed by the Health Communication Research Laboratory at St. Louis University in Missouri. In response to the fact that less than half of children ages 2 and younger are fully immunized in most major U.S. cities, the ABC Immunization Calendar program was developed to raise immunization rates among children from families in lower socioeconomic groups—the targeted audience (Zell et al., 1994). Based on evidence that more patient-oriented approaches by providers have been recommended and that computer-generated educational materials that are tailored to individuals are more likely to be read, remembered, saved, and discussed and to lead to changes in behavior, especially among poor and underserved populations, the program provides computer-made immunization promotion calendars tailored to each child (National Vaccine Advisory Committee, 1992; Skinner et al., 1994; Brug et al., 1996; Bull et al., 1999). The calendar includes the child's name, picture, height, and weight as well as room to track his or her growth, family birth dates, helpful hints, interesting facts about the child's living environment (e.g., use of car seats, limiting exposure to smokers, and the presence of smoke detectors in the house), the most recent and next immunization appointment, and appointments for future well-baby checkups.

The calendars were developed on the basis of interviews and focus group meetings with mothers of young children from communities of lower socioeconomic status who strongly supported the inclusion of a color photo of their child on the calendar. Because many families could not afford to have professional pictures taken of their child, the calendar fulfilled this need and was seen as a valuable and prized addition to the home. The calendars were printed on brightly colored paper and laminated for durability. Mothers would receive calendars for each of the months leading up to their children's next immunization appointment. When the child was vaccinated, new calendars were generated for the next appointment. As a result, the calendars provided an incentive for the family to keep appointments, come to the clinic, and have the child immunized.

To monitor the program's effectiveness, mothers who were given calendars, as well as the providers at participating health clinics, were asked about the perceived value and utility of the calendars, enrollment in the program, adherence to the immunization schedule in terms of keeping appointments, and overall immunization behavior. In the clinics and communities where the ABC Immunization Calendar program has been implemented, great strides have been made in increasing the number of immunized children. Multiple strategies at the state, clinic, and family or community levels, however, are needed to more effectively increase the rate of childhood immunization among families in lower socioeconomic groups. An immunization tracking database at the state level can help health care providers identify children who are not yet immunized, whereas clinics can offer immunizations during the evenings and weekends or at facilities in the community, such as a house of worship or community center, so that more parents have opportunities to have their children vaccinated. Coupled with these two components, the ABC Immunization Calendar program uses the focus and strategies of social marketing to more effectively engage parents and ensure higher rates of childhood immunization among low-income and underserved families.

The national Turning Point Initiative[3] understood the potential impact that social marketing initiatives can have on improving population health and formed a collaborative of partners to review and widely disseminate social marketing information to improve community health. A resource guide on social marketing is available from the Turning Point (2002) website.

A clear tension exists between social marketing and corporate marketing, especially when corporate advertising messages result in audience confusion. Corporation-sponsored ads that are health promoting can undermine public health media campaigns. Farrelly and colleagues (2002) found that corporation-sponsored "don't smoke" campaigns that target youth were associated with an increase in the intention to smoke in the next year. Landman and colleagues (2002) also concluded that tobacco industry programs that target youth do more harm than good for tobacco control. In Florida, tobacco program evaluators noted that Philip Morris ads confused youth viewers and interfered with the state-sponsored antismoking campaign.

> Since its commercials, which are preachy and poorly done, run in the same demographic buy as the "truth" commercials, which have already been established as irreverent and effective, Philip Morris' efforts have proven problematic. Many teens assume the Philip Morris ads are "truth" ads and have asked why the campaign has "gone lame." (Florida Department of Health, 1999)

As a result of such findings, antismoking associations such as the America Legacy Foundation (www.americanlegacy.org) have called for the removal of tobacco industry-supported "don't smoke" campaigns.

---

[3] The national Turning Point Initiative is sponsored by the Robert Wood Johnson Foundation and the Kellogg Foundation. Turning Point has established 21 state and 41 community-level partnerships to improve and strengthen the public health system. The Social Marketing Collaborative is a partnership of Turning Point members.

Media Advocacy

As discussed in Chapter 2, an increasing science base links social determinants to the health status of populations. Health behavior, in particular, has been shown to be linked to the larger social, political, and economic environments (Smedley and Syme, 2000). Media advocacy is a developing strategy that seeks to change social determinants of health, primarily public policy, rather than personal habits or behaviors. Specifically, media advocacy is defined as the strategic use of mass media and its tools, in combination with community organizing, to advance healthy public policies. The primary focus is on the role of the news media, with secondary attention to the use of paid advertising (DHHS, 1989; Wallack and Sciandra, 1990, 1991; Wallack et al., 1993; Chapman, 1994; Wallack, 1994; Wallack and Dorfman, 1996; Winett and Wallack, 1996). Media advocacy seeks to create a loud voice for social change and shape the message so that it resonates with social justice values that are the presumed basis of public health (Beauchamp, 1976; Mann, 1977). A wide range of grassroots community groups, public health leadership groups, public health and social advocates, and public health researchers have used media tools to effect social change that would influence health (Wallack et al., 1993, 1999; Woodruff, 1996).

Media advocacy differs in many ways from traditional public health campaigns. In particular, it emphasizes the following: [4]

- Linking public health and social problems to inequities in social arrangements rather than to flaws in the individual;
- Changing public policy rather than personal health behavior;
- Focusing primarily on reaching opinion leaders and policy makers rather than on those who have the problem (the traditional audience of public health communication campaigns);
- Working with groups to increase participation and amplify their voices rather than providing health behavior change messages; and
- Having a primary goal of reducing the power gap rather than just filling the information gap.

Media advocacy is generally seen as a part of a broader strategy rather than as a strategy per se and focuses on four primary activities in support of community organizing, policy development, and advancing policy:

---

[4] This section was previously published in *Speaking About Health: Assessing Health Communication Strategies for Diverse Populations* (IOM, 2002).

1. *Developing an overall strategy*: Media advocacy relies on critical thinking to understand and respond to problems as social issues rather than personal problems. Following problem definition, the focus is on elaborating policy options; identifying the person, group, or organization that has the power to create the necessary change; and identifying organizations that can apply pressure to advance the policy and create change. Finally, various messages for the different targets of the campaign are developed.

2. *Setting the agenda*: Getting an issue in the media can help set the agenda and provide legitimacy and credibility to the issue and the group. Media advocacy involves understanding how journalism works to increase access to the news media. This includes maintaining a media list, monitoring the news media, understanding the elements of newsworthiness, pitching stories and holding news events, and developing editorial strategies for reaching key opinion leaders.

3. *Shaping the debate*: The news media generally focuses on the plight of the victim, whereas policy advocates emphasize the social conditions that create victims. Health advocates frame policy issues using public health values that resonate with broad audiences. Some of the steps include "translat[ing] personal problems into public issues" (Mills, 1959); emphasizing social accountability as well as personal responsibility; identifying individuals and organizations that must assume a greater burden for addressing the problem; presenting a clear and concise policy solution; and packaging the story by combining key elements such as visuals, expert voices, authentic voices (those with experience with the problem), media bites, social math (creating a context for large numbers that is interesting to the press and understandable to the public), research summaries, fact sheets, policy papers, and so forth.

4. *Advancing the policy*: Policy battles are often long and contentious, and it is important to develop strategies to maintain the media spotlight on the policy issue on a continuing basis. This means identifying opportunities to reintroduce the issue to the media, such as on key anniversaries of relevant dates, upon publication of new reports, by providing notice of significant meetings or hearings, and by linking the policy solution to breaking news (Wallack, 2000; Dorfman and Woodruff, 2002).

To demonstrate when media advocacy is an appropriate strategy, Wallack and Dorfman (2000) provide the example given in Box 7–5. This example emphasizes that economic conditions had to change before individual behaviors could be expected to change.

The Coalition on Alcohol Outlet Issues (CAOI) in Oakland, California, is one group that has used media tools to secure passage and implementation of legislation designed to reduce crime around liquor stores (Seevak, 1997). Formed in 1993, the citywide coalition included a broad range of

---

BOX 7–5
Wallack and Dorfman's Example

5-a-Day campaigns have as their goal improving health status by increasing consumption of fruit and vegetables. This worthy goal will remain unattainable, despite the most persuasive communications campaign, if fruit and vegetables are not easily available and affordable. One local group in California wanted to initiate a local 5-a-Day campaign to improve the outcomes of teen pregnancies. When they sought our advice on administering a 5-a-Day campaign, we asked, "Where will the young women get the fruit and vegetables?" The major supermarkets have abandoned the inner-city neighborhoods that were home to the teens they wanted to reach, leaving nothing but corner liquor stores that stocked old and expensive fruit and vegetables, if they stocked them at all. We suggested they frame this from an economic development perspective and involve the teens in a campaign to demand the return of the grocers, to initiate a community garden, or other effort to create an environment in which they could make healthy choices for themselves and their families. In this example, a 5-a-Day social marketing campaign would make sense only after a campaign had been carried out to ensure the local availability of fruits and vegetables.

SOURCE: Wallack and Dorfman (2000).

---

community-based organizations and residents whose goals were to educate the community about alcohol outlet issues and to organize and generate support for Ordinance 11625. This ordinance would require liquor stores to pay an annual fee of $600 to cover the cost of an education, monitoring, and enforcement program to reduce problems associated with alcohol outlets such as violence, drug dealing, gambling, prostitution, vandalism, and other public health and safety problems. Ultimately, this ordinance would give the city authority to revoke the business permits of noncompliant liquor stores.

CAOI's membership included all racial and ethnic groups and mirrored the population mix of the city, especially the "flatland" areas with the lowest median household income; the largest number of public housing projects; the fewest grocery stores, community centers, and job opportunities; and three to five times as many liquor stores as the wealthier parts of the city. From the beginning, CAOI committed itself to keeping its members engaged in a well-organized and clear strategy to secure passage of the ordinance. The strategy also called for reaching out to the community and building support among members who would actively participate in CAOI's initiatives. The coalition used media tools to educate community members about the ordinance, demonstrate unity of opinion to policy makers, and identify "holes" in the arguments of the opposing side (i.e., the liquor industry's desire for profits over social and environmental improvements in the city). CAOI's strategy included meeting with public officials, testifying at hearings, providing well-prepared spokespersons, and holding demonstrations and rallies to which the media was always invited.

The coalition developed close relationships with journalists and other media outlets by providing newsworthy information, storylines, and testimonials. CAOI also prepared media or press kits for all journalists and easy access to coalition contacts. As a result, dozens of print, television, and radio stories were generated that secured the attention of policy makers and helped frame the issue as one of public safety and local control.

CAOI incorporated media tools with each step of the political process, including drafting the ordinance, securing passage by the City Council, and implementing the legislation. The coalition also helped fight off the legal and legislative tactics employed by the liquor industry, which sought to derail the ordinance by arguing that the city had overstepped its authority and had no legal right to pass such requirements on alcohol outlets. In the end, the California Supreme Court upheld the ordinance and ensured that cities and counties across California had tools to better regulate alcohol availability.

HEALTH COMMUNICATION CAMPAIGNS: THEORY, EVALUATION, AND RESEARCH NEEDS

In the twentieth century, large-scale health communication campaigns focused on the promotion of hygiene behaviors, safety and accident prevention, substance abuse prevention, adoption of healthy lifestyles and eating habits, family planning and contraceptive use, and many other topics (Valente and Schuster, 2002). Through mass media campaigns, health promoters try to accelerate behavioral change by informing the public (increasing knowledge), changing attitudes, and directly encouraging individuals to adopt healthy behaviors.

Theories Used to Understand Media Impact

Behavioral change theory plays an important role in the promotion of health by use of communication strategies (Valente, 2002). Theory indicates the types of messages that will more likely be successful by specifying how behavioral change occurs. For example, if theory indicates that adolescents smoke because they incorrectly perceive smoking to be popular, then successful programs will have to change these norms. In short, theory guides program and message design. Theory is also used to estimate how much impact can be expected from a health communication program. Estimates of impact are important for determining the sample size needed to conduct an appropriate evaluation to assess whether the program worked. Finally, theory can help determine why and how a health promotion program did or did not work (Valente, 2002). A short synopsis of relevant behavioral change and media impact theories follows.

Social Influence, Social Comparison, and Convergence Theories

Social influence, social comparison, and convergence theories proposed by social scientists specify that one's perception and behavior are influenced by the perceptions and behaviors of the members of groups to which one belongs. Peer group influences and social influences such as those presented through television and radio can affect the process of change and eventual conversion of behavior (Johns Hopkins University, 2003).

Health Belief Model

The health belief model is one of the oldest models developed to understand health-related behavioral change (Becker, 1974). It reflects a conscious decision-making process (Peterson and DiClemente, 2000). The model posits that two major factors influence the likelihood that a person will adopt a recommended health-protective behavior. First, the person must feel susceptible or threatened by the disease or condition, and a high level of severity must characterize the condition. Second, the person must believe that the benefits of taking the recommended action outweigh the perceived barriers (or costs) to performing the preventive action (IOM, 2002). The health belief model is believed to have been used more than any other health-related behavioral change model over the past decade (Peterson and DiClemente, 2000).

Diffusion of Innovation Theory

The diffusion of innovation theory describes the process by which an innovation, new ideas, opinions, attitudes, and behaviors are communicated through certain channels over time and spread among the members of a social system or community (Ryan and Gross, 1943; Katz et al., 1963; Rogers and Kincaid, 1981; Valente, 1993, 1995; Rogers, 1995; Valente and Rogers, 1995). Diffusion theory has been used to examine the spread of new computer technology, educational curricula, farming practices, family planning methods, medical technology, and many other innovations. Diffusion theory has five major assumptions: (1) adoption takes time; (2) people pass through various stages in the adoption process; (3) they can modify the innovation and sometimes discontinue its use; (4) the perceived characteris-

---

BOX 7–6
Critical Steps in Persuasion

1. Exposure and attention to the message
2. Comprehension of the message
3. Yielding to the message (personalizing the behavior to fit one's life and accepting the change)
4. Retaining the message
5. Acting to make the change and accepting the behavior in one's life

---

tics of the innovation influence its adoption; and (5) individual characteristics influence its adoption (Valente and Schuster, 2002). Rogers (1995) suggests that the mass media are quick, effective routes for introducing new information, especially in the early stages and with audiences that are predisposed to accepting new ideas.

Input–Output Persuasion Model

Formulated by William McGuire in 1969, the input–output persuasion model identifies five steps that are critical to how successful persuasion attempts will be in effecting change (see Box 7–6). The theory also considers how various aspects of communication such as the message design, source, and channel, as well as receiver characteristics, affect the behavioral outcome of communication (McGuire, 1969, 1981).

Theory of Reasoned Action

Proposed by Fishbein and Azjen in 1975, the theory of reasoned action specifies that the adoption of a behavior is a function of a person's intention to perform that behavior. The intention to perform a given behavior is, in turn, a function of a person's attitude toward performing the behavior (belief that performing the behavior will lead to certain outcomes and the expected value of the outcome) and of perceived social norms (belief that a specific individual or groups thinks that one should or should not perform the behavior in question) and motivations to comply (the degree to which, in general, one wants to do what the referent thinks one should do) (IOM, 2002).

Social Learning (Cognitive) Theory

According to the social learning (cognitive) theory model, four components are critical if behavioral change is to occur. First, an information component is needed to increase awareness and knowledge and to convince people that they have the ability to change behavior. Second, a motivational component is needed to develop social and self-regulatory skills to practice the new behavior. A third component enhances the development of social and self-regulatory skills (through the promotion of self-efficacy), and a fourth component develops or engages social supports for the individual making the change. Applied to communication through the mass media, the message gives audiences an opportunity to identify with characters who demonstrate (different or new) behaviors and allows them to engage the emotions and mentally rehearse and model the new behavior (Bandura, 1977, 1986; Peterson and DiClemente, 2000; IOM, 2002).

Theories of Emotional Response

As described by Zajonc, emotional response is believed to precede and condition cognitive and attitudinal effects. For communication strategies, this means that highly emotional messages would be more readily accepted by audience members and would more likely lead to behavioral change than messages that are low in emotional content.

Stages-of-Change Theory

The stages-of-change theory posits that several psychological stages can be observed in individuals who are making a behavioral change (Prochaska et al., 1992). Changes in behavior are believed to result when the psyche moves through several iterations of a spiral process. This process begins with precontemplation (not really considering making the change); continues with contemplation of making the change, preparation (intention to make the change), and action (making the change); and finally, ends with maintenance of the new behavior.

Cultivation Theory of Mass Media

George Gerbner proposed the cultivation theory of mass media in 1973. The theory proposes that repeated and intense exposure to definitions of "reality" in television and other mass media messages can lead to the perception of that reality as normal. The social legitimization of the reality presented can thus affect behavior (Gerbner, 1973, 1977; Gerbner et al., 1980).

Agenda Setting

The agenda-setting theory was made prominent by McCombs and Shaw (1972) and, more recently, by Dearing and Rogers (1996). The theory provides a framework for understanding how media influences the salience of an issue in the minds of audiences. The theory suggests that the pervasiveness of mass media and the passivity of audiences allow the media to shape opinions. Furthermore, the theory allows consideration of how media attention to specific issues (e.g., violent crime) that is disproportionate to objective measures (e.g., statistics on violence) can influence what an audience thinks.

Framing Theory

Drawing from the political and social sciences, framing theory suggests that the way in which information is framed can have a significant impact on the way that people process information and on their subsequent actions. As explained by Kinder and Berinsky (1999), "frames" are verbal, visual, or image devices used to focus and define a topic or issue in a particular way.

In the context of health communication, framing theory is used to develop strategies that will result in individual behavioral change or changes in public policy. For example, framing genetically linked cancers as a family issue as opposed to an individual issue could increase the impact of screening not only for the individual but also for the individual's blood relatives, allowing a "family-centered approach" to cancer screening (Sheila Murphy, Annenberg School of Communication, University of Southern California, personal communication, 2002). Similarly, different public policy options are required if violent actions are framed as isolated, random incidents or as a public health problem that takes into consideration population-based violence statistics in the context of other community indicators, such as the availability of firearms and alcohol and the degree of unemployment.

The theories reviewed here are the most common ones used in the health and medical fields (Glanz et al., 1997), and most of them acknowledge that the media can play some role in influencing human behavior. These theories can be used to understand how health information in the media affects the public's health, whether the information is received from deliberate media programming or from day-to-day behavior (IOM, 2002).

Evaluation and Research

Regardless of the media channels used to promote health, all health communication and promotion programs should be accompanied by evaluation and research activities designed to determine the impacts of the health promotion messages. This section provides a discussion of evaluation and research issues.

Evaluation

Evaluations of health communication and promotion programs should be systematic and participatory and should be designed to provide information that is useful for understanding whether the program worked, for whom, and to what degree and to provide information useful for deciding the appropriate next steps.

Evaluation frameworks such as Green and Kreuter (1991) and Valente (2002) can be used to plan evaluation activities. These frameworks generally call for needs assessment, formative research, monitoring, and summative research. The evaluation can be both qualitative and quantitative, but most importantly, it should be tailored so that it is appropriate to the intervention being evaluated. The tailoring requires that the evaluation be integrated into the design and implementation of the health communication activities.

Media-led interventions pose certain challenges for evaluation. First, for example, media communication cannot usually be restricted in its dissemination; thus, creating control groups can be challenging. Community-level evaluations have been conducted, but these often suffer from low statistical power. A second challenge is that media communication is often designed for specific audiences (e.g., teens, African Americans, or Hispanics) and so often cannot be replicated for other audiences or settings. A third challenge is to have the research and implementation teams integrated enough so that the evaluation team can respond to creative changes that occur in the intervention. McKenna and Williams (1993), for example, found that a CDC counteradvertising strategy based on subtle portrayal of the tobacco industry as manipulating teens to smoke did not communicate the message clearly to young teens. About 38 percent of those who viewed a campaign television spot believed that the main message promoted smoking. In conclusion, CDC researchers learned that it is important to obtain input from the target audience throughout the creative process and that more research is needed to better execute messages to target audiences.

Naturally, many other challenges face evaluators as they try to determine what works in the deliberate and not-so-deliberate communication of health information to the public (Valente, 2002). Behavioral change theory is useful for setting program goals and objectives, as these theories attempt to explain the motivations for human behavior. These objectives are then used to determine the study sample sizes needed to demonstrate program effectiveness. Selecting an appropriate study design (experimental versus quasiexperimental, community versus individual level) is a challenge and is often dictated by the planned intervention. For example, a program that uses billboards to communicate its message is delivered at the community level; thus, it is not possible to assign individuals randomly to the intervention.

The difficulty in health promotion program evaluation lies in the fact that every evaluation presents its own demands in terms of the trade-off between rigor and cost. Although randomized control trials are the "gold standard" for evaluating the impact of an intervention, they are rarely feasible for community- or population-based programs. Trade-offs between rigor and feasibility are inevitable and are best addressed by informed researchers who can control relevant threats to validity. Thus, there is a need not only to evaluate health promotion interventions but also to develop an evidence base for what works, among whom, and to what degree.

Research

Research on the effectiveness of media promotions for changing health-related behavior has been conducted for some time. The most commonly researched topics have been tobacco use, alcohol abuse, screening for cancer and other diseases, seat belt use, and the promotion of contraceptives and methods to prevent STDs. These studies have shown that the media can be used to increase knowledge about appropriate behaviors, create more positive attitudes toward the health behaviors, and lead to behavioral change among audience members. This triad of outcomes, knowledge (K), attitudes (A), and practices (P), has provided a convenient shorthand for guiding research on the effectiveness of media-driven health promotions. The degree of evidence for KAP models of behavioral change, however, is limited (Valente et al., 1998). Further research is needed to determine whether the KAP model is a useful one for understanding the impacts of media communication and what other models can or should be developed to understand media-generated behavioral change.

Regardless of the steps that precede behavioral change, media communication has been found to influence behavioral change. In a series of meta-analyses, Snyder (2001) has discovered that media communication about health have been shown to create about an 8-percentage-point change in behavior. Media communication creates more change when it promotes the adoption of new behavior (condom promotion) than when it attempts to get people to quit addictive behaviors (tobacco use). Research by Flynn and colleagues (1992, 1994) also suggests that media campaigns combined with other strategies such as school smoking prevention programs are effective in changing behavior. Thus, although the mechanisms for their effectiveness are not entirely understood, the media play a vital role in assuring the health of the public in the twenty-first century.

The top priority for the research agenda on the effect of media communication on health behavior is to conduct basic research on how the media influence individual health decisions as well as the public's health (Logan et al., 1999). This research would attempt to understand how media communications affect health-related behavior by understanding the steps to behavioral change and comparing different theories of behavioral change within a media intervention framework.

A second priority is to determine which media vehicles should be used for which purposes to determine the most effective way to communicate health information to the public. Most research has been conducted with the understanding that the mass media is useful for raising awareness and driving the public agenda, but behavioral decisions are also influenced by interpersonal communication. The interaction between interpersonal communication and media messages, however, is not well understood (Valente and Saba, 1998, 2001). For example, do the media prompt interpersonal discussions that then set in motion a series of behavioral change steps?

A third priority is to develop the evidence base for how health communication can better influence public policy. Research is needed particularly on the overall strategies of media advocacy and social marketing for effecting policy changes, in particular changes that may shape the social determinants of health. Research that can tease out the effects of media communication from community organizing and policy advocacy is also needed. Furthermore, a deeper understanding of which strategies are most appropriate and suited to which goals would be useful to public health practitioners. **The committee recommends that public health and communication researchers develop an evidence base on media influences on health knowledge and behavior, as well as on the promotion of healthy public policy.**

CONCLUDING OBSERVATIONS

In this age of information, there is good reason to acknowledge the potential of the mass media in assuring population health. Print and broadcast news media outlets, entertainment television, and the Internet constitute immensely influential channels through which people gather their information, accurate or not, about health. Given the speed and diversity of media outlets, they cannot be considered mere commentators in dialogues on popular culture about health, health risk, and health behaviors. They can foster and participate in informal interfaces (e.g., professional connections and contact points) and formal interfaces (e.g., fellowships and other cross-training for media and public health professionals) with academia. Also, the media and governmental public health agencies can enhance their understanding of each other's methods and perspectives (e.g., through communication between health officials and journalists or reporters). It is time that media outlets acknowledge their role in the public health system, the strength of their influence, and their potential for assuring the public's health.

REFERENCES

AAP (American Academy of Pediatrics). 2001. Children, Adolescents, and Television Policy Statement RE0043. Pediatrics 107(2):423–426.

AdAge. 2001. 100 leading national advertisers: ranked by total U.S. advertising spending in 2001. Available online at www.adage.com.

AHCJ (Association of Health Care Journalists). 2002a. Joint statement from the Association of Health Care Journalists and the National Association of Science Writers regarding proposed reorganization of Department of Health and Human Services. Minneapolis, MN. Available online at http://www.ahcj.umn.edu/cont.htm. Accessed October 16, 2002.

AHCJ. 2002b. Covering the Quality of Health Care—A Resource Guide for Journalists. Available online at http://www.ahcj.umn.edu/qualityguide/. Accessed March 18, 2003.

AIDS Project Los Angeles. 2001. Timeline of the AIDS epidemic. Available online at http://www.apla.org/apla/ed/TIMELINE.HTM. Accessed October 16, 2002.

American Opinion Research. 2002. Study of American Journalism and Public Issues. Princeton, NJ: Foundation for American Communications.

APA (American Psychological Association), Commission on Youth Violence. 1993. Violence and Youth: Psychology's Response. Washington, DC: American Psychological Association

Atkin C. 2001. Impact of Public Service Advertising: Research Evidence and Effective Strategies. Project conducted for Kaiser Family Foundation.

Balbach ED, Glantz SA. 1998. Tobacco control advocates must demand high-quality media campaigns: the California experience. Tobacco Control 7(4):397–408.

Bandura A. 1977. Social Learning Theory. Englewoods Cliffs, NJ: Prentice-Hall.

Bandura A. 1986. Social Foundations of Thought and Action. Englewood Cliffs, NJ: Prentice-Hall.

Bayer R, Gostin L, Javitt GH, Brandt A. 2002. Tobacco advertising in United States. Journal of the American Medical Association 287(22):2990–2995.

Beauchamp D. 1976. Public health as social justice. Inquiry 13:3–14.

Becker MH (Ed.). 1974. The health belief model and personal health behavior. Health Education Monographs 2(4):409–419.

Berger W. 2002. Shouting to be heard. Public Service Advertising in a New Media Age. Menlo Park, CA: The Henry J. Kaiser Family Foundation. Available online at http://www.kff.org/content/2002/20020221a/. Accessed March 15, 2002.

Berland G, Elliot M, Morales L, Algazy J, Kravitz RL, Broder MS, Kanouse DE, Munoz JA, Puyol JA, Lara M, Watkins KE, Yang H, McGlynn EA. 2001. Health information on the Internet: accessibility, quality, and readability in English and Spanish. Journal of the American Medical Association 285(20):2612–2621.

Bly L. 1999. A network of support. USA Today, July 14, pp. D1, D2.

Boodman SG. 1999. Medical web sites can steer you wrong. Washington Post, August 10, Health Section, p. 7.

Brodie M, Flournoy R, Altman D, Blendon R, Benson J, Rosenbaum M. 2000. Health information, the Internet, and the digital divide. Health Affairs 19(6):255–265. Available online at www.digitaldivide.gov.

Brodie M, Foehr U, Rideout V, Baer N, Miller C, Flournoy R, Altman D. 2001. Communicating health information through the entertainment media: a study of the television drama ER lends support to the notion that Americans pick up information while being entertained. Health Affairs 20(1):192–199.

Brug J, Steenhaus I, Van Assema P, de Vries H. 1996. The impact of a computer-tailored nutrition intervention. Preventive Medicine 25:236–242.

Bull F, Kreuter M, Scharff D. 1999. Effects of tailored, personalized, and general materials on physical activity. Patient Education and Counseling 36:181–192.

Cannon T. 1986. Basic Marketing: Principles and Practice. London: Holt, Rinehart and Winston.

CDC (Centers for Disease Control and Prevention). 1981a. Pneumocystis pneumonia—Los Angeles. Morbidity and Mortality Weekly Report 30:1–3.

CDC. 1981b. Kaposi's sarcoma and Pneumocystis pneumonia among homosexual men—New York City and California. Morbidity and Mortality Weekly Report 30:305–308.

CDC. 1981c. Follow-up on Kaposi's Sarcoma and Pneumocycstis Pneumonia. Morbidity and Mortality Weekly Report 30:409–410.

CDC. 1982. Epidemiologic Notes and Reports Possible Transfusion-Associated Acquired Immune Deficiency Syndrome (AIDS)—California. Morbidity and Mortality Weekly Report 31(48):652.

CDC. 2000. 1999 Healthstyles Survey: soap opera viewers and health information. Avilable online at http://www.cdc.gov/communication/healthsoap.htm. Accessed March 18, 2002.

CDC. 2001a. 1999 Healthstyles survey. Available online at www.cdc.gov/communication/healthsoap.htm. Accessed October 16, 2002.

CDC. 2001b. A glimpse at the colorful history of TB: its toll and its effect on the U.S. and the world. TB Notes 2000. Available online at HtmlResAnchor www.cdc/nchstp/ tb/notes.

CDC. 2002a. Smallpox Response Plan and Guidelines. Available online at www.cdc.gov/ smallpox. Accessed November 1, 2002.

CDC. 2002b. Communication at CDC: Entertainment Education. Available online at http:// www.cdc.gov/communication/entertainment_education.htm. Accessed March 31, 2002.

CDC Foundation. 2002. The Knight Public Health Journalism Fellowships. Website, Available online at http://www.cdcfoundation.org/programs/fellowships/ knight_leadership. html. Accessed March 18, 2002.

Chapman L. 1994. The Fight for Public Health: Principles and Practice of Media Advocacy. London: BMJ Publishing Group.

Clinton WJ. 2000. Improving access to services for persons with limited English proficiency. Executive Order 13166.

Dearing JW, Rogers EM. 1996. Agenda-Setting. Thousand Oaks, CA: Sage.

Dejong W, Wallack L. 1992. The role of designated driver programs in the prevention of alcohol-impaired driving: a critical reassessment. Health Education Quarterly 19:429–442.

Department of Health, Education, and Welfare. 1964. Smoking and Health: Report of the Advisory Committee to the Surgeon General of the Public Health Service. Office of the Surgeon General Publication 1103. Washington, DC: U.S. Public Health Service.

Department of Transportation. 1999. 8,500 billboards across America to remind motorists to buckle up. Available online at http://www.dot.gov/ affairs/1999/nhtsal299.htm. Accessed January 17, 2002.

DHHS (Department of Health and Human Services). 1989. Media Strategies for Smoking Control: Guidelines. DHHS Publication 89-3013. Washington, DC: Department of Health and Human Services.

DHHS. 2001. The public health infrastructure. In Healthy People 2010. Available online at http://www.health.gov/healthypeople/document/HTML/Volume. Accessed March 14, 2002.

DHHS. 2002. Healthfinder Espanol. Website. Available online at www.healthfinder.gov/ espanol. Accessed October 10, 2002.

Dorfman L, Wallack L. 1993. Advertising health: the case for counter-ads. Public Health Reports 108(6):716–726.

Dorfman L, Thorson E. 1998. Measuring the effects of changing the way violence is reported. Nieman Reports (Nieman Foundation for Journalism, Harvard University) 52(4):42–43.

Dorfman L, Woodruff K. 2002. Media Advocacy: A Tool for Changing Environments to Promote Public Health. Berkeley, CA: Berkeley Media Studies Group.

Dorfman L, Thorson E, Stevens JE. 2001. Reporting on violence: bringing a public health perspective into the newsroom. Health Education and Behavior 28(4):402–419.

Eng T, Maxfield A, Patrick K, Deering MJ, Ratzan SC, Gustafson DH. 1998. Access to health information and support—a public highway or a private road. Journal of the American Medical Association 280(15):1371–1375.

FACSNET (Foundation for American Communications). 2002. Journalist rate themselves 'not well prepared' to cover major issues. Available online at http://www.facsnet.org/about/survey.php3. Accessed July 29, 2002.

Farrelly MC, Healton CG, Davis KC, Messeri P, Hersey JC, Haviland ML. 2002. Getting to the truth: evaluating national tobacco countermarketing campaigns. American Journal of Public Health 92(6):901–907.

Fishbein M, Ajzen I. 1975. Belief, Attitude, Intention and Behavior: An Introduction to Theory and Research. Reading, MA: Addison-Wesley.

Fisher J, Fisher W. 2000. Theoretical approaches to individual-level change in HIV risk behavior, pp. 3–55. In Handbook of HIV Prevention. Peterson J, DiClemente R (Eds.). New York: Kluwer Academic/Plenum Publishers.

Florida Department of Health. 1999. Tobacco Pilot Program Progress Report. October 1, 1998 to December 31, 1998. Issued February 4, 1999.

Flynn BS, Worden JK, Secker-Walker RH, Badger GJ, Geller BM, Costanza MC. 1992. Prevention of cigarette smoking through mass media intervention and school programs. American Journal of Public Health 82(6):827–834.

Flynn BS, Worden JK, Secker-Walker RH, Pirie PL, Badger GJ, Carpenter JH, Geller BM. 1994. Mass media and school interventions for cigarette smoking prevention: effects 2 years after completion. American Journal of Public Health 84(7):1148–1150.

Foote S, Etheredge L. 2002. Strategies to Improve Consumer Health Information Services. Washington, DC: Health Insurance Reform Project.

Fox S. 2001. More online, doing more. The peer internet and American life project, Washington DC. Available online at http://www.pewinterest.org/. Accessed July 29, 2002.

GAO (General Accounting Office). 1996. Consumer Health Informatics: Emerging Issues. Report number AIMD-96-86. Washington, DC: Government Printing Office.

Gerbner G. 1977. Mass media policies in changing cultures. New York: Wiley.

Gerbner G, Gross LP, Melody WH. 1973. Communications Technology and Social Policy. New York: Wiley.

Gerbner G, Gross L, Morgan M, Signorelli N. 1980. The "mainstreaming" of America: violence profile no. 11. Journal of Communication 30(3):10–29.

Gilliam F. 1995. The color of crime in California: trends in arrests, dispositions, and victimization. Unpublished manuscript. University of California, Los Angeles.

Glanz K, Lewis FM, Rimer B. 1997. Health Behavior and Health Education: Theory, Research, and Practice. San Francisco, CA: Jossey-Bass.

Gottlieb M, Eichenwald K, Barbanel J. 1997. Health care's giant: powerhouse under scrutiny—a special report: biggest hospital operator attracts federal inquiries. New York Times, July 29, 2002.

Green LW, Kreuter MW. 1991. Health Promotion Planning. Mountain View, CA: Mayfield Publishing Company.

Gustafson DH, Wise M, McTavish F, Taylor JO, Wolberg W, Stewart J, Smalley RV, Bosworth K. 1993. Development and pilot evaluation of a computer-based support system for women with breast cancer. Journal of Psychosocial Oncology 11(4):69–93.

Harris LM. 1995. Health and the New Media: Technologies Transforming Personal and Public Helath. Mahwah, NJ: Lawrence Erlbaum Associates.

Harris Interactive. 2002. Cyberchondriacs continue to grow in America. Health Care News 2(9):1. Available online at http://www.harrisinteractive.com/news/newsletters/healthnews/HI_HealthCareNews2002Vol2_Iss09.pdf. Accessed May 22, 2003.

Hartz J, Chappell C. 1997. Worlds apart. First Amendment Center, Nashville, TN. Available online at www.freedomforum.org. Accessed October 5, 2002.

Harvard School of Public Health Center for Health Communication. 1999. The Harvard Alcohol Project's designated driver campaign. Available online at http://www.hsp.harvard.edu/chc/alcohol.html. Accessed January 10, 2002.

Hastings G, Haywood A. 1991. Social marketing and communication in health promotion. Health Promotion International 6(2):135–145.

Hu T, Sung H, Keeler TE. 1995. Reducing cigarette consumption in California: tobacco taxes vs. an anti-smoking media campaign. American Journal of Public Health 85(9):1218–1222.

IOM (Institute of Medicine). 2002. Introduction, pp. 22–23. In Speaking of Health: Assessing Health Communication Strategies for Diverse Populations. Washington, DC: The National Academies Press.

Johns Hopkins University. 2003. Theoretical Framework. Website. Available online at http://www.jhuccp.org/research/theory.shtml. Accessed March 18, 2003.

Joseph SC. 2002. Improving public health capabilities in interacting with the media: an urgent issue in the current context of terrorism. Summary proceedings of a discussion conference convened at the Columbia Graduate School of Journalism, June 17–18, 2002.

Kaiser Family Foundation. 1996. Covering the epidemic: AIDS in the media 1985–1996: a content analysis. Princeton Survey Research Associates. Available online at www.kff.org/content/archive/1157. Accessed January 14, 2002.

Kaiser Family Foundation. 2002a. Shouting to Be Heard: Public Service Advertising in a New Media Age. Menlo Park, CA: Kaiser Family Foundation.

Kaiser Family Foundation. 2002b. Kaiser media fellowships in health. Website. Available online at http://www.kff.org/docs/fellowships. Accessed October 18, 2002.

Katz E, Levine ML, Hamilton H. 1963. Traditions of research on the diffusion of innovation. American Sociological Review 28:237–253.

Kees B. 2002. Newsroom training: where's the investment?. Survey Context, Analysis and Commentary, November 22, 2002. The Poynter Institute. Available online at http://www.poynter.org/content/content_view.asp?id=10841. Accessed March 18, 2003.

Kinder D, Berinsky A. 1999. Making sense of issues through frames. The Political Psychologist 4(2):3–8.

Koop CE. 2002. Virtual Office of the Surgeon General C. Everett Koop (1982–1989). Available online at http://www.surgeongeneral.gov/library/history/biokoop.htm. Accessed January 16, 2002.

Kotler P, Zaltman G. 1971. Social marketing: an approach to planned social change. Journal of Marketing 35:3–12.

Kotler P, Roberto E. 1989. Social Marketing: Strategies for Changing Public Behavior. New York: Free Press.

Kotler P, Roberto N, Lee N. 2002. Social Marketing: Improving the Quality of Life. Thousand Oaks, CA: Sage Publications.

LaMay A. 2002. Shouting to be heard: public service advertising in a new media age. Background Papers, February 2002. Menlo Park, CA: Kaiser Family Foundation. Available online at http://www.kff.org/content/2002/3153a/BackgroundPapers.KaiserPSAs.pdf.pdf. Accessed March 13, 2003.

Landman A, Ling PM, Glantz SA. 2002. Tobacco industry youth smoking prevention programs: protecting the industry and hurting tobacco control. American Journal of Public Health 92(6):917–930.

Langlieb AM, Cooper CP, Gielen A. 1999. Linking health promotion with entertainment television. American Journal of Public Health 89(7):1116–1117.

Larsson A, Oxman AD, Carling C, Herrin J. 2001. Journalist and doctor: different aims, similar constraints. PressWise, Available online at http://www.presswise.org.uk/Health%20report%20survey.htm. Accessed October 11, 2002.

Leaman L. 1998. Motel Families Report. Orange County, CA: Social Services Administration.

Leathar DS, Hastings GB, O'Reilly KM, Davies JK (Eds.). 1986. Health Education and the Media II. New York: Pergamon Press.

Lewitt E, Coate D, Grossman M. 1981. The effects of government regulation on teenage smoking. Journal of Law and Economics 24(3):541–573.

Locke SE, Kowaloff HB, Hoff RG, Safran C, Popovsky MA, Cotton DJ, Finkelstein DM, Page PL, Slack WV. 1992. Computer-based interview for screening blood donors for risk of HIV transmission. Journal of the American Medical Association 268(10):1301–1305.

Logan RA, Longo DR. 1999. Rethinking antismoking media campaigns: two generations of research and issues for the next. Journal of Health Care Finance 25:77–90.

Lynch BS, Bonnie R (Eds.). 1994. Growing up Tobacco Free. Washington, DC: National Academy Press.

Mann JM. 1997. Medicine and public health, ethics and human rights. Hastings Center Report 27(3):6–13.

McCombs M, Shaw D. 1972. The agenda-setting function of mass media. Public Opinion Quarterly 36(2):176–187.

McGuire, W. 1981. Theoretical foundations of campaigns. pp. 41–70. In Rice R, Paisley W (Eds.). Public Communication Campaigns. Beverly Hills, CA: Sage.

McGuire WJ. 1969. Attitudes and attitude change. In Lindzey G, Aronson E (Eds.). Handbook of Social Psychology. Vol. 2. Reading, MA: Addison-Wesley.

McKenna JW, Williams KN. 1993. Crafting effective tobacco counteradvertisements: lessons from a failed campaign directed at teenagers. Public Health Reports 108(Suppl. 1):85–89.

Mills C. 1959. The Sociological Imagination. New York: Oxford University Press.

Mitretek Systems. 2002. Information Quality Tool. Website. Available online at http://hitiweb.mitretek.org/iq/. Accessed March 18, 2003.

NACCHO (National Association of County and City Health Officials). 2003. Community Status Indicators Project. Available online at http://www.naccho.org/project2.cfm. Accessed May 22, 2003.

National Center for Tobacco-Free Kids. 2002. Research and facts. Washington, DC. Available online at www.tobaccofreekids.org. Accessed July 29, 2002.

National Vaccine Advisory Committee. 1992. Access to Childhood Immunizations: Recommendations and Strategies for Action. Washington, DC: Department of Health and Human Services.

NCI (National Cancer Institute). 2002. Mass communication, and social marketing theories, models, and practices. Available online at http://rex.nci.nih.gov/ NCI_Pub_Interface/HCPW/INREO.HTM. Accessed May 3, 2001.

Nelkin D. 1996. Medicine and the media: an uneasy relationship: the tensions between medicine and the media. Lancet 347:1600–1603.

Nelkin D. 1998. Scientific journals and public disputes. Lancet 352(Suppl. 2):25–28.

Nelson D, Weiss R. 2000. Gene test deaths not reported promptly. Washington Post, January 31, p. A1.

NIMH (National Institute of Mental Health). 1982. Television and Behavior: 10 Years of Scientific Progress and Implications for the Eighties. Washington, DC: Government Printing Office.

NRC (National Research Council). 2000. Networking Health: Prescriptions for the Internet. Committee on Enhancing the Internet for Health Applications: Technical Requirements and Implementation Strategies. Washington, DC: National Academy Press.

NTIA (National Telecommunications and Information Administration). 2002. A Nation Online: How Americans Are Expanding Their Use Of The Internet. Washington, DC: NTIA. Available online at http://www.ntia.doc.gov/ntiahome/dn/index.html. Accessed March 18, 2003.

Paisley W. 2001. Public communication campaigns, pp. 3–21. In Rice R, Atkin C (Eds.). Public Communication Campaigns, 3rd ed. Thousand Oaks, CA: Sage.

Patrick K, Robinson TN, Alemi F, Eng T. 1999. Policy issues relevant to evaluation of interactive health communication applications. American Journal of Preventive Medicine 16(1):35–42.

Peterson JL, DiClemente RJ. 2000. Handbook of HIV Prevention, pp. 3–48. New York: Kluwer Academic/Plenum Publishers.

Pingree S, Hawkins RP, Gustafson DH, Boberg E, Bricker E, Wise M, Behre H, Hsu E. 1996. Will the disadvantaged ride the information highway? Hopeful answers from a computer-based health crisis system. Journal of Broadcasting and Electronic Media 40(3):331–353.

Proschaska JO, DiClemente CC, Norcross JC. 1992. In search of how people change: application to addictive behaviors. American Psychology 47:110–114.

Roberts DF. 2000. Media and youth: access, exposure, and privatization. Journal of Adolescent Health 27(2 Suppl):8–14.

Robinson TN, Patrick, K, Eng T, Gustafson D. 1998. An evidence-based approach to interactive health communication: a challenge to medicine in the information age. Journal of the American Medical Association 280(14):1264–1269.

Robinson TN. 1989. Community health behavior change through computer network health promotion: preliminary findings from Stanford Health-Net. Computer methods and programs in biomedicine 30(2–3):137–144.

Rogers E. 1983. Diffusion of Innovations. New York: Free Press.

Rogers EM. 1995. Diffusion of Innovations, 4th ed. New York: Free Press.

Rogers EM, Kincaid DL. 1981. Communication Networks: A New Paradigm for Research. New York: Free Press.

Rogers EM, Storey JD. 1987. Communication campaigns, pp. 817–846. In Berger CR, Chafee SH (Eds.). Handbook of Communication Science. Beverly Hills, CA: Sage.

Ruggiero D. 2000. A Glimpse at the Colorful History of TB: Its Toll and Its Effect on the U.S. and the World. In TB Notes, prepared by the Division for Tuberculosis Elimination, Centers for Disease Control and Prevention. Available online at http://www.cdc.gov/nchstp/tb/notes/TBN_1_00/TBN2000Ruggiero.htm. Accessed March 18, 2003.

Ryan B, Gross N. 1943. The diffusion of hybrid seed corn in two Iowa communities. Rural Sociology 8(1):15–24.

Saari L. 1998. Growing Up in "Toxic Communities." Orange County Register, August 2, 1998.

Schuman M. 2002. Journalists as change agents in medicine and health care. Journal of the American Medical Association 287:776–777.

Seevak A. 1997. Oakland shows the way: the coalition on alcohol outlet issues and media advocacy as a tool for change. Issue 3. Berkeley, CA: Berkeley Media Studies Group.

Sharf B, Freimuth V, Greenspan P, Plotnick C. 1996. Confronting cancer on Thirtysomething: audience response to health content on entertainment television. Journal of Health Communication 1(2):157–172.

Shine, KI (President, Institute of Medicine, the National Academies). 2001. Testimony at a Hearing on Risk Communication: National Security and Public Health, Subcommittee on National Security, Veteran Affairs, and International Relations, Committee on Government Reform, U.S. House of Representatives, Washington, DC, November 29.

Shuchman M. 2002. Journalists as change agents in medicine and health care. Journal of the American Medical Association 287(6):776.

Siegel M, Biener L. 2000. The impact of an antismoking media campaign on progression to established smoking: results of a longitudinal youth study. American Journal of Public Health 90:380–386.

Signorelli N. 1990. Television and health: images and impact, p. 96–113. In Atkin C, Wallack L (Eds.). Mass Communication and Public Health: Complexities and Conflicts. London: Sage.

Skinner CS, Strecher VJ, Hospers H. 1994. Physician's recommendations for mammography: do tailored messages make a difference? American Journal of Public Health 84(1):43–49.

Smedley BD, Syme SL. 2000. Promoting Health: Intervention Strategies from Social and Behavioral Research. Washington, DC: National Academy Press.

Snyder L. 2001. How effective are mediated health campaigns?, pp. 181–190. In Rice R, Atkin C (Eds.). Public Communication Campaigns, 3rd ed. Thousand Oaks, CA: Sage.

Stevens JE. 1998. The violence reporting project: a new approach to covering crime. Nieman Reports (The Nieman Foundation for Journalism, Harvard University) 52(4). Available online at http://www.nieman.harvard.edu/reports/98-4NRwint98/Stevens.html. Accessed June 13, 2002.

Taylor H. 2002. Internet penetration at 66% of adults (137 million) nationwide. Harris Interactive. Access online at www.harrisinteractive.com/harris_poll/ index.asp. Accessed October 11, 2002.

The Media Project. 2002. The Media Project-Entertainment Media's Sexual & Reproductive Health Resource. Website. Available online at http://www.themediaproject.com/shine/index.htm. Accessed March 18, 2003.

Turning Point. 2002. Turning Point, Collaborating for a New Century in Public Health. Social Marketing Resource Guide. Seattle, WA: Turning Point National Program Office, University of Washington. Available online at www. turningpointprogram.org. Accessed March 18, 2002.

TVinsite. 2001. Radio repeats for PSA title. Available online at http://www.tvinsite.com/08/13/2001&stt=001&display=searchResults. Accessed February 5, 2002.

University of North Carolina. 2002. Website. Available online at www.publichealthgrand rounds.unc.edu. Accessed October 18, 2002.

University of Southern California. 2002. Public Health Expertise Brought to Entertainment Industry by USC Annenberg's Norman Lear Center. Press release, April 2, 2002. Available online at http://ascweb.usc.edu/news.php?storyID=12. Accessed March 18, 2003.

U.S. Surgeon General's Scientific Advisory Committee on Television and Social Behavior. 1972. Television and Growing Up: The Impact of Televised Violence. Rockville, MD: National Institute of Mental Health.

Valente T. 2001. Evaluating communication campaigns, p. 105–124. In Rice R, Atkin C (Eds.). Public Communication Campaigns, 3rd ed. Thousand Oaks, CA: Sage.

Valente T, Schuster D. 2002. The public health perspective for communicating environmental issue. In Diets T, Stern P (Eds.). The Human Dimension of Global Change. Washington, DC: National Academy Press.

Valente TW. 1993. Diffusion of innovations and policy decision-making. Journal of Commu-
nication 43(1):30–41.
Valente TW. 1995. Network Models of the Diffusion of Innovations. Cresskill, NJ: Hampton
Press.
Valente TW. 2002. Evaluating Health Promotion Programs. New York: Oxford University
Press.
Valente TW, Rogers EM. 1995. The origins and development of the diffusion of innovations
paradigm as an example of scientific growth. Science Communication: An Interdiscipli-
nary Social Science Journal 16(3):238–269.
Valente TW, Saba W. 1998. Mass media and interpersonal influence in a reproductive health
communication campaign in Bolivia. Communication Research 25:96–124.
Valente TW, Saba W. 2001. Campaign recognition and interpersonal communication as
factors in contraceptive use in Bolivia. Journal of Health Communication 6(4):1–20.
Valente TW, Paredes P, Poppe PR. 1998. Matching the message to the process: The relative
ordering of knowledge, attitudes and practices in behavior change research. Human
Communication Research 24:366–385.
Versky A, Kahneman D. 1981. The framing decisions and the psychology of choice. Science
211:453–458.
Voss M. 2002. Checking the pulse: Midwestern reporters' opinions on their ability to report
health care news. American Journal of Public Health 92(7):1158–1160.
Wallack L. 1990. Improving health promotion: media advocacy and social marketing ap-
proaches, pp. 147–163. In Atkin C, Wallack L (Eds.). Mass Communication and Public
Health: Complexities and Conflicts. London: Sage.
Wallack L. 1994. Media advocacy: a strategy for empowering people and communities. Jour-
nal of Public Health Policy 15(4):420–435.
Wallack L. 2000. The role of mass media in creating social capital: a new direction for public
health. In Smedley B, Syme L (Eds.). Promoting Health: Intervention Strategies from
Social and Behavioral Research. Washington, DC: National Academy Press.
Wallack L, Dorfman L. 1996. Media advocacy: a strategy for advancing policy and promoting health. Health Education Quarterly 23(3):293–317.
Wallack L, Dorfman L. 2000. Putting policy into health communication: The role of media
advocacy, pp. 389–401. In Rice R, Atkin C (Eds.). Public Communication Campaigns,
3rd ed. Thousand Oaks, CA: Sage.
Wallack L, Sciandra R. 1990. Media advocacy and public education in the community trial to
reduce heavy smoking. International Quarterly of Community Health Education
11(3):205–222.
Wallack L, Dorfman L, Jernigan D, Themba M. 1993. Media Advocacy and Public Health:
Power for Prevention. Newbury Park, CA: Sage.
Wallack L, Woodruff K, Dorfman L, Diaz I. 1999. News for a Change: An Advocate's Guide
to Working with the Media. Thousand Oaks, CA: Sage.
Walsh Chapman D, Rudd R, Moeykens BA, Moloney TW. 1993. Social marketing for public
health. Health Affairs 12(2):104–119.
Warner K. 1979. Clearing the airwaves: the cigarette ban revisited. Policy Analysis 5:435–
450.
Weinreich NK. 1999. What is social marketing? Weinreich Communications. Available online
at http://www.social-marketing.com. Accessed February 11, 2002.
Whitaker R, Kong D, Globe Staff. 1998. Doing harm: research on the mentally ill. Boston
Globe, November 15, p. A1.
White House. 2000. Executive Order 13166: Improving Access to Services for Persons with
Limited English Proficiency. Available online at http://www.usdoj.gov/crt/cor/pubs/
eolep.htm. Accessed October 10, 2002.

Willman D. 2000. The new FDA: how a new policy led to seven deadly drugs. Los Angeles Times, December 20, p. 1.

Winnett L, Wallack L. 1996. Advancing public health goals through mass media. Journal of Health Communication 1(2):173–196.

Winsten JA, DeJong W. 2001. The Designated Driver Campaign. In RE Rice and CK Atkin (Eds.). Public Communication Campaigns Thousand Oaks, CA: Sage Publications.

Woloshin S, Schwartz LM. 2002. Press releases: translating research into news. Journal of the American Medical Association 287(21):2856–2858. (Reprinted.)

Woodruff K. 1996. Alcohol advertising and violence against women: a media advocacy case study. Health Education Quarterly 23(3):330–345.

Zell ER, Dietz V, Stevenson J, Cochi S, Bruce RH. 1994. Low vaccination levels of U.S. preschool and school-age children. Journal of the American Medical Association 271:833–839.

Zucker D, Hopkins R, Sly D, Urich J, Kershaw J, Solari S. 2001. "Florida truth" campaign: a counter-marketing, anti tobacco media campaign. Journal of Public Health Management Practice 6(3):1–6.

8

Academia

The health of the public during the twenty-first century can be assured only through the cooperation and collaboration of many individuals in diverse institutional settings, each of which has important contributions to make to this important and challenging endeavor. Among the recommendations in *The Future of Public Health* (IOM, 1988), several focused on needed improvements in academia regarding the education of public health professionals. The report called for the following changes:

- Creating new linkages among public health schools and programs and public health agencies at the federal, state, and local levels;
- Developing new relationships within universities between public health schools and programs and other professional schools and departments;
- Formulating more extensive approaches to education that encompass the full scope of public health practice;
- Strengthening the knowledge base in the areas of international health and the health of minority groups;
- Conducting a wide range of research that includes basic and applied research, as well as research on program evaluation and implementation; and
- Developing new training opportunities for professionals who are already practicing in public health.

There has been progress in most of these areas. For example, collaborations and partnerships are receiving increased emphasis, practice-based research efforts are expanding, and certificate programs and distance-learning programs aimed at providing lifelong learning to practicing public health workers have grown. Much more can be achieved, but these improvements are dependent on a critical analysis of the functions of academia, an examination of academia's potential contributions to the public health system, and a discussion of recommendations made to enhance academia's capacity to make these contributions.

Academia performs three important functions within the public health system. These are to (1) educate and train public health workers; (2) conduct basic and applied research in disciplines pertinent to public health; and (3) engage in community, public, and professional service. Of course, academia is not the only institution that provides education, research, and service. Federal, state, and local public health agencies, for example, provide training to public health workers. Public health agencies and the Centers for Disease Control and Prevention (CDC) conduct community-based research. Federal and state health agencies collect and disseminate valuable, credible information and statistics for the nation through vehicles such as the National Health Interview Survey, the Vital Statistics system, and the publication *Morbidity and Mortality Weekly Report*. The Public Health Faculty/Agency Forum, convened by CDC and the Health Resources and Services Administration (HRSA), illustrates one way in which nonacademic institutions convene and foster cooperation and coordination between academia and public health agencies in support of community health.

Although numerous federal, state, and local agencies make important contributions through education and training, information dissemination, collaborative activities, and research, these functions are central to the mission of academia. These functions are not, however, mutually exclusive. For example, service learning (defined as a method by which students learn through active participation in organized service experiences that meet actual community needs [Rhoads and Howard, 1998]) can be classified under the education and training function as well as the service function. Community-based participatory research is another example. Although it is clearly classified under the research function of academia, this approach to research is also a component of the service function because it is conducted in a collaborative fashion with the community and addresses problems identified as important by the community.

The emphasis of this chapter is on how academia fulfills its responsibilities for assuring the health of the public through education (and training), research, and service. For the purposes of this discussion, "academia" refers to all units within community and 4-year colleges and universities that contribute to assuring the health of the population.

EDUCATION AND TRAINING

The "most distinctive role of public health education lies in the preparation of public health professionals" (Fineberg et al., 1994). Because of the critical role of education in preparing public health professionals to function effectively, the Institute of Medicine (IOM) convened the Committee on Educating Public Health Professionals for the 21st Century that, concurrent with the work of the Committee on Assuring the Health of the Public in the 21st Century, has conducted an in-depth examination of the future needs of public health professional education and developed a framework and recommendations for how, over the next 5 to 10 years, education, training, and research in programs and schools of public health can be strengthened to prepare future public health professionals to improve population health.

Given the in-depth examination and analysis of public health education that was undertaken by the IOM Committee on Educating Public Health Professionals for the 21st Century, the present report will not go into detail about the future of public health education but, rather, will briefly describe the kinds of degree and professional development programs available, discusses the current workforce and its training needs, identifies problems and barriers to providing public health education, and makes recommendations for maximizing academia's contributions to the education of the current and future public health workforce.

People who work as professionals in the public health system receive their education and training in a wide range of disciplines and in diverse academic settings, including schools of public health, medicine, nursing, dentistry, social work, allied health professions, pharmacy, law, public administration, veterinary medicine, engineering, environmental sciences, biology, microbiology, and journalism.

The master of public health (MPH) is the basic professional degree traditionally earned by public health workers, but many college graduates who work in public health are educated in other health professions. For example, nurses make up about 10.9 percent of the total public health workforce, whereas physicians comprise about 1.3 percent (HRSA, 2000a). The doctor of public health (DrPH) is offered for advanced training in public health leadership. Individuals with academic degrees (e.g., a master of science or doctorate) in the public health disciplines such as epidemiology, biostatistics, environmental health, health services and administration, nutrition, and the social and behavioral sciences also may be found in the larger state and local public health agencies and in the health care delivery system.

The 32 accredited schools of public health, along with the 45 accredited MPH programs, supply the bulk of public health graduates. The Association of Schools of Public Health (ASPH), the organization that represents accredited schools of public health, reports that in 1998–1999, the 29 accredited schools of public health graduated 5,568 students. Of all degree recipients, 89.9 percent received a master's degree (61.5 percent received an MPH degree) and 10.1 percent received doctoral degrees (of these, 6.7 percent received a doctor of philosophy [PhD] degree and 2 percent received a DrPH degree) (ASPH, 2000). It is estimated that accredited graduate programs in community health and preventive medicine and in community health education graduate an additional 700 to 800 master's degree students each year (Davis and Dandoy, 2001). Many of these graduate programs in public health are represented by the Association of Teachers of Preventive Medicine. Additionally, in 1997–1998 there were 9,947 master's graduates of programs of public administration and public affairs, many of whom emphasized health policy and management and public health in their training (National Association of Schools of Public Affairs and Administration, 1998). The Association of University Programs in Health Administration reports that in 2000 there were 1,778 graduates who received master's degrees (in health administration); some (an unknown number) of them received the MPH and master of science degrees (Association of University Programs in Health Administration, 2000). Many public health workers also receive undergraduate training from 4-year institutions that offer programs in the environmental sciences or in health education and health promotion. These programs can offer valuable continuing education to health workers by providing current scientific information in many specialized areas.

Those who graduate with training in public health are only a small part of the public health workforce. Although it is unclear exactly how many public health workers there are in the United States today, it is estimated that about 450,000 people are employed in salaried positions in public health and that an additional 2.85 million people volunteer their services (HRSA, 2000a). This is probably an undercount because, according to HRSA, states reporting the number of workers within their jurisdictions almost never include information about public health workers found in nongovernmental and community partner agencies. Additionally, limited information is obtained regarding the numbers of volunteers and salaried staff in voluntary agencies.

Kennedy and colleagues (1999), in an 18-month study of the Texas public health workforce, counted nearly 17,700 professional public health workers in that state. Only one-third of the professional public health workforce identified in that study was employed in official public health agencies, and only an estimated 7 percent had formal education in public health. Nationally, it is estimated that about 80 percent of public health workers lack basic training in public health (CDC, 2001a). Furthermore, only 22 percent of chief executives of local health departments have graduate degrees in public health (Turnock, 2001).

Public Health Education and Training

Basic public health training has changed over the years. Early public health efforts in the United States were directed toward improving sanitation and ensuring the safety of the food and water supply, controlling infectious diseases, and providing immunizations to children. Thus, in the early 1900s, the public health workforce was trained primarily in medicine, nursing, and the biological sciences (Brandt and Gardner, 2000; Garrett, 2000; Mullan, 2000). Basic public health training now requires an approach that incorporates understanding of the following:

• Health problems must be examined in the context of defined populations;
• Many problems of public health are deeply rooted in the behavior of individuals and in their social context;
• Public health problems of the twenty-first century are rooted in the technologies of economic development; and
• Public health problems continue to require the engagement of the body politic, in the form of government participation, for their solution (Fineberg et al., 1994).

Additionally, changing demographics in the United States and the importance of community engagement in problem solving contribute to the need for a more broadly trained and diverse workforce. Involvement in global health issues also argues for increased attention to workforce diversity, but achieving such diversity in the workforce is a major challenge for governmental public health agencies and other public health entities because of the inadequate number of students and faculty from ethnic minority groups. Without high school and undergraduate degree programs in public health, there is little exposure of potential minority candidates to public health as a career option. A related issue is the lack of ethnic minority faculty in programs and schools of public health. Public health agencies, schools and programs of public health, professional organizations, and other components of the public health system need to devote major efforts to identify and facilitate, through funding and other mechanisms, approaches to increase cultural diversity, as well as to enhance awareness of global health issues among public health faculty, students, and staff. For example, many schools of public health have established programs that provide students with practical experiences working abroad, offer short-term international internships as well as fellowship programs related to global health, and engage in international research collaboration on major global health issues.

Recent efforts directed toward achieving the goal of a broadly trained workforce have focused on identifying basic competencies in public health and developing curricula that teach the information and skills necessary to meet those competencies. A number of different organizations have tackled this task. For example, the Pew Health Professions Commission (O'Neil, 1998) has developed a set of 21 competencies for successful practice that apply to physicians, nurses, and allied health professionals. The Council on Linkages Between Academia and Public Health Practice has developed a set of core competencies for public health professionals that apply to three job categories: frontline staff, senior-level staff, and supervisory management staff (Council on Linkages, 2001).

The ASPH has endorsed the core competencies developed by the Council on Linkages and plans to develop additional and complementary competencies for MPH students. Furthermore, the CDC Office of Workforce Policy and Planning (CDC, 2001b) has developed a table of competency sets (see Appendix E), differentiated into the categories of

- Core-basic public health (addresses the essential services of public health);
- New topical areas (emergency response, genomics, law, informatics);
- Functional areas (leadership, management, supervisory, secretarial);
- Discipline-specific areas (professional, technical, entry-level students); and
- Other topical areas (e.g., maternal and child health, environmental health, health communication, sexually transmitted diseases).

The preparation of students and workers to engage in effective public health practice requires not only a definition of competencies but also an educational approach that encompasses a necessarily broad range of skills and information. Integrated approaches to education and training are crucial.

Integrated Interdisciplinary Learning

One example of an effort to promote an integrated approach to education is the Medicine/Public Health Initiative, a national consortium created in 1994 under the joint leadership of the American Medical Association and the American Public Health Association and involved in efforts to improve the working relationship and bridge the gap between medical and public health practitioners. The initiative has the following seven primary goals:

1. To engage the community and change existing thinking to focus on improving the health of the community.

2. To change the educational process so that public health and medicine can enhance their understanding of each other's practices.

3. To create joint research efforts by developing a common research agenda for public health and medicine by using the threefold approach of relaying advantages of joint research, using preventive medicine certification and training as a form of integrated learning, and supporting the funding of research that links medicine and public health.

4. To devise a shared view of health and illness so that public health and medicine can use a common conceptual framework of health and illness.

5. To work together in health care provision and integrate health promotion and prevention into clinical health care delivery systems.

6. To jointly develop health care assessment measures such as quality, effectiveness, and outcome evaluations.

7. To translate Initiative ideas into action.

The Initiative's work led to the development of a program that funded 19 collaborative projects around the country (Phillips, 2000). The Agency for Health Care Policy and Research also funded three projects aiming to enhance cooperation between the medical and public health communities in the context of community-based health programs (AHCPR, 1997).

Preventive medicine certification and training is another example of integrated interdisciplinary learning. In preventive medicine training, the primary emphasis is on disease prevention and health promotion. There are currently 6,091 certified preventive medicine specialists in the United States, but the proportion of these specialists among all U.S. physicians is on the decline. The decline has been greatest among those training in public health, with the primary reason for the decline being inadequate funding (Lane, 2000).

In addition, it is critical for public health education to cross traditional boundaries and link more effectively with the educational programs for other health professionals. In 1998, the Josiah Macy, Jr., Foundation sponsored a conference entitled Education for More Synergistic Practice of Medicine and Public Health (Hager, 1999). The goal of the conference was to develop recommendations on how public health practitioners and physicians can be trained to collaborate with one another. During the conference, Lasker (1999) emphasized the importance of public health education for medical students, whereas Lumpkin (1999) discussed what to teach students of public health about medical practice. He pointed out that because of the changes in the issues facing public health, enrolling students no longer come primarily from the medical or nursing profession. This, in turn, means that those students do not have a working knowledge of the biomedical basis of medical treatment or of the medical treatment system.

To gain needed exposure to the academic disciplines and the actual practices of their counterparts, medical students must become acquainted with epidemiology, biostatistics, public health policy, the elements of prevention, and other essentials of public health, whereas students of public health require familiarization with the workings of the health care delivery system, the pharmacological and therapeutic treatment of disease, and techniques of dealing with individual patients (Hagar, 1999).

Nursing education is another area for integrated interdisciplinary learning, such as linkages with education in public health. Although schools of nursing require course work in community and public health nursing at the bachelor's level, there is a great deal of variation in the content of these programs. In 2001, there were 85 schools of nursing that offered master's degrees in community health and/or public health nursing (Berlin, 2002). Model curricula incorporating public health content into bachelor's nursing curricula are lacking; an insufficient number of nursing faculty are prepared in public health; and access to public health agencies for population-based clinical experience is often a problem, as is access to continuing education in population-based public health and public health nursing. For additional information about preparing nurses to enter the public health workforce, refer to *Who Will Keep the Public Healthy?* (IOM, 2003).

Unfortunately, efforts to integrate teaching across schools and departments face several institutional barriers. First, most schools and colleges are departmentalized, with the resources provided for teaching distributed among the departments. Departmental priorities lie with ensuring that courses for majors and service courses are taught within the department's discipline. Faculty who teach departmental, discipline-based courses are provided with both monetary support for teaching such courses and recognition by their departmental colleagues for contributing to the department's teaching load.

At present, either integrated interdisciplinary courses must receive funding from sources outside the various departments involved, or each department supporting the disciplines involved in integrated interdisciplinary courses must agree to contribute faculty teaching time to the teaching efforts. Even when such agreements among departments can be reached, faculty are still reluctant to participate because the development and teaching of integrated interdisciplinary courses usually require more time than that required to teach a course in one's own discipline. This additional time is usually not recognized in either commensurate pay or teaching credit.

A second disincentive for faculty participation in integrated interdisciplinary educational approaches relates to promotion and salary review. Faculty teaching integrated interdisciplinary courses may be penalized during promotion and salary merit review because their departmental colleagues know little of their interdisciplinary teaching activities or do not value such activities as highly as they value contributions to the department's curriculum. Because integrated interdisciplinary teaching is important to the preparation of a well-trained workforce that is capable of addressing today's broad array of public health issues, academic institutions must ensure that funds are available for integrated interdisciplinary teaching activities and must provide incentives in their reward structures for faculty participating in such activities.

The emerging focus of a broad education based on competencies, both basic and discipline specific, is important. However, the need for public health students to understand medical practice and for physicians to understand public health practice, including the ethical and legal foundations of public health, must be kept in mind. The committee endorses the findings of the Macy Foundation conference—that there must be greater synergy between education for medicine and education for public health—and extends that endorsement of synergy to education in other clinical health science professions.

Therefore, **the committee recommends that academic institutions increase integrated interdisciplinary learning opportunities for students in public health and other related health science professions. Such efforts should include not only multidisciplinary education but also interdisciplinary education and appropriate incentives for faculty to undertake such activities.** Additional discussion of the need to increase collaboration and education between public health and other health professions can be found in the report *Who Will Keep the Public Healthy?*, developed by the IOM Committee on Educating Public Health Professionals for the 21st Century (IOM, 2003).

Public health workers should be trained in a set of core public health competencies and should have opportunities for practical experience; and additional education and training must be tailored to and depend on the experiences, activities, and functions of particular groups. For example, current MPH students have training needs that differ from those of past graduates of such programs who have been practicing for many years in a public health agency. The training needs of public health nurses differ in critical ways from the training needs of health educators, administrators, and environmental professionals. Identification of these specific training needs requires assessment and evaluation.

Solloway and colleagues (1997) reported on a study funded by HRSA to assess state agency-based health workforce capacity and examine state training and educational needs in five states: Illinois, Maryland, Missouri, Oregon, and Rhode Island. The authors report that most state public health workers have no formal education or training in the field of public health, lack a good understanding of the goals and mission of public health, and do not have a full understanding of the activities carried out by public health workers outside their own units or departments. They identified educational and training needs in eight areas:

1. Information systems and computer skills
2. Technical writing and presentation skills
3. Research and policy development skills
4. Management and administrative skills
5. Grantsmanship
6. Public relations
7. Transition skills
8. Leadership skills

The study also found that states need federal support to obtain technical assistance for the acquisition and use of new technologies for distance-based or remote-site learning, ongoing financial support, and symbolic support demonstrating that training and education are valued and are priorities.

Another study conducted by Reder and colleagues (1999) assessed the training needs of public health professionals in Washington State. They found that communication was the area in which public health professionals require the most training, with the four most highly rated topics being interpersonal communication, cross-cultural and cross-age communication, electronic communication, and participatory teaching and training skills.

The educational and training needs of the current public health workforce are enormous and multifaceted. Academia has an essential and unique role to play in ensuring that broad-based educational and training opportunities are available on a regional basis. All accredited MPH programs, school based or otherwise, are required to provide some continuing education; however, what is offered varies widely depending on the available resources and expertise. With the advent of new and expanding information technologies, the opportunity for schools and programs to provide education and training to a broader audience via distance learning is increasing rapidly. The means for achieving this are discussed further in the chapter on the governmental public health infrastructure (Chapter 3). Although academia can play a leadership role in the coordination of various educational and training opportunities for the public health workforce, it cannot meet all of these needs. In some cases, practitioners in the field can best provide in-service training.

Funding of Public Health Professional Education and Training

A current lack of funding is a major problem in providing training and education for both students seeking degrees and those already in the public health workforce. According to Gebbie (1999), the primary barrier to workforce development is the "incredibly weak" budget allocated for training. This has not always been the case, however. Over the past five decades, the major sources of funds for the training of students in public health were HRSA and CDC. Table 8–1 provides a chronology of legislation authorizing funds for health professional training in public health between 1956 and 1976 (DHHS, 1980).

In 1976, Congress passed the Health Professions Educational Assistance Act (P.L. 94–484). This act provided for a number of programs in health professions education, including

- Extensions of existing public health traineeships.
- Grants to accredited schools of public health for student traineeships.
- A separate program of grants to public or nonprofit private educational entities (excluding schools of public health) that offered an accredited program in health administration, hospital administration, or health policy analysis and planning.
- Funding to public or nonprofit private educational entities (excluding schools of public health) for graduate programs in health administration.
- Grants to assist accredited schools of public health and other public or nonprofit educational entities with accredited graduate programs in health administration, health planning, or health policy analysis and planning in meeting costs of special projects to develop new programs or expand existing ones in the same four public health disciplines mentioned above.
- A requirement for the Secretary of Health and Human Services, in coordination with the National Center for Health Statistics, to continuously develop and disseminate statistics and other information on the supply of and need for different types of public and community health personnel.

Between 1980 and 1987, spending by the Bureau of Health Professions (which is part of HRSA in the Department of Health and Human Services [DHHS]) for education in all health professions declined yearly, from a high of $411,469,000 in 1980 to $189,353,000 in 1987. General-purpose traineeship grants to schools of public health went from $6,842,000 in 1980 to $2,958,000 in 1987. Curriculum development grants, funded at $7,456,000 in 1980, were not funded at all in 1981 and 1982; but the funding recovered slowly in 1983, with funding at $1,740,000, and increased in 1984 to $2,856,000 and reached $9,787,000 in 1987. Grants for graduate programs in health administration were

TABLE 8–1 Funding Legislation for Health Professional Training

Legislation	Description
P.L. 84–911. Health Amendments Act of 1956	Authorized a 3-year program of grants to public or other nonprofit institutions or to individuals for traineeship awards for graduate or specialized training in public health.
P.L. 85–544. Public Health—Training and Services—Grants-in-Aid	Authorized awards of not more than $1 million in grants-in-aid for provision in public or nonprofit accredited schools of public health of comprehensive professional training, specialized consultative services, and technical assistance in the fields of public health and the administration of state and local public health programs.
P.L. 86–106. An Act to Extend Certain Traineeship Provisions of the Health Amendments Act of 1956	Extended for 5 years (through fiscal year [FY] 1964) the authority for traineeship awards for graduate or specialized training in public health.
P.L. 86–720. An Act to Amend Title III of the Public Health Service Act to Authorize Project Grants for Graduate Training in Public Health	Authorized the award of project grants to schools of public health and to schools of nursing and engineering that provide graduate or specialized training in public health for nurses or engineers, for the purpose of strengthening or expanding graduate public health training in such schools. Appropriation authorizations for the grants were $2 million a year for FY 1961 through 1965.
P.L. 87–395. Community Health Services and Facilities Act of 1961	Extended for FY 1962 through 1966 the authority for grants-in-aid to schools of public health and increased the authorization from $1 million to $2.5 million.
P.L. 88–497. Graduate Public Health Training Amendments of 1964	Extended for 5 years (through FY 1969) the authority for traineeship awards for professional public health personnel. Dollar limitations were $4.5 million for FY 1965, $7 million for FY 1966, $8 million for FY 1967, and $10 million each for FYs 1968 and 1969. Also increased authorization for project grants for graduate or specialized training in public health to $2.5 million for FY 1965 and extended the program for 4 additional years.
P.L. 89–109. Community Health Services Extension Amendments of 1965	Extended through FY 1967 the grants-in-aid for schools of public health.

continued on next page

TABLE 8-1   Continued

Legislation	Description
P.L. 89–749. Comprehensive Health Planning and Public Health Services Amendments of 1966	Transferred authority for grants-in-aid to schools of public health and extended authority to FY 1968, with a $5 million appropriation authorized.
P.L. 90–174. Partnership for Health Amendments of 1967	Extended for 2 years (through FY 1970) the authority for grants-in-aid to schools of public health, with up to $7 million authorized for 1970.
P.L. 90–490. Health Manpower Act of 1968	Extended for 2 years (through FY 1971) authority for traineeship awards for professional public health personnel, with up to $14 million authorized for FY 1971, and extended through FY 1971 authority for project grants for graduate or specialized training in public health, with up to $12 million authorized for 1971.
P.L. 91–208. Public Health Service Act Amendments	Extended through FY 1973 authority for traineeship awards, with up to $18 million authorized for 1973. Also extended through FY 1973 authority for project grants for graduate or specialized training in public health, with up to $14 million authorized for FY 1971. Also extended through FY 1973 the authority for grants-in-aid, with up to $15 million authorized for FY 1973.
P.L. 93–45. Health Programs Extension Act	Extended through FY 1974 authority for traineeship awards, for project grants for graduate or specialized training in public health, and for grants-in-aid to schools of public health. For FYs 1975 and 1976, Congress passed continuing appropriations acts providing continuing authority and funding for public health training programs that would otherwise have expired on June 30, 1974.

SOURCE: DHHS (1980).

funded at $2,967,000 in 1980, dropped to $726,000 in 1981, and rose to $1,416,000 in 1982, where they remained fairly steady, with funding in 1987 being $1,482,000 (DHHS, 1988).

The 1990s saw funding levels remain approximately constant, so that increases in tuition and other costs have actually resulted in a reduction in the amount of public health professional education provided.

The Bureau of Health Professions has begun to create a nationwide network of Public Health Training Centers (HRSA, 2000b). The purpose of the program is to improve the nation's public health system by strengthening the technical, scientific, managerial, and leadership competence of the current and future public health workforce. Each of the Public Health Training Centers for each respective state or region will work to

- Assess the educational needs of and training materials and facilities available to local and state public health agencies;
- Use distance-learning technology and other new educational approaches to provide both basic and specialized public health education;
- Improve public health providers' ability to interpret and make informed decisions based on relevant data and information;
- Establish on-site educational programs in underserved areas;
- Develop field-based educational opportunities for students from traditional on-campus graduate public health programs;
- Develop new curricula for public health practitioners on emerging public health issues such as bioterrorism, behavioral and mental health, domestic and societal violence, and environmental health issues; and
- Train lay workers from local boards of health and community health offices.

The centers are designed to offer training and continuing education programs to about 100,000 public health students and professionals each year. To date, 14 centers have been funded. These centers involve 35 academic institutions and more than 42 states. Funding levels range from about $250,000 to $500,000 per year per center, although the recommended levels were $1 million. Although this is a needed program, funds are insufficient to compensate for the reduction in training funds experienced over the past two decades. Adequate funding, especially in states with small and medium populations, would create the opportunity to release staff to prepare and provide training programs and to increase the number of sessions provided. Additionally, adequate funding would allow the training center to hire distance-learning specialists to aid in the preparation of courses.

CDC has also been a major supporter of education for public health professionals. The CDC Graduate Certificate Program (GCP) was a federally sponsored initiative directed primarily toward CDC field officers, state health department personnel, and selected others with at least 3 to 5 years of experience in public health practice. The programs were designed for midcareer professionals in public health practice who desired to further their professional standing. The program provided the means by which Public Health Advisors working in state and local health departments across the country could earn a graduate certificate in public health from one of four accredited schools of public health: Tulane University School of Public Health and Tropical Medicine, Emory University Rollins School of Public Health, Johns Hopkins University Bloomberg School of Public Health, and University of Washington School of Public Health and Community Medicine.

Although originally designed for CDC staff, the GCP was later opened to all interested public health professionals. Core courses in epidemiology, health policy, health management, biostatistics, behavioral sciences, and health education were typically delivered in the first half of the program. In the later phase, students focused on one of the following specialty tracks: epidemiology and surveillance, health policy and management, or community health. The Graduate Certificate Program in Public Health began in 1996 and ended in January 2001, leaving programs with no resources to continue the training program.

In recent years, schools of public health have made praiseworthy efforts to form critical links with practice and community sectors. Most schools of public health now require practicums of their students; the development of collaborations and partnerships has received increasing emphasis (discussed below in the section Service); practice-based research efforts have been expanded (discussed in the section Research); and certificate programs and distance-learning programs aimed at providing lifelong learning to practicing public health workers have grown.

Development of certificate programs that emphasize core public health concepts is one response to the 1988 recommendation for programs aimed at educating the current workforce. This type of certificate is an abbreviated version of the MPH. The content of the program tends to emphasize the concepts from the five core content areas of knowledge basic to public health taught in MPH programs. Some schools also offer certificate programs that follow courses of study in the specific content areas of public health. Admissions standards and completion requirements vary with each certificate program. Courses within certificate programs generally must be taken for academic credit. The certificate is issued by the sponsor upon satisfactory completion of course work.

Academic institutions also offer summer institutes and courses aimed at the current workforce. A variety of subjects are covered in this manner, from basic biostatistics, epidemiology, and geographic information system applications to management and administration for middle to upper managers. Such programs can range in length from a 1-day course to weeklong offerings. At present, the majority of students pursuing degrees in professional public health programs are educated via classroom-based instruction. Such face-to-face contact in teaching is important for a number of reasons, not the least of which is that these close and continuing relationships help break down racial, cultural, and class barriers and promote trust and a sense of community (Citrin, 2001). Additionally, most planning and collaborative work is best done at meetings and work sessions that physically bring people together.

Many academic institutions, along with state health agencies and CDC, offer short courses, seminars, or workshops addressing specific public health training needs. One approach taken to meet the demand for distance-based training is the Public Health Training Network. This network has provided training to nearly 1 million people on a wide range of subjects in a variety of formats: print-based self-instruction, interactive multimedia, videotapes, two-way audio conferences, and interactive satellite videoconferences (CDC, 2001c).

As distance-learning technology improves and new electronic delivery modalities become more widespread, online in-service training opportunities will be more accessible. These new approaches under development will assist in providing training opportunities for public health workers who are not able to participate in classroom-based educational programs. The use of web-based tools for education is referred to as *distance learning* (Riegelman and Persily, 2001). Distance-learning programs and new information technologies are perceived to be a boon to meeting the educational needs of the public health workforce in the United States (Cannon et al., 2001). Although this development builds on more than two decades of computer networking activities (e.g., e-mail and bulletin board systems), increased access to the Internet has produced phenomenal growth in the extent and scope of online education. Teaching and learning on the World Wide Web demand new and special skills from teachers and learners alike.

Another educational approach attracting attention is service learning, defined as the "method under which students learn and develop through active participation in thoughtfully organized service experiences that meet actual community needs, that are integrated into the student's academic curriculum or provide structured time for reflection, and that enhance what is taught in school by extending student learning beyond the classroom and into the community" (Rhoads and Howard, 1998). According to Porter and Monard (2001) "understanding and fostering reciprocity is a central aim of service-learning programs," meaning that service-learning programs differ from other practical educational approaches in that their intent is to benefit both the provider and the recipient of the service and to emphasize equally the provision of service and the learning experience (Cauley et al., 2001).

According to Howard (2001), three criteria must be met for a course to be considered service learning:

1. Service that is both relevant and meaningful to all stakeholder parties must be provided in the community.

    2. The service must not only serve the community but also enhance student academic learning.

    3. The service must also directly and intentionally prepare students for active civic participation in a diverse democratic society.

    Service-learning programs benefit the community, the student, and academia. Academia depends on this type of learning to teach students about real-world public health. Students are able to translate their academic learning into practice activities. The community, particularly in rural and inner-city areas that may be experiencing a shortage of health professionals, is able to reap the benefit of services provided by students in these learning situations.

    On the basis of the findings detailed in the preceding pages, the committee identifies the need for increased funding of public health training and education. Funding is needed to support existing and emerging mechanisms for training and education of public health students, public health workers, and others. **The committee recommends that Congress increase funding for HRSA programs that provide financial support for students enrolled in public health degree programs through mechanisms such as training grants, loan repayments, and service obligation grants. Funding should also be provided to strengthen the Public Health Training Center program to effectively meet the educational needs of the existing public health workforce and to facilitate public health worker access to the centers. Support for leadership training of state and local health department directors and local community leaders should continue through funding of the National and Regional Public Health Leadership Institutes and distance-learning materials developed by HRSA and CDC.**

    The following section discusses the second important contribution of academia, research.

RESEARCH

    Relevant, high-quality research is essential to health assessment, policy development, and assurance. Such research provides fresh insights and creative solutions to health problems and supplies the evidence base necessary for policy development and assurance activities. Public health practice is grounded in science, both the traditional medical and natural sciences (e.g., biology, microorganisms, vectors, and risks in the physical environment) and, increasingly, the social and behavioral sciences (e.g., anthropology, sociology, and psychology) that "affect our understanding of human culture and behaviors influencing health and illness" (Turnock, 2001). It is in academia that most such research is conducted. In addition to basic biomedical research and epidemiological studies that contribute to an understanding of what makes people healthy, research on the multiple determinants of health has begun to enrich the understanding of the numbers and complexities of factors that determine the health of the population (see Chapter 2 for a more comprehensive discussion of the determinants of health).

Increased understanding of the determinants of health has demonstrated the importance of social and behavioral factors to health. McGinnis and Foege (1993) reported that about half of all causes of mortality in the United States are linked to social and behavioral factors and accidents. Several studies have shown the relationship between unintentional injuries and certain risk factors: for example, accessibility to firearms, use of alcohol and tobacco, and use of seat belts (Turnock, 2001). Other research has shown the influence of psychological risk factors on disease; for example, the management of diabetes is influenced by coping skills and family stresses; other research demonstrates that acute stress may trigger myocardial ischemia (IOM, 2001).

Another important area for increased research is public health systems research. Bialek (2000) makes the point that there is little scientific evidence about what constitutes effective public health departments. He defines public health systems research as "a field of inquiry using quantitative or qualitative methodology to examine the impact of the organization, financing, staffing, and management of systems on the access to, delivery, cost, outcomes, and quality of population-based services." Turnock (2001) states that improving public health practice requires research that explicates the links and relationships of key processes, programs, and services or outputs. The limited amount of public health systems research conducted to date has produced some important findings, such as the findings that the effectiveness of local health departments does not appear to be influenced by jurisdiction size and full-time leadership appears to positively influence effectiveness (Bialek, 2000). The committee believes that public health systems research is an important area for increased attention.

Despite the many achievements of research, much remains to be accomplished. The vast majority of the nation's health research resources have been directed toward biomedical research endeavors that cannot, by themselves, address the most significant challenges to improving the public's health (IOM, 2000). Past and current research funding priorities focus especially on risk factor identification through either large- or small-scale epidemiological studies. Comparatively few resources have been devoted to supporting prevention research, community-based research, or the translation of research findings into practice. For example, in the area of obesity, a great deal of research is needed about causes and about appropriate and effective interventions. Despite a significant reduction since 1990 in the amount of dietary fat consumed by the population, the rate of obesity has increased significantly. Clearly, achieving a reduction in obesity is not as simple as changing one risk factor, but will require interventions on multiple determinants at various levels.

Only 1 to 2 percent of the U.S. health care budget is spent on prevention, and a like imbalance exists between funding for basic biomedical research and for population-based prevention research (Scrimshaw et al., 2001). As a consequence, although the scientific literature includes an enormous amount of information about physical and biological risk factors for disease and disability, as well as more limited information about social and behavioral determinants of health, little of this knowledge has been translated into forms that are accessible or useful to local public health practitioners or to the community.

Although many scholars agree on the importance of prevention research, exact definitions of the term vary. According to Scrimshaw and colleagues (2001), this "lack of a consistent definition for prevention research decreases the conceptual clarity of the term and impedes the development of a clear understanding of prevention research." Brownson and Simoes (1999) assert that prevention research focuses on determining the underlying causes of death, injury, and disability; research discoveries are then applied at the community level. CDC defines prevention research as research directly applicable to public health practice (Doll et al., 2001). Sattin (2001) states that prevention research is a multidisciplinary approach to discovering new ways to prolong the health, well-being, and self-sufficiency of all Americans; it focuses on preventing disease, injury, and disability. Scrimshaw and colleagues (2001) describe how prevention is frequently defined in terms of the self-interest of the person giving the definition.

Prevention is frequently categorized into three levels: primary, secondary, and tertiary. Primary prevention in public health is aimed at preventing an illness or disability from occurring. Secondary prevention efforts include interventions in illness to prevent continued illness or disability, whereas tertiary prevention activities attempt to limit further progression of illness or disability or to postpone death. Clinical preventive services are generally considered secondary or tertiary preventions. To increase the clarity of its discussion, the committee has chosen to define population-based prevention research using a modified version of the definition developed by the Association of Schools of Public Health (Spencer, 2000) for population-based prevention research, which

- Addresses health problems that affect large numbers of people;
- Involves a definable population and operates at the level of the whole person;
- Evaluates the application and impacts of new discoveries on the actual health of the population; and

• Focuses on behavioral or environmental (social, economic, cultural, physical) factors associated with primary and secondary prevention of disease in populations; the behavioral, biological, or clinical variations among populations; or the integration of behavioral, biological, and environmental factors.

As discussed previously, prevention research (including clinical preventive services research) has been underfunded and undervalued, yet it is crucial to understanding how to improve health. The following section of this chapter discusses the specific research approaches that the committee believes will, if properly funded, contribute greatly to the understanding of the determinants of health and to evaluation of the effectiveness of public health interventions.

Population-Based Research

The term *population-based research* means that the research focuses on groups or populations rather than individuals (Scrimshaw et al., 2001). Population-based research draws on populations or random samples of populations at a national, state, or local level. In general, it builds on an understanding of the determinants of health that includes multiple levels of influence, from environmental (both social and physical) to behavioral to individual (biological, genetic). Although all research does not incorporate all potential levels, increased understanding of etiology and prevention will come about by working at multiple levels. Examples of well-known population-based research include the Framingham Heart Study, which continues to yield new insights, and the Woman's Health Initiative (see Box 8–1).

Although population-based studies are often used to generate hypotheses about the potential risk factors for disease, population studies can also test hypotheses developed in earlier studies. Most of the earlier population-based data collection focused on the biological and environmental risk factors for disease. There is, however, an increasingly rich amount of data about the social determinants of health (see Chapter 2), and investigators are poised on the brink of being able to link these social risk factors with biomedical factors, thereby developing a more complex model of disease and health through population-based studies.

Community-Based Research

Community-based research is an overarching concept of collaborative research that encompasses many different types of studies (e.g., applied, descriptive, and evaluative). Community-based participatory research is defined as research that involves all stakeholders in each aspect of a study

---

BOX 8–1
Research Definitions for Academia

The term *population based* means that the research focuses on groups or populations rather than individuals (Scrimshaw et al., 2001). The following definitions are used in this report:

- *Basic (or fundamental) research*—research conducted for the purpose of advancing knowledge with little concern for any immediate or practical benefits.
- *Applied research*—research designed to use the results of other research (e.g., basic research) to solve real-world problems. This type of research is also called *translational research* by the National Institutes of Health.
- *Evaluative research*—the use of scientific research methods to assess the effectiveness of a program or initiative.
- *Descriptive research*—research that attempts to discover facts or describe reality (Sullivan, 2001). This includes hypothesis-generating studies, epidemiological studies, observational studies, and surveys.
- *Community-based research*—a collaborative approach to research that equitably involves community members, organizational representatives, and researchers in all aspects of the research process (Israel et al., 1998). This definition is similar to that used by Green and Mercer (2001) in defining *participatory research* as an approach that entails the involvement of all potential users of the research and other stakeholders in the formulation as well as the application of the research.

---

designed to evaluate the application and impact of new discoveries aimed at improving the health of a defined population, frequently involving the evaluation of interventions designed to promote health in community settings.

Community-based research is often divided into three distinct phases: formative, process, and summative (Valente, 2002). The length and nature of each of these stages vary depending on the type of project and type of study, but some general parameters can be described. Community-based research requires active partnerships between the community and researchers who may or may not be members of that community (Green et al., 2001). Partnerships and coalitions are necessary because no one agency has the resources, access, and trust relationships to address the wide range of community determinants of public health problems (Green et al., 2001). Clark (1999) states that research needs a three-way partnership of academia, public health practice groups, and community-based organizations. A key factor in establishing successful partnerships is trust (Nelson et al., 1999). Lack of trust and perceived lack of respect are frequently perceived to hinder effective community-based research (Israel et al., 1998).

The Formative Phase

In the first or formative phase, researchers and the community engage in activities that lay the groundwork for a successful partnership (Valente, 2002). Such activities include defining and agreeing on the mission, goals, and outcomes of the research; identifying strengths and assets within the community and the research institution; determining responsibilities; and establishing the decision-making process. Although some relations may already exist among potential partners, further developmental activities must be undertaken for each new project. For example, an existing network or coalition on tobacco prevention may be expanded to include nutrition activities. This network would then have to conduct a formal needs assessment that involves both the researchers and the community to identify health needs and set goals and objectives. The formative phase, whether it entails expanding an existing partnership or developing new relations among researchers and the community, is time-consuming and cannot be carried out without sufficient funds to support the activities described.

The Process Phase

During the process phase, potential intervention strategies and research instruments are designed and pilot tested among small community samples (Valente, 2002). Agreement must be reached on the health promotion strategies, specific media and messages, and research instruments after repeated iterations. Once agreement is reached, baseline data are collected and the intervention is implemented. Depending on the nature of the intervention, this phase could be short (e.g., 3 months) or quite long (years).

The Summative Phase

The summative phase of research begins after the intervention is completed or at a point when some assessment is needed (Valente, 2002). The summative phase includes collection of follow-up data and interviews with key stakeholders (such as project administrators or program recipients). This phase includes data analysis to determine the impact, specify the lessons learned, and develop recommendations for future activities (e.g., whether to expand the program and whether or how to modify the program). The summative phase is iterative because results need to be shared with key stakeholders. If the program is expanded and disseminated to other communities or settings, effectiveness evaluation is needed to determine whether the program can be generalized to these other settings and what lessons are learned as the program is implemented elsewhere.

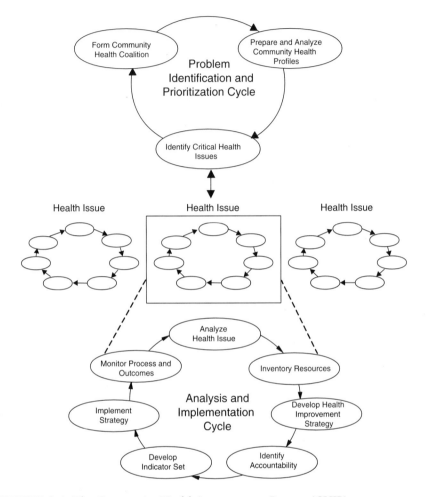

FIGURE 8–1 The Community Health Improvement Process (CHIP).
SOURCE: IOM (1997b).

Time Estimates for Research

Time estimates for each of these phases are imprecise, but experience has shown that, at a minimum, each phase will take at least 2 years in a modest-size program. A specific example of community-based research in which academia has the potential to contribute in many ways is the Community Health Improvement Process discussed in Chapter 4 (see Figure 8–1).

Unfortunately, academic institutions have undervalued community-based participatory research. It is sometimes perceived as lacking in rigorous methodology because it cannot use the randomized, single-intervention evaluation approach. However, practice research demonstrates increased relevance to social goals with the translation of research findings into community action, thereby demonstrating the value to the nation of the use of public resources devoted to academic research; communities benefit from a program based on knowledge of evidence-based practice and community-relevant issues. Therefore, **the committee recommends that federal funders of research and academic institutions recognize and reward faculty scholarship related to public health practice research.**

Funding of Prevention Research

The Centers for Disease Control and Prevention

CDC, in collaboration with local, state, and other federal health and education agencies, plays a major role in prevention activities in the United States. In terms of research, CDC defines prevention research as research that is directly applicable to public health practice and views it as an important part of the CDC mission (Doll et al., 2001).

CDC has both intramural and extramural research programs. *Intramural research* (or CDC-directed research) is carried out within its laboratories or in the field in collaboration with state and local health departments. *Extramural research*, in which decision making regarding the study approach rests with the grantee, was, until the early 1970s, a relatively small grants program. During the next two decades it became decentralized, with programs developed and administered independently through CDC's Centers, Institutes, and Offices (CIOs). More recently, CDC has begun to expand further as a supporter of extramural research (Doll et al., 2001).

CDC has three categories of extramural research programs: (1) program- or CIO-generated research; (2) investigator-initiated research; and (3) research centers of excellence. The following descriptions and examples of these types of research are taken from Doll et al. (2001).

Program- or CIO-Generated Research In program- or CIO-generated research, the topic (and perhaps the research approach as well) is determined by the CIO, which then publishes a request for application (RFA). Proposals are submitted to the CIO and then reviewed. Research topics in program-generated research have included the influence of folic acid on neural tube defects in China and the effectiveness of an intervention to reduce dating violence.

Another approach to program-generated research is to enter into cooperative agreements with health-related professional organizations with which CDC has agreements (e.g., the Association of the Schools of Public Health, the Minority Health Foundation, and the Association of American

Medical Colleges). Funding announcements are mailed to members of these organizations. Funds for the projects are provided by the CIOs and are administered by CDC's Public Health Practice Program Office (PHPPO).

Investigator-Initiated Research at CDC   In the investigator-initiated approach to research, applicants propose research in topic areas of their choosing or under broad topic areas provided by the CIOs. The Extramural Prevention Research Program (also known as the Prevention Research Initiative [PRI]) is one of the largest investigator-initiated research efforts at CDC and is administered by PHPPO. In 1999, with a budget of $12.5 million, CDC began the PRI and funded 50 research service endeavors at academic health centers, research centers, and university-affiliated programs. The average grant was approximately $250,000, and most service endeavors were funded for 3 years. Awards covered a range of subjects and included prevention of specific diseases (e.g., asthma and sexually transmitted diseases) and injury prevention (Sattin, 2001).

All grants and cooperative agreements in this program are externally peer reviewed and are administered by the scientifically appropriate CIOs. Plans for 2002 called for emphasizing investigator-initiated research grants in topic areas that cross-cut diseases, injuries, and conditions and that address gaps in individual CIO agendas. Awards are to be for larger amounts to allow evaluation of service endeavors targeting large populations or the subgroups at highest risk (Doll et al., 2001). A major problem, however, is the lack of a central, organized focus for investigator-initiated research. There is no defined unit to which applications are submitted, and there is no single source of information on the availability of grants.

All applications submitted to CDC requesting research funding are subject to review. CDC uses two approaches to review applications: (1) objective review and (2) external peer review. *Objective review* is a process that includes an independent assessment of the technical or scientific merit of research by panels composed of federal reviewers only, predominantly from CDC. The *peer review* process includes an independent assessment of the technical or scientific merit of research by predominantly nonfederal reviewers, scientists with knowledge and expertise equal to that of the researchers whose work they review (Sattin, 2001).

Although CDC has been active and is a leader in prevention research, there are several barriers to maximizing its investigator-initiated prevention research. First, although CDC has recently funded increased numbers of investigator-initiated research projects, this remains a relatively small endeavor that is too dependent on CIO-specific programs. Another barrier relates to the fact that CDC staff frequently play a more directive role than is acceptable for academic research. Additionally, project funding is often for too short a time, and indirect cost allowances (which are based on the assumption that funding is for a health department that already receives substantial CDC funds) are too low to attract researchers from academic institutions with higher indirect rates.

Although CDC has strengthened its peer review process for investigator-initiated proposals, problems still exist. For example, administrative staff with no scientific training or scientists with no extramural program training frequently manage the peer review process and monitor funded projects (Doll et al., 2001). Finally, because CDC has no centralized office for the planning and coordinating of extramural peer review research programs, it is frequently difficult to know where to submit investigator-initiated proposals.

Prevention Research Centers The Prevention Research Center (PRC) program was authorized by Congress (P.L. 98–551) and established by CDC. This program, the largest research center program at CDC, is administered by the National Center for Chronic Disease Prevention and Health Promotion (Doll et al., 2001). To be funded as a PRC, a university must have a school of public health or a school of medicine or osteopathy with an accredited preventive medicine residency program, and the center must collaborate with individuals and organizations in the communities to determine research priorities (Doll et al., 2001). Each PRC focuses on projects related to a specific public health theme. The 24 currently funded PRCs and their research themes are listed in Table 8–2.

According to Scrimshaw and colleagues (2001), PRCs are the locus of leadership in community-based prevention efforts. They are intended to serve as bridges between science and practice and from academia to state and local health departments, health care providers and provider organizations, and community organizations, as well as CDC. Evaluation research is embedded in many of the PRC interventions; the centers also train public health professionals in applied prevention research (IOM, 1997a). Scrimshaw and colleagues (2001) attribute the successes of the PRCs to the fact that their research is collaborative, community based, interdisciplinary and multidisciplinary, problem solving and solution oriented, and "disseminative" and translatable.

Unfortunately, according to the IOM report (1997a) *Linking Research and Public Health Practice*, PRCs have not achieved the vision for which they were created, in large part because of insufficient funding. None were funded at their initially recommended level of $1 million per year. Most PRCs received only half of this amount, even though annual inflation increases would suggest the need for funding at levels higher than the original $1 million per year. Thus, the PRCs have not been able to build the infrastructure necessary to sustain the prevention research initiatives for which they were intended.

TABLE 8–2   Prevention Research Centers, 2001

Institution	Year First Funded	Research Theme
University of Alabama, Birmingham	1993	Bridging the gap between public health science and practice in underserved communities
University of Arizona, Tucson	1998	Promoting the health of multiethnic communities of the Southwest
University of California, Berkeley	1993	Chronic disease prevention: partnerships for action with families, neighborhoods, and communities
University of California, Los Angeles	1998	Starting adolescent health promotion and risk reduction at home
University of Colorado, Denver	1998	Promoting healthy lifestyles in rural communities
Columbia University, New York City	1990	Putting health promotion into action through community collaboration
Harvard University, Boston	1998	Nutrition and physical activity in children and youth
University of Illinois, Chicago	1990	A life-span approach to chronic disease prevention
The Johns Hopkins University, Baltimore	1993	Promoting adolescent health through families and communities
University of Kentucky, Lexington	2000	Controlling cancer in central Appalachia
University of Michigan, Ann Arbor	1998	Closing gaps and improving health through families and communities
University of Minnesota, Minneapolis	1996	Teen pregnancy prevention and youth development
Morehouse School of Medicine, Atlanta	1998	Risk reduction and early detection in African-American and other minority communities
University of New Mexico, Albuquerque	1995	Partnerships with Native American communities to improve health and well-being
University of North Carolina, Chapel Hill	1986	Improving community health through workplace health promotion

TABLE 8–2   Continued

Institution	Year First Funded	Research Theme
University of Oklahoma, Oklahoma City	1994	Promoting healthy behavior in Native American populations
St. Louis University, St. Louis	1994	Chronic disease prevention in high-risk communities
University of South Carolina, Columbia	1993	Promoting health through physical activity
University of South Florida, Tampa	1998	Community-based marketing for disease prevention and health promotion
University of Texas, Houston Health Science Center	1986	From healthy children to healthy adults
Tulane Medical Center, New Orleans	1998	Environmental agents and the health of communities
University of Washington, Seattle	1986	Keeping older adults healthy and independent by using community partnerships
West Virginia University, Morgantown	1994	Health promotion and disease prevention in rural Appalachia
Yale University, New Haven	1998	Public health initiatives across the prevention spectrum

SOURCE: Doll et al. (2001).

The committee recommends that the U.S. Congress provide funds for CDC to enhance its investigator-initiated program for prevention research while maintaining a strong CIO-generated research program. CDC should take steps that include

• Expanding the external peer review mechanism for review of investigator-initiated research;
• Allowing research to be conducted over the more generous time lines often required by prevention research; and
• Establishing a central mechanism for coordination of investigator-initiated proposal submissions.

Furthermore, CDC should authorize an analysis of the funding levels necessary for effective Prevention Research Center functioning, taking into account the levels authorized by P.L. 98–551 as well as the amount of prevention research occurring in other institutions and organizations.

National Institutes of Health

The National Institutes of Health (NIH) is the single largest source of health research funding, with a fiscal year 2000 research budget of nearly $20 billion (compared to CDC's total research budget of $570 million) (IOM, 2002). Although NIH emphasizes biomedical research, it is increasingly funding what it terms prevention research. It has invested in large-scale community trials (Green et al., 2001), conducts research on risk factors for disease, and evaluates drugs for secondary prevention of disease.

The National Institute of Environmental Health Sciences (NIEHS) developed a program in collaboration with the Environmental Protection Agency and CDC to "promote translation of basic research findings into applied intervention and prevention methods." NIEHS conducts multidisciplinary basic, applied research, and "community-based prevention research," including studies on the causes and mechanisms of children's disorders having an environmental etiology; studies to identify relevant environmental exposures; intervention studies to reduce hazardous exposures and their adverse effects; and studies to decrease the prevalence, morbidity, and mortality of environmentally related childhood diseases (NIH, 2002a).

Eight Centers for Children's Environmental Health and Disease Prevention Research were funded to conduct the first set of studies that will focus on respiratory disease and growth and development. The National Institute of Child Health and Human Development web page (NIH, 2002b) describes several prevention research projects, which include studies designed to conduct the following activities:

- Test the efficacy of a multicomponent program of school-based interventions for the primary prevention of problem behavior in a sample of middle school students;
- Identify determinants of the lack of age-appropriate immunizations;
- Examine the efficacy of an integrated system of office-based primary pediatric care interventions for the prevention of medically attended injuries;
- Assess determinants of parent-to-child transfer of responsibility for asthma self-management;
- Determine whether parent and teen expectations predict teens' driving behaviors during their first year of driving; and
- Determine relevant factors and effective interventions for family management of type 1 diabetes.

Despite the many NIH-funded research activities labeled as prevention research, these efforts tend to focus on individual health and on secondary prevention and risk factor analysis rather than on the health of populations

(Scrimshaw et al., 2001). This committee has defined community-based prevention research as a collaborative approach that involves all stakeholders in each aspect of a study designed to evaluate the application and impact of new discoveries aimed at improving the health of a defined population. The findings detailed in this section demonstrate that assuring adequate funding for prevention research is a population health priority and is particularly relevant to the work of the nation's federal agencies engaged in public health research. Therefore, **the committee recommends that NIH increase the portion of its budget allocated to population- and community-based prevention research that**

- Addresses population-level health problems;
- Involves a definable population and operates at the level of the whole person;
- Evaluates the application and impacts of new discoveries on the actual health of the population; and
- Focuses on the behavioral and environmental (social, economic, cultural, physical) factors associated with primary and secondary prevention of disease and disability in populations.

Furthermore, the committee recommends that the Director of NIH report annually to the Secretary of DHHS on the scope of the population- and community-based prevention research activities undertaken by the NIH centers and institutes.

SERVICE

Although service has traditionally been viewed as a responsibility of academic faculty, it has been seen as less important than the functions of teaching and research. However, in public health there is growing discussion about the importance of service as a scholarly activity that contributes not only to the knowledge base but also to improving the health of the public. This section examines the role of academia in providing service to the community through collaborative efforts (participation in training centers and institutes, service learning, and other mechanisms). Next, barriers to active participation in service are discussed, and a recommendation for overcoming the impediments to faculty participation in scholarly service activities is made.

A Pew Health Professions Commission report (O'Neil, 1998) stated, "The nation and its health professionals will be best served when public service is a significant part of the typical path to professional practice." The academic community provides three kinds of service:

1. *Community service*, that is, service to state and local health departments, community organizations, and individuals;

2. *Policy guidance*, that is, helping to inform the public debate; and

3. *Service to the profession*, for example, providing peer review for professional journals, serving as officers of professional associations, and serving on committees both within academia and for professional organizations.

As the center of expertise in research and teaching, academia is uniquely positioned to provide technical assistance and service, based on credible evidence from its research and the expertise of its faculty and students, for the development and implementation of programs and policies designed to assure and improve the health of the public. For example, state public health departments might use academically developed information about computer technology and health informatics to implement a statewide surveillance and information system. Community workers might use the results of research on nutrition and behavior modification to organize a campaign designed to address the current obesity epidemic. Health care delivery systems use information and expertise developed in academia to design and implement smoking cessation programs and to coordinate efforts aimed at preventing and managing diabetes. Businesses and employers rely on academia for consultation on the design, implementation, and analysis of therapeutic intervention studies. Policy makers might respond to information emerging from academia that points to the need for new legislative or regulatory programs, for example, the presence of toxic residues in children resulting from exposure to residential pesticide use. Finally, the media use evidence developed in academia to inform the public regarding the impact of global infections on health.

Collaboration

As communities try to address their health issues in a comprehensive manner, all of the stakeholders will need to sort out their roles and responsibilities, which will vary from community to community. These interdependent sectors must address issues of shared responsibility for various aspects of community health and individual accountability for their actions. They also must participate in the process of communitywide social change that is necessary for health improvement efforts and related performance monitoring to succeed (IOM, 1997b).

Fundamental to effective service is effective collaboration. Emerging emphasis is being placed on academia's participation in collaborations, partnerships, and coalitions as mechanisms for improving the health of the public. Nelson and colleagues (1999) define collaboration as "a purposive relationship between partners committed to pursuing both an individual and a collective benefit." According to Berkowitz (2000), collaboration is "a method used by members of communities when developing coalitions, by organizations when doing strategic planning, and by researchers who desire the partnership of those being studied." Feighery and Rogers (1990) define a coalition as "an organization of individuals representing diverse organizations, factions or constituencies who agree to work together in order to achieve a common goal."

Collaborations are attractive for a number of reasons. They emphasize communitywide behavioral change through the use of a "multicomponent, multisector" approach to changing the environments that establish and maintain behaviors (Roussos and Fawcett, 2000). Success in affecting today's public health problems and their determinants requires the resources and trust relationships of a broad-based coalition of partners (Green et al., 2001). Bringing together people with different perspectives increases the potential to identify new and better ways of thinking about health issues (Lasker, 2000). Additionally, governmental financial and programmatic constraints require health partnerships, coalitions, and shared resources to achieve public health objectives (Baker et al., 1994).

What makes for a successful collaboration? The results of a study conducted by Kegler and colleagues (1998) to identify factors that contribute to coalition effectiveness suggest that coalitions with higher-quality action plans are better able to mobilize resources and implement activities, and that good communication, devotion of sufficient staff time to the coalition, a sense of cohesion, and a defined structure with multiple task forces appear to be related to the ability to implement activities. Such findings support the idea that developmental or formative activities are important for project success. Butterfoss and colleagues (1993) suggest that coalitions develop in stages (formation, implementation, maintenance, and outcomes) and that different sets of factors may be important to coalition functioning at each stage. For example, articulation of a clear mission, a spirit of cooperation, and positive expectations of outcomes are important during the formation stage, whereas formalization or definition of operational procedures, a strong central leadership, pooling of member assets (e.g., staff support, fundraising capability, meeting space, and access to relevant policy makers), the degree of membership participation, the continued perception of the partners that the benefits outweigh the costs of participation, and skills training are important during the implementation and maintenance stages.

Active involvement by many different parts of the community is believed to increase the likelihood of success for collaborative efforts (Feighery and Rogers, 1990; Israel et al., 1998; Lantz et al., 2001; Seifer and Krauer, 2001). Coalitions take time to coalesce; and the issues to be addressed immediately include agreement on a mission statement with goals and objectives, clarification of roles and relationships, definition of a decision-making process, development of an organizational structure, the frequency and length of meetings, and the benefits for each member of the coalition (Feighery and Rogers, 1990).

The benefits of successful collaborative efforts and partnerships are many. Collaborations can reduce disparity in access to information, resources, and skills; increase public health's understanding of community needs and assets; and lead to the development of a process for continual improvement in public policy and health systems (Berkowitz, 2000). Additional benefits include the freedom to become involved in new issues without bearing sole responsibility for managing or developing those issues; developing widespread public support for issues, actions, or unmet needs; developing a critical mass for action; minimizing duplication of effort and services; mobilizing a broad array of talents, resources, and approaches to problem solving; providing a mechanism for recruiting participants with diverse backgrounds and beliefs; and having flexibility in providing an opportunity to exploit new resources in changing situations (Butterfoss et al., 1993; Green et al., 2001).

Centers and Institutes

Academia engages in service to the community in many ways. One approach to service is through various centers and institutes. For example, in 2002 the University of Washington's Center for Ecogenetics and Environmental Health conducted a town meeting to engage in discussions with the community on racial disparity, poverty, and pollution. Activities brought together researchers, legislators, and community members to discuss the health risks of pesticides to agricultural workers and their families, contamination of seafood by marine toxins and chemical pollutants, hazardous waste sites, culturally appropriate research strategies, and links between indoor and outdoor air pollution and asthma. These discussions led to a number of projects designed to address community-identified concerns and needs.

The three newly funded CDC Centers for Genomics and Public Health, located at the University of Michigan, University of North Carolina, and University of Washington, are another mechanism through which service to the community can be provided. Each center will develop a regional hub of expertise for the use of genetic information to improve health and prevent disease. In addition to contributing to the knowledge base on genomics and public health and providing training for the public health workforce, the centers are to provide technical assistance to regional, state, and local public health organizations. "With this collaborative approach, CDC hopes to

... demonstrate—through real examples—the translation of gene discoveries into disease prevention and improved health" (CDC, 2001d).

Of primary importance in providing service to the working public health community is the Public Health Leadership Institute. The institute was developed as a collaborative effort of CDC and the Western Consortium for Public Health to provide leadership training for senior public health officers in state and local health departments. The University of North Carolina now coordinates its efforts. Each year a cohort of senior public health officials is selected to participate in a 12-month program that includes self-study, teleconferences, electronic seminars, action-learning projects, and an intensive on-campus week. The curriculum is centered around four modules concerning the challenges to public health: the study of the future, leadership and vision, communication and information, and political and social change (Scutchfield et al., 1995). The institute has spawned the development and growth of regional leadership training efforts aimed at increasing the leadership skills of public health practitioners at various levels of the system. Other approaches to service include the summer institutes and courses discussed above in the section Education and Training. These institutes and courses provide education and training to state and local health departments and other members of the community.

Academia's contributions to service also can be seen in the work of the Centers for Public Health Preparedness funded by CDC. There are academic centers, specialty centers, and local exemplar centers (see Table 8–3).

Academic centers aim to increase individual preparedness at the front line by linking schools of public health, state and local public health agencies, and other academic and community health partners. Specialty centers focus on a topic, professional discipline, core public health competency, practice setting, or application of learning technology. Local exemplar centers develop advanced applications at the community level in three areas: integrated communications and information systems, advanced operational readiness assessment, and comprehensive training and evaluation. Table 8–3 lists the centers in existence as of the writing of this report.

The centers work in collaboration with partners across their regions to assure a well-trained and prepared public health workforce, informed health care providers, and an alert citizenry to protect against terrorism. In September 2000, CDC, the Association of Schools of Public Health, state and local public health agencies, and other academic communities entered into a partnership to begin development of a national system of Centers for Public Health Preparedness (DHHS, 2002).

Service learning (also discussed above in the section Education and Training) is another way in which academic institutions engage in community service. Academic service-learning organizations and activities are growing and include the following: (1) service-learning centers on college

TABLE 8–3   Centers for Public Health Preparedness

Type	Location
Academic centers	University of Illinois at Chicago School of Public Health
	University of North Carolina, Chapel Hill, School of Public Health
	University of Washington School of Public Health and Community Medicine
	Columbia University Mailman School of Public Health
	University of Iowa College of Public Health
	University of South Florida College of Public Health
	St. Louis University School of Public Health
Specialty centers	Dartmouth College Medical School Interactive Media Laboratory
	Saint Louis University School of Public Health
	The Johns Hopkins University Bloomberg School of Public Health and the Georgetown University Law Center
	University of Findlay (Ohio) National Center of Excellence for Environmental Management
Local exemplar centers	DeKalb County Health Department
	Denver Public Health
	Monroe County Health Department

campuses across the United States that support and facilitate student and faculty work in communities; (2) the National Service-Learning Exchange, which provides training and technical assistance to service-learning programs; (3) campus compact (a national organization of more than 750 college and university presidents), which offers workshops, tool kits, and publications aimed at encouraging student and faculty involvement in community and public service; (4) research opportunities and studies; and (5) a planned National Center for Service-Learning Research (Howard, 2001).

Barriers and Solutions

There are barriers to establishing successful collaborations and partnerships. Clark (1999) outlined four barriers or gaps:

- *Communication*—a lack of a shared language and emphases;
- *Access*—little access to skilled public health faculty by some practitioners and communities;
- *Credibility*—practitioner skepticism of academic understanding and vice versa; and

- *Expectations*—the failure of what it takes to operate in the real world to meet academic standards of scientific rigor.

Other investigators include as barriers perceived threats to a sense of autonomy, disagreement about community needs, conflicts over funding decisions, a lack of consensus about membership criteria or coalition structure, failure to include relevant constituencies, and a lack of leadership (Feighery and Rogers, 1990; Kreuter et al., 2000).

A continuing barrier to scholarly service and one of great concern relates to faculty rewards, promotion, and tenure. Public health practice activities are not generally valued or rewarded by most academic institutions. Israel and colleagues (2001) write that multiple means are needed to provide evidence and recognition of the scholarship of public health practice. They list a number of matters that must be addressed to overcome this barrier. For example, peer-reviewed journals must recognize difficult methodological issues associated with conducting community-based participatory research and should be willing to publish such articles. Universities need to expand their evaluation of reputable journals. Because faculty members may assist communities in preparing grant proposals, these activities should be recognized and valued by academic institutions. Similarly, training activities for and technical assistance to community partners should be given credit toward tenure and promotion.

Practice Scholarship

Efforts are in progress to overcome the institutional lack of recognition of public health practice and service as scholarly endeavors. Maurana and colleagues (2000) report on two evidence-based models for documenting and assessing community scholarship activities. The first model, the Points of Distinction Project, is part of the Outreach Committee of Michigan State University. This model identified quantitative and qualitative indicators of success for four dimensions of quality outreach. The service must have significance, in that the issues addressed are of importance and value to project goals. The context of the service is crucial, in that it should have a close fit with the environment, use appropriate expertise and methods, have a substantial degree of collaboration, and use resources sufficiently and creatively. The scholarship of the service should demonstrate appropriate application, generation, and use of knowledge. Lastly, the service should be able to demonstrate that it has influence on issues, institutions, and individuals.

The second model is the Competency-Based Model of Alverno College in Milwaukee, Wisconsin. This model divides scholarly activity into four competencies, each of which specifies skills, activities, and requirements that faculty must master for promotion. These skills include being able to teach effectively, work responsibly in the college community, develop and pursue a research agenda, and serve the wider community.

The model proposed by Maurana and colleagues (2000) defines community scholarship as "the products that result from active, systematic engagement of academics with communities for such purposes as addressing a community-identified need, studying community problems and issues, and engaging in the development of programs that improve health." They offer standards and criteria for assessment of this scholarship. Criteria evaluate goals, preparation, methods, results presentation, and reflective critique. The model also describes four types of community scholarship products:

1.   Resources, such as how-to manuals, technical assistance, and tools and strategies to assess community strengths and assets or concerns;

2.   Program outcomes, such as improved community health outcomes, increased community leadership and funding for health, and integration of students and residents into community-based efforts or creative education;

3.   Dissemination, such as presentations, journal articles, and leadership at the national, state, and community levels; and

4.   Other products, such as new or strengthened partnerships and coalitions and program development grants.

In *Demonstrating Excellence,* ASPH (1999: 9) discusses the issue of service as scholarship:

> Service is relevant as scholarship if it requires the use of professional knowledge, or general knowledge that results from one's role as a faculty member. This knowledge is applied as consultant, professional expert, or technical advisor to the university community, the public health practice community, or professional practice organizations. The dimension of scholarship distinguishes practice-based service from a form of service known traditionally as the general responsibilities of citizenship.

To meet the requirements of scholarship as defined by ASPH, academic service must be provided through community-based participatory research, service learning or the work of the Prevention Research Centers, Centers for Genomics and Public Health, and Centers for Public Health Preparedness. Such activities to improve the health of the community not only fulfills academia's obligation of service but also expands the knowledge base and contributes to improvements in the health of the public. The value of these contributions is great and should be acknowledged by academic institutions in their promotion and tenure policies.

For these reasons, **the committee recommends that academic institu-**

tions develop criteria for recognizing and rewarding faculty scholarship related to service activities that strengthen public health practice.

CONCLUDING OBSERVATIONS

Academia, as one component of the public health system, provides important contributions to the health of the public in three ways: educating and training public health workers; conducting research in disciplines pertinent to public health; and engaging in community, public, and professional service. Numerous activities have been undertaken to educate and train the current and future public health workforce through methods such as classroom-based instruction, distance-learning programs, and training and leadership institutes. Stagnant and shrinking resources allocated to public health training are, however, impeding the ability of academic institutions to address today's new and emerging health problems. If it is true that the public health workforce is at the heart of the nation's ability to respond to new challenges such as emerging infections and preparedness against terrorist attacks, then that public health workforce must be adequately educated and trained to successfully face those challenges. This cannot be accomplished without making the training and education of public health workers the number one priority as demonstrated through adequate funding.

Academia has made major contributions to prolonging life and increasing the quality of life through research. Basic research has provided the knowledge necessary to develop precious vaccines that protect against debilitating and deadly diseases, whereas research on the determinants of health has demonstrated the importance of social and behavioral factors to health. However, comparatively few resources have been devoted to supporting prevention research, community-based research, or the translation of research findings into practice. Such resources must be found and allocated if academia is to continue to have a major impact on the health of communities. With the collaboration and partnership of academia, scholarly service has the potential to make great strides in engaging the community in improving its own health. However, without a restructuring of the reward system within universities and colleges, this most promising approach to change encounters barriers that are difficult to surmount.

Improvement of the public's health faces great challenges. Academia is committed to working in partnership with other components of the public health system to meet these challenges. Yet, to be successful, the role of academia must be valued, and funding must be available to develop the programs and approaches needed for education and training, research, and service to improve the public's health.

REFERENCES

AHCPR (Agency for Health Care Policy and Research). 1997. AHCPR funds project to foster collaboration between medicine and public health. In Research Activities Newsletter, No. 202. AHCPR Publication 97–0024. Rockville, MD: AHCPR.

ASPH (Association of Schools of Public Health). 1999. Demonstrating Excellence. Washington, DC: ASPH. Available online at http://www.asph.org/uploads/demon.pdf. Accessed March 17, 2002.

ASPH. 2000. 1999 Annual Data Report: Applications, New Enrollments & Students, and Fall 1999 Graduates, 1998–99 with Trends, 1989–1999. Washington, DC: ASPH.

Association of University Programs in Health Administration. 2000. Health Services Administration Education Director of Programs 2001–2002. Washington, DC: Association of University Programs in Health Administration.

Baker EL, Melton RJ, Stange PV, Fields ML, Koplan JP, Guerra FA, Satcher D. 1994. Health reform and the health of the public: forging community health partnerships. Journal of the American Medical Association 272(160):1276–1282.

Berkowitz B. 2000. Collaboration for health improvement: models for state, community, and academic partnerships. Journal of Public Health Management and Practice 6(1):67–72.

Berlin L. 2002. Special tabulation from the American Association of Colleges of Nursing 2001–2002 database. Washington, DC: American Association of Colleges of Nursing.

Bialek, R. 2000. Building the science base for public health practice. Journal of Public Health Management and Practice 6(5):51–58.

Brandt AM, Gardner M. 2000. Antagonism and accommodation: interpreting the relationship between public health and medicine in the United States during the 20th century. American Journal of Public Health 90(5):707–715.

Brownson RC, Simoes EJ. 1999. Measuring the impact of prevention research on public health practice. American Journal of Preventive Medicine 16(3 Suppl.):72–79.

Butterfoss FD, Goodman RM, Wandersman A. 1993. Community coalitions for prevention and health promotion. Health Education Research: Theory & Practice 8(3):315–330.

Cannon MM, Umble KE, Steckler A, Shay S. 2001. "We're living what we're learning": student perspectives in distance learning degree and certificate programs in public health. Journal of Public Health Management and Practice 7(1):49–59.

Cauley K, Canfield A, Clasen C, Dobbins J, Hemphill S, Jaballas E, Walbroehl G. 2001. Service learning: integrating student learning and community service. Education for Health 14(2):173–181.

CDC (Centers for Disease Control and Prevention). 2000. Proceedings from the Public Health Workforce Development Expert Panel Workshop, November 1–2, 2000, Calloway Gardens, GA. Atlanta, GA: CDC.

CDC. 2001a. A Global Life-Long Learning System: Building a Stronger Frontline Against Health Threats. A Global and National Implementation Plan for Public Health Workforce Development. Revision date: January 5, 2001. Atlanta, GA: CDC.

CDC. 2001b. A collection of competency sets of public health-related occupations and professions. Available online at www.phppo.cdc.gov/workforce. Accessed August 30, 2001.

CDC. 2001c. What is PHTN? The history. Available online at http://www.phppo.cdc.gov/phtn/history.asp. Accessed October 31, 2002.

CDC. 2001d. Centers for Disease Control and Prevention (CDC) Awards Funds for Genetics Programs. CDC National Center for Environmental Health (NCEH) news release, October 18, 2001. Available online at www.cdc.gov/genomics/activities/fund2001.htm. Accessed October 31, 2002.

CDC and Agency for Toxic Substance and Disease Registry (ATSDR). 1999. Strategic Plan for Public Health Workforce Development: Toward a Life-Long Learning System for Public Health Practitioners. Atlanta, GA: CDC.

Citrin T. 2001. Enhancing public health research and learning through community-academic partnerships: the Michigan experience. Public Health Reports 116:74–78.

Clark, NM. 1999. Community/practice/academic partnerships in public health. American Journal of Preventive Medicine 16(3 Suppl.):18–19

Council on Linkages. 2001. Core Competencies for Public Health Professionals. Washington, DC: Public Health Foundation.

Davis MV, Dandoy S. 2001. Survey of Graduate Programs in Public Health and Preventive Medicine and Community Health Education. Washington, DC: Association of Teachers of Preventive Medicine and the Council on Education for Public Health.

DHHS (Department of Health and Human Services). 1980. Chronology of Health Professions Legislation: 1956–1979. Washington, DC: Office of Program Development, Bureau of Health Professions, Health Resources Administration.

DHHS. 1988. Bureau of Health Professions: Selected Summary Data on Fiscal Years 1980–87 Awards. ODAM Report 3–88. Washington, DC: Office of Data Analysis and Management, Bureau of Health Professions, Health Resources and Services Administration.

DHHS. 2002. HHS announces new funding for academic centers. Press release, February 6. Available online at www.hhs.gov/news. Accessed March 2, 2002.

Doll L, Berkelman R, Rosenfield A, Baker E. 2001. Extramural prevention research at the Centers for Disease Control and Prevention. Public Health Reports 116(Suppl. 1):10–19.

Feighery E, Rogers T. 1990. Building and Maintaining Effective Coalitions, 2nd ed. Palo Alto, CA: Stanford Health Promotion Resource Center.

Fineberg HV, Green GM, Ware JH, Anderson BL. 1994. Changing public health training needs: professional education and the paradigm of public health. Annual Review of Public Health 15:237–257.

Garrett L. 2000. Betrayal of Trust: The Collapse of Global Public Health. New York: Hyperion.

Gebbie KM. 1999. The public health workforce: key to public health infrastructure. American Journal of Public Health 89(5):660–661.

Green LW, Mercer SL. 2001. Can public health researchers and agencies reconcile the push from funding bodies and the pull from communities? American Journal of Public Health 91(12):1926–1929.

Green L, Daniel M, Novick L. 2001. Partnerships and coalitions for community based research. Public Health Reports 116(Suppl. 1):20–30.

Hager, M. 1999. Education for More Synergistic Practice of Medicine and Public Health. New York: Josiah Macy, Jr., Foundation.

Howard J (Ed.). 2001. Service-Learning Course Design Workbook. Ann Arbor, MI: OCSL Press.

HRSA (Health Resources and Services Administration). 2000a. The public health workforce: enumeration 2000. Prepared for HRSA by Kristine Gebbie, Center for Health Policy, Columbia University School of Nursing, December. Washington, DC: HRSA.

HRSA. 2000b. Public health training centers. Available online at http://bhpr.hrsa.gov/publichealth/phtc.htm. Accessed October 31, 2002.

IOM (Institute of Medicine). 1988. The Future of Public Health. Washington, DC: National Academy Press.

IOM. 1997a. Linking Research and Public Health Practice: A Review of CDC's Program of Centers for Research and Demonstration of Health Promotion and Disease. Washington, DC: National Academy Press.

IOM. 1997b. Improving Health in the Community: A Role for Performance Monitoring. Washington, DC: National Academy Press.

IOM. 2000. Promoting Health: Intervention Strategies from Social and Behavioral Research. Washington, DC: National Academy Press.

IOM. 2001. Health and Behavior: The Interplay of Biological, Behavioral, and Societal Influences. Washington, DC: National Academy Press.

IOM. 2002. The National Clinical Research Enterprise: Draft Discussion Paper of the Clinical Research Roundtable. Washington, DC: National Academy Press.

IOM. 2003. Who Will Keep the Public Healthy? Educating Public Health Professionals. Washington, DC: National Academy Press.

Israel BA, Schulz AJ, Parker EA, Becker AB. 1998. Review of community-based research: assessing partnership approaches to improve public health. Annual Review of Public Health 19:173–202.

Israel BA, Schulz AJ, Parker EA, Becker AB. 2001. Community-based participatory research: policy recommendations for promoting a partnership approach in health research. Education for Health 14(2):182–197.

Kegler MC, Steckler A, McLeroy K, Malek SH. 1998. Factors that contribute to effective community health promotion coalitions: a study of 10 project ASSIST coalitions in North Carolina. Health Education & Behavior 25(3):338–353.

Kennedy VC, Spears WD, Loe HD, Jr., Moore FI. 1999. Public health workforce information: a state-level study. Journal of Public Health Management Practice 5(3):10–19.

Kreuter MW, Lezin NA, Young LA. 2000. Evaluating community-based collaborative mechanisms: implications for practitioners. Health Promotion Practice 1(1):49–63.

Lane DS. 2000. A threat to the public health workforce: evidence from trends in preventive medicine certification and training. American Journal of Preventive Medicine 18(1):87–96.

Lantz PM, Viruell-Fuentes E., Israel BA, Softley D, Guzman R. 2001. Can communities and academia work together on public health research? Evaluation results from a community-based participatory research partnership in Detroit. Journal of Urban Health: Bulletin of the New York Academy of Medicine 78(3): 495-507.

Lasker RD. 1999. What to teach medical students about public health for synergistic practice, pp. 148–158. In Hager M (Ed.). Education for More Synergistic Practice of Medicine and Public Health. New York: Josiah Macy, Jr., Foundation.

Lasker RD. 2000. Promoting Collaborations that Improve Health. Prepared for Discussion at Community-Campus Partnerships for Health's 4th Annual Conference. New York: The New York Academy of Medicine Division of Public Health

Lumpkin J. 1999. What to teach students of public health about medical practice. In Hager M (Ed.). Education for More Synergistic Practice of Medicine and Public Health. New York: Josiah Macy, Jr., Foundation.

Maurana C, Wolff M, Beck BJ, Simpson DE. 2000. Working with Communities: Moving from Service to Scholarship in the Health Professions. Prepared for Discussion at Community-Campus Partnerships for Health's 4th Annual Conference. San Francisco, CA: Community-Campus Partnerships for Health.

McGinnis JM, Foege WH. 1993. Actual causes of death in the United States. Journal of the American Medical Association 170(18):2207–2211.

Mullan F. 2000. Public health then and now. American Journal of Public Health 90(5):702–706.

National Association of Schools of Public Affairs and Administration. 1998. Survey of Enrollment and Degrees—Academic Year 1997–1998. Washington, DC: National Association of Schools of Public Affairs and Administration.

Nelson JC, Rashid H, Galvin VG, Essien JDK, Levine LM. 1999. Public/private partners: key factors in creating a strategic alliance for community health. American Journal of Preventive Medicine 16(3 Suppl.):94–102.

NIH (National Institutes of Health). 2002a. Centers for Children's Environmental Health and Disease Prevention Research. Division of Extramural Research and Training (DERT) website. Available online at www.niehs.nih.gov/dert/. Accessed October 31, 2002.

NIH. 2002b. Current research. Prevention Research Branch, National Institute for Child Health and Human Development (NICFD), NIH. Available online at www.nichd.nih. gov/ about/despr/prbrsh.htm. Accessed October 31, 2002.

O'Neil EH, Pew Health Professions Commission. 1998. Recreating Health Professional Practice for a New Century. San Francisco, CA: Pew Health Professions Commission.

Phillips DF. 2000. Medicine–public health collaboration tested. Journal of the American Medical Association 283(4):465–467.

Porter M, Monard K. 2001. Ayni in the global village: building relationships of reciprocity through international service-learning. Michigan Journal of Community Service Learning Fall 5–17.

Reder S, Gale JL, Taylor J. 1999. Using a dual method needs assessment to evaluate the training needs of public health professionals. Journal of Public Health Management and Practice 5(6):62–69.

Rhoads R, Howard J (Eds.). 1998. Academic Service Learning: A Pedagogy of Action and Reflection. San Francisco, CA: Josey-Bass Publishers.

Riegelman R, Persily NA. 2001. Health information systems and health communications: narrowband and broadband technologies as core public health competencies. American Journal of Public Health 91(8):1179–1195.

Roussos ST, Fawcett SB. 2000. A review of collaborative partnerships as a strategy for improving community health. Annual Review of Public Health 21:369–402.

Sattin RW. 2001. The Prevention Research Initiative and the peer review process at CDC. Public Health Reports 116(Suppl. 1):254–256.

Scrimshaw SC, White L, Koplan J. 2001. The meaning and value of prevention research. Public Health Reports 116(Suppl. 1):4–9.

Scutchfield FD, Spain C, Pointer DD, Hafey JM. 1995. The Public Health Leadership Institute: leadership training for state and local health officers. Journal of Public Health Policy 16(3):304–323.

Seifer S, Krauer P. 2001. Toward a policy agenda for community-campus partnerships. Education for Health 14(2):156–162.

Solloway M, Haack M, Evans L. 1997. Assessing the Training and Education Needs of the Public Health Workforce in Five States. Washington, DC: Center for Health Policy Research, Workforce Study Group, The George Washington University Medical Center.

Spencer HC. 2000. Testimony before the IOM Committee on Assuring the Health of the Public in the 21st Century. Washington, DC: Institute of Medicine.

Sullivan TJ. 2001. Methods of Social Research. Fort Worth, TX: Harcourt Brace and Co.

Turnock BJ. 2001. Public Health: What It Is and How It Works. Gaithersburg, MD: Aspen Publishers, Inc.

Valente TW. 2002. Evaluating Health Promotion Programs. New York: Oxford University Press.

APPENDIXES

A

Models of Health Determinants

As noted in Chapter 2, several models have been developed to describe the social or ecological determinants of health—the ways in which elements of the social, economic, and physical environments interact with individual biological factors and behaviors and shape health status. Some representative examples are provided below. An additional model, not pictured below, was developed by Keating and Hertzman (1999).

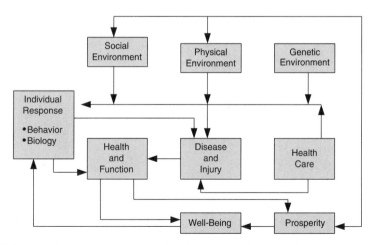

FIGURE A–1 A comprehensive model of the determinants of health.
SOURCE: Evans and Stoddart (1990). Used with permission from Elsevier Science.

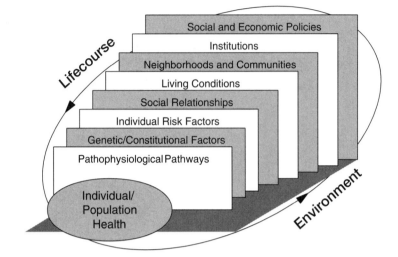

FIGURE A–2 Multilevel approach to epidemiology.
SOURCE: Institute of Medicine (2000).

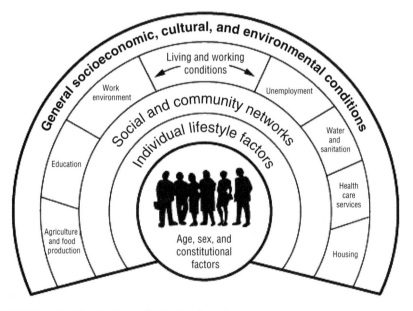

FIGURE A–3 The Dahlgren-Whitehead model.
SOURCE: Dahlgren and Whitehead (1991). Used with permission of the Institute
for Futures Studies, Stockholm, Sweden.

REFERENCES

Dahlgren G, Whitehead M. 1991. Policies and Strategies to Promote Social Equity in Health. Stockholm, Sweden: Institute for Futures Studies.

Evans RG, Stoddart GL. 1990. Producing health, consuming healthcare. Social Science and Medicine 31:1347–1363.

IOM (Institute of Medicine). 2000. Promoting Health: Intervention Strategies from Social and Behavioral Research, p. 43. Washington, DC: National Academy Press.

Keating DP, Hertzman C. 1999. Developmental Health and the Wealth of Nations: Social, Biological, and Educational Dynamics, p. 30. New York: Guilford Press.

B

Models for
Collaborative Planning in Communities

Chapter 4 discusses the models available to guide collaborative planning for communities. Three examples are provided below.

The MAPP Model

The MAPP (Mobilizing for Action through Planning and Partnership) tool was developed by the National Association of County and City Health Officials (NACCHO) in collaboration with the Centers for Disease Control and Prevention (CDC). MAPP (see Figure B–1) was built on the foundation of the Assessment Protocol for Excellence in Health, or APEXPH. APEXPH was developed as a tool to guide local health officials in conducting assessment and planning (NACCHO and CDC, 2000). The MAPP work group vision is "Communities achieving improved health and quality of life by mobilizing partnerships and taking strategic action." MAPP is targeted to communities, and its goal is to equip them with a structured framework for planning health programs. The MAPP process is centered on community organizing and partnership development and includes four assessments: assessing community themes and strengths, assessing the local public health system, assessing the community's health status, and assessing the forces of change. Next, MAPP involves the identification of strategic issues, the formulation of goals and strategies, and a continuous cycle of planning, implementation, and evaluation.

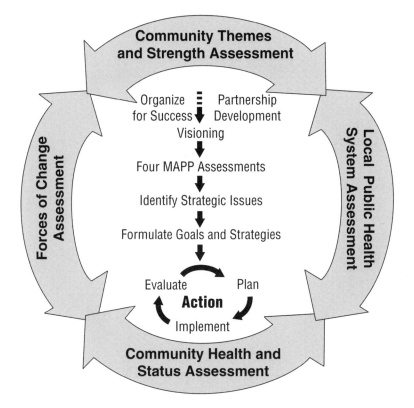

FIGURE B–1 The MAPP (Mobilizing for Action through Planning and Partnerships) model.
SOURCE: NACCHO and CDC (2000).

The PATCH Model

PATCH, the Planned Approach to Community Health, is a community health planning model developed by CDC in 1983. PATCH was created for application among diverse partners at the local level, but also within the context of vertical collaboration within the governmental public health infrastructure (federal, state, and local levels) and horizontal collaborations with voluntary organizations, academia, and other partners at all levels (Kreuter, 1992; CDC, 1997; Green et al., 2001). PATCH has five critical elements or phases (see Figure B–2). These include (1) community member participation, (2) data-based program development, (3) collaborative development of a comprehensive health promotion strategy, (4) evaluation for feedback and improvement, and (5) the enhancement of community capac-

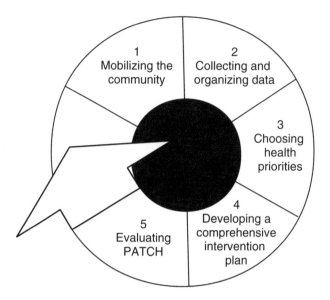

FIGURE B–2 The PATCH (Planned Approach to Community Health) model.
SOURCE: CDC (1997).

ity for health promotion. In a survey conducted by NACCHO between 1992 and 1993, 239 local health agencies were using PATCH (NACCHO and CDC, 1995). Although PATCH encourages the active engagement of local governmental health agencies, it recognizes that these may not always be the "most appropriate and/or effective focal point for PATCH" and "primary care clinics, university groups, businesses, and other nongovernmental organizations may be in a better position to exercise leadership for a PATCH program" with the support and facilitation of the local health agency (Kreuter, 1992). The implementation of PATCH highlighted several elements that seem to be associated with successful community-based public health planning and action. These include the existence of a core of community support and participation, data collection and analysis, setting of objectives and standards to help with planning and evaluation, the adoption of multiple strategies on multiple fronts, sustained monitoring and progress evaluation to fine-tune projects, and the support of the governmental public health infrastructure nationally and locally (Kreuter, 1992). One of the major applications of PATCH is carrying out the assessment function of public health, described in the 1988 IOM report (IOM, 1988). Assessment is a core function of the public health infrastructure, but public health activities in the private sector and the efforts of communities can also contribute to the process of assessing population health status.

The CHIP Model

CHIP, the Community Health Improvement Process, is a tool for community health planning and evaluation through inventory taking and performance monitoring. CHIP (Figure B–3) has two interacting cycles: the problem identification and prioritization cycle, which includes phases of community organizing, assessment, and selection of priority areas, and the analysis and implementation cycle, which includes seven phases that range from planning, through implementation, to evaluation (IOM, 1997). CHIP's

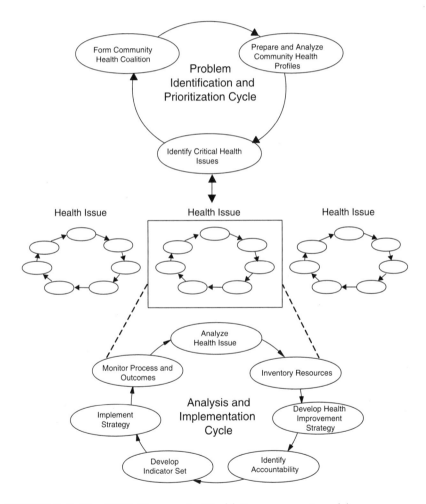

FIGURE B–3 The CHIP (Community Health Improvement) model.
SOURCE: IOM (1997).

resource inventory step is related to the concepts of asset-based community development (identifying strengths on which to build) and ultimately addresses health problems and needs (Kretzmann and McKnight, 1993). CHIP also uses the performance measurements provided by *Healthy People 2000* (USPHS, 1991) and Healthy Communities 2000 Model Standards (IOM, 1997; APHA, 1999). CHIP's process of developing indicators has been further elaborated in CDC's Principles of Community Engagement and incorporated in a wide range of community and regional health report cards (CDC, 1997).

REFERENCES

APHA (American Public Health Association). 1999. Healthy Communities 2000: Model Standards. Washington, DC: APHA.

CDC (Centers for Disease Control and Prevention). 1997. Principles of Community Engagement. CDC/ATSDR Committee on Community Engagement. Atlanta, GA: CDC.

Green L, Daniel M, Novick L. 2001. Partnerships and coalitions for community-based research. Public Health Reports 116(Suppl. 1):20–31.

IOM (Institute of Medicine). 1997. Improving Health in the Community: A Role for Performance Monitoring. Washington, DC: National Academy Press. Available online at http://www.nap.edu/catalog/5298.html.

IOM. 1988. The Future of Public Health. Washington, DC: National Academy Press.

Kretzmann JP, McKnight JL. 1993. Building Communities from the Inside Out: A Path Toward Finding and Mobilizing a Community's Assets. Evanston, IL: Institute for Policy Research.

Kreuter MW. 1992. PATCH: its origin, basic concepts, and links to contemporary public health policy. Journal of Health Education 23(3):135–139. Available online at http://www.cdc.gov/nccdphp/patch/.

NACCHO (National Association of County and City Health Officials) and CDC (Centers for Disease Control and Prevention). 1995. 1992–1993 National Profile of Local Health Departments. Atlanta, GA: CDC.

NACCHO and CDC. 2000. A strategic approach to community health improvement: MAPP. Available online at http://mapp.naccho.org/MAPP_Home.asp. Accessed October 16, 2002.

USPHS (U.S. Public Health Service). 1991. Healthy People 2000: National Health Promotion and Disease Prevention Objectives. DHHS Publication 91–50212. Washington, DC: U.S. Public Health Service.

C

Recommendations from
*The Future of Public Health**

Objective: To provide a set of directions for public health that can attract the support of the total society, the committee made three basic recommendations dealing with:

- The mission of public health
- The governmental role in fulfilling the mission
- The responsibilities unique to each level of government

THE PUBLIC HEALTH MISSION, GOVERNMENTAL ROLE, AND LEVELS OF RESPONSIBILITY

Mission

The committee defines the mission of public health as fulfilling society's interest in assuring conditions in which people can be healthy.

The Governmental Role in Public Health

- The committee finds that the core functions of public health agencies at all levels of government are assessment, policy development, and assurance.

---

* Institute of Medicine. 1988. The Future of Public Health. Washington, DC: National Academy Press.

Assessment

 • The committee recommends that every public health agency regularly and systematically collect, assemble, analyze, and make available information on the health of the community, including statistics on health status, community health needs, and epidemiologic and other studies of health problems.

Policy Development

 • The committee recommends that every public health agency exercise its responsibility to serve the public interest in the development of comprehensive public health policies by promoting use of the scientific knowledge base in decision making about public health and by leading in developing public health policy. Agencies must take a strategic approach, developed on the basis of a positive appreciation for the democratic political process.

Assurance

 • The committee recommends that public health agencies assure their constituents that services necessary to achieve agreed upon goals are provided, either by encouraging action or by other entities (private or public sector), by requiring such action through regulation, or by providing services directly.
 • The committee recommends that each public health agency involve key policymakers and the general public in determining a set of high-priority personal and communitywide health services that governments will guarantee to every member of the community. This guarantee should include subsidization or direct provision of high-priority personal health services for those unable to afford them.

Levels of Responsiblity

States

The committee believes that the states are and must be the central force in public health, They bear primary public sector responsibility for health.

The committee recommends that the public health duties of states should include the following:

 • Assessment of health needs within the state based on statewide data collection;

• Assurance of an adequate statutory base for health activities in the state;

• Establishment of statewide health objectives, delegating power to localities as appropriate and holding them accountable;

• Assurance of appropriate organized statewide effort to develop and maintain requisite personal, educational, and environmental health services; provision of access to necessary services; and solution of problems inimical to health;

• Guarantee of a minimum set of essential health services; and

• Support of local service capacity, especially when disparities in local ability to raise revenue and/or administer programs require subsidies, technical assistance, or direct action by the state to achieve adequate service levels.

Federal

The committee recommends the following as federal public health obligations:

• Support of knowledge development and dissemination through data gathering, research, and information exchange;

• Establishment of nationwide health objectives and priorities, and stimulation of debate on interstate and national public health issues;

• Provision of technical assistance to help states and localities determine their objectives and to carry out action on national and regional objectives;

• Provision of funds to states to strengthen state capacity for services, especially to achieve an adequate minimum capacity, and to achieve national objectives; and

• Assurance of actions and services that are in the public interest of the entire nation such as control of AIDS and similar communicable diseases, interstate environmental actions, and food and drug inspections.

Localities

The committee recommends the following functions for local public health units:

• Assessment, monitoring, and surveillance of local health problems and needs and of resources for dealing with them;

• Policy development and leadership that foster local involvement and a sense of ownership, that emphasize local needs, and that advocate equitable distribution of public resources and complimentary private activities commensurate with community needs; and

• Assurance that high-quality services, including personal health services, needed for the protection of public health in the community are available and accessible to all persons; that the community receives proper consideration in the allocation of federal and state as well as local resources for public health; and that the community is informed about how to obtain public health, including personal health, services, or how to comply with public health requirements.

FULFILLING THE GOVERNMENT ROLE: IMPLEMENTING RECOMMENDATIONS

Statutory Base

The committee recommends that states review their public health statutes and make the revisions necessary to accomplish the following two objectives:

• Clearly delineate the basic authority and responsibility entrusted to public health agencies, boards, and officials at the state and local levels and the relationships between them; and
• Support a set of modern disease control measures that address contemporary health problems such as AIDS, cancer, and heart disease, and incorporate due process safeguards (notice, hearings, administrative review, right to counsel, standards of evidence).

Structural/Organizational Steps

States

• The committee recommends that each state have a department of health that groups all primarily health-related functions under professional direction—separate from income maintenance. Responsibilities of this department should include disease prevention and health promotion, Medicaid and other indigent health care activities, mental health and substance abuse, environmental responsibilities that clearly require health expertise, and health planning and regulation of health facilities and professions.
• The committee recommends that each state have a state health council that reports regularly on the health of the state's residents, makes health policy recommendations to the governor and legislative [branch], promulgates public health regulations, reviews the work of the state health department, and recommends candidates for director of the department.

• The committee recommends that the director of the department of health be a cabinet (or equivalent-level) officer. Ideally, the director should have doctoral-level education as a physician or in another health profession, as well as education in public health itself and extensive public-sector administrative experience. Provisions for tenure in office, such as a specific term of appointment, should promote needed continuity of professional leadership.

• The committee recommends that each state establish standards for local public health functions, specifying what minimum services must be offered, by what unit of government, and how services are to be financed. States (unless providing local services directly) should hold localities accountable for these services and for addressing statewide health objectives.

Localities

• The committee finds that the larger the population served by a single multipurpose government, as well as the stronger the history of local control, the more realistic the delegation of responsibility becomes: for example, to a large metropolitan city, county, or service district. Two attributes of such a locally responsible system are strongly recommended:

— To promote clear accountability, public health responsibility should be delegated to only one unit of government in a locality.

— Where sparse population or scarce resources prevail, delegation to regional single-purpose units, such as multicounty health districts, may be appropriate.

• The committee recommends that mechanisms be instituted to promote local accountability and assure the maintenance of adequate and equitable levels of service and qualified personnel.

• The committee finds that the need for a clear focal point at the local level is as great as at the state level, and for the same reasons. Where the scale of government activity permits, localities should establish public health councils to report to elected officials on local health needs and on the performance of the local health agency.

Federal

• The committee recommends that the federal government identify more clearly, in formal structure and actual practice, the specific officials and agencies with primary responsibility for carrying out the federal public health functions recommended earlier.

• The committee recommends the establishment of a task force to consider what structure or programmatic changes would be desirable to enhance the federal government's ability to fulfill the public health leadership responsibilities recommended in this report.

Special Linkages

Environmental Health

- The committee recommends that state and local health agencies strengthen their capacities for identification, understanding, and control of environmental problems as health hazards. The agencies cannot simply be advocates for the health aspects of environmental issues, but must have direct operational involvement.

Mental Health

- The committee recommends that those engaged in knowledge development and policy planning in public health and in mental health, respectively, devote a specific effort to strengthening linkages with the other field, particularly in order to identify strategies to integrate these functions at the service delivery level.
- The committee recommends that a study of the public health/mental health interface be done in order to document how the lack of linkages with public health hampers the mental health mission.

Social Services

- The committee recommends that public health be separated organizationally from income maintenance, but that public health agencies maintain close working relationships with social service agencies in order to act as effective advocates for, and to cooperate with, social service agency provision of social services that have an impact on health.

Care of the Indigent

- The committee endorses the conclusion of the President's Commission for the Study of Ethical Problems in Medical Care and Biomedical and Behavioral Research that the ultimate responsibility for assuring equitable access to health care for all, through a combination of public- and private-sector action, rests with the federal government.
- The committee finds that, until adequate federal action is forthcoming, public health agencies must continue to serve, with quality and respect and to the best of their ability, the priority personal health care needs of uninsured, underinsured, and Medicaid clients.

Strategies for Capacity Building

Technical

• The uniform national data set should be established that will permit valid comparison of local and state health data with those of the nation and of other states and localities and that will facilitate progress toward national health objectives and implementation.

• There should be an institutional home in each state and at the federal level for development and dissemination of knowledge, including research and the provision of technical assistance to lower levels of government and to the academic institution and voluntary organizations.

• Research should be conducted at the federal, state, and local levels into population-based health problems, including biological, environmental, and behavioral issues. In addition to conducting research directly, the federal government should support research by states, localities, universities, and the private sector.

Political

• Public health agency leaders should develop relationships with and educate legislators and other public officials on community health needs, on public health issues, and the rationale for strategies advocated and pursued by the health department. These relationships should be cultivated on an ongoing basis rather than being neglected until a crisis develops.

• Agencies should strengthen the competence of agency personnel in community relations and citizen participation techniques and develop procedures to build citizen participation into program implementation.

• Agencies should develop and cultivate relationships with physicians and other private-sector representatives. Physicians and other health professionals are important instruments of public health by virtue of such activities as counseling patients on health promotion and providing immunizations. They are important determinants of public attitudes and of the image of the public health. Public health leaders should take the initiative to seek working relationships and support among local, state, and national medical and other professional societies and academic medical centers.

• Agencies should seek stronger relationships and common cause with other professional and citizen groups pursuing interests with health implications, including voluntary health organizations, groups concerned with improving social services or environment, and groups concerned with economic development.

• Agencies should undertake education of the public on community health needs and public health policy issues.

- Agencies should review the quality of "street-level" contacts between department employees and clients and where necessary conduct inservice training to ensure that members of the public are treated with cordiality and respect.

Managerial

- Greater emphasis in public health curricula should be placed on managerial and leadership skills, such as the ability to communicate important agency values to employees and enlist their commitment; to sense and deal with important changes in the environment; to plan, mobilize, and use resources effectively; and to relate the operation of the agency to its larger community role.
- Demonstrated management competence as well as technical/professional skills should be a requirement for upper-level management posts.
- Salaries and benefits should be improved for health department managers, especially health officers, and systems should be instituted so that they can carry retirement benefits with them when they move among different levels of jurisdictions of government.

Programmatic

- The committee recommends that public health professionals place more emphasis on factors that influence health-related behavior and develop comprehensive strategies that take these factors into account.

Fiscal

The committee recommends the following policies with respect to intergovernmental strategies for strengthening the fiscal base of public health:

- Federal support of state-level health programs should help balance disparities in revenue-generating capacities and encourage state attention to national health objectives. Particular vehicles for such support should include "core" funding with appropriate accountability mechanisms, as well as funds targeted for specific uses.
- State support of local-level health services should balance local revenue-generating disparity, establish local capacity to provide minimum levels of service, and encourage local attention to state health objectives; support should include "core" funding. State funds could be furnished with strings attached and sanctions available for noncompliance, and/or general support could be provided with appropriate accountability requirements

built in. States have the obligation in either case to monitor local use of state funds.

Education for Public Health

•   Schools of public health should establish firm practice links with state and/or local public health agencies so that significantly more faculty members may undertake professional responsibilities in these agencies, conduct research there, and train students in such practice situations. Recruitment of faculty and admission of students should give appropriate weight to prior public health experience as well as to academic qualifications.

•   Schools of public health should fulfill their potential role as significant resources to government at all levels in the development of public health policy.

•   Schools of public health should provide students an opportunity to learn the entire scope of public health practice, including environmental, educational, and personal health approaches to the solution of public health problems; the basic epidemiological and biostatistical techniques for analysis of those problems; and the political and management skills needed for leadership in public health.

•   Research in schools of public health should range from basic research in fields related to public health, through applied research and development, to program evaluation and implementation research.

•   Schools of public health should take maximum advantage of training resources in their universities, for example, faculty and courses in schools of business administration, and departments of physical, biological, and social sciences.

•   Schools of public health should extend their expertise to advise and assist with the health content of the educational programs of other schools and departments of the university.

•   Schools of public health should undertake an expanded program of short courses to help upgrade the competence of these personnel. In addition, short course offering should provide opportunities for previously trained public health professionals, especially health officers, to keep up with advances in knowledge and practice.

•   Schools of public health should encourage and assist other institutions to prepare appropriate, qualified public health personnel for positions in the field. When educational institutions other than schools of public health undertake to train personnel for work in the field, careful attention to the scope and capacity of the educational program is essential.

•   Schools of public health should strengthen their response to the needs for qualified personnel for important, but often neglected aspects of public health such as the health of minority groups and international health.

- Schools of public health should help develop, or offer directly in their own universities, effective courses that expose undergraduates to concepts, history, current context, and techniques of public health to assist in the recruitment of able future leaders into the field.
- Education programs for public health professionals should be informed by comprehensive and current data on public health personnel and their employment opportunities and needs.

D

*Healthy People 2010** Objectives for the Public Health Infrastructure

Goal: Ensure that federal, tribal, state, and local health agencies have the infrastructure to provide essential public health services effectively.

Data and Information Systems

1. Increase the proportion of Tribal, State, and local public health agencies that provide Internet and e-mail access for at least 75 percent of their employees and that teach employees to use the Internet and other electronic information systems to apply data and information to public health practice.

2. (Developmental) Increase the proportion of Federal, Tribal, State, and local health agencies that have made information available to the public in the past year on the Leading Health Indicators, Health Status Indicators, and Priority Data Needs.

3. Increase the proportion of all major national, State, and local health data systems that use geocoding to promote nationwide use of geographic information systems (GIS) at all levels.

4. Increase the proportion of population-based *Healthy People 2010* objectives for which national data are available for all population groups identified for the objective.

5. Increase the proportion of Leading Health Indicators, Health Status Indicators, and Priority Data Needs for which data—especially for select populations—are available at the Tribal, State, and local levels.

6. Increase the proportion of *Healthy People 2010* objectives that are tracked regularly at the national level.

---

* Department of Health and Human Services. 2000. Public health infrastructure. In Healthy People 2010. Available online at www.health.gov/healthypeople/document/tableofcontents. htm#volume2.

7. Increase the proportion of *Healthy People 2010* objectives for which national data are released within 1 year of the end of data collection.

Workforce

8. Increase the proportion of Federal, Tribal, State, and local agencies that incorporate specific competencies in the essential public health services into personnel systems.

9. Increase the proportion of schools for public health workers that integrate into their curricula specific content to develop competency in the essential public health services.

10. Increase the proportion of Federal, Tribal, State, and local public health agencies that provide continuing education to develop competency in essential public health services for their employees.

Public Health Organizations

11. Increase the proportion of State and local public health agencies that meet national performance standards for essential public health services.

12. Increase the proportion of Tribes, States, and the District of Columbia that have a health improvement plan and increase the proportion of local jurisdictions that have a health improvement plan linked with their State plan.

13. Increase the proportion of Tribal, State, and local health agencies that provide or assure comprehensive laboratory services to support essential public health services.

14. Increase the proportion of Tribal, State, and local public health agencies that provide or assure comprehensive epidemiology services to support essential public health services.

15. Increase the proportion of Federal, Tribal, State, and local jurisdictions that review and evaluate the extent to which their statutes, ordinances, and bylaws assure the delivery of essential public health services.

Resources

16. Increase the proportion of Federal, Tribal, State, and local public health agencies that gather accurate data on public health expenditures, categorized by essential public health service.

Prevention Research

17. Increase the proportion of Federal, Tribal, State, and local public health agencies that conduct or collaborate on population-based prevention research.

E

Competencies for Public Health Workers: A Collection of Competency Sets for Public Health-Related Occupations and Professions

The Public Health Practice Program Office, Centers for Disease Control and Prevention (CDC) (www.phppo.cdc.gov/OWPP) developed this table of competency sets of public health-related occupations and professions for its Annual Public Health Workforce Development Meeting (June 2001, revised January 2003).

Purpose

The competency sets are intended to be a resource for persons interested in public health workforce development. It includes online sources for all documents listed. The information listed can be used as an aid to curriculum developers and instructional designers in planning training programs for the Nation's public health workers. This resource document also provides relevant examples of competency statements from other occupations and professions that share in the work of public health. Used as a starting point, this list may help avoid duplication of efforts and will build on existing activities across the U.S.

Methodology

This report on competency sets was developed using print and electronic references and experts in workforce development. Sources included: Council on Linkages, Core Competencies (Public Health Foundation), and competency sets from other professions, United Kingdom, Australia and other countries. Other sources also used were Institute of Medicine Reports: *The Future of Public Health*, 1988, 2002; *Who Will Keep the Public Healthy: Educating Public Health Professionals for the 21st Century* (2003, The National Academies Press, Washington, DC); and *Public Health in America*, 1994 (http://www.health.gov/phfunctions/public.htm). Where competencies sets are lacking, selected resources are listed if appropriate.

Ms. Kimberley Geissman, M.S., M.Ed., and Dr. Anil Patel, M.D., M.P.H. conducted the primary research.

The Competency Sets

The competency sets can be grouped and differentiated several ways:

- Core: Basic Public Health Skills (skills needed to perform the essential functions of public health)
- Function-specific: e.g., leadership, management, supervisory, support staff
- Discipline-specific: e.g., community dentistry for public health dentists, other professionals or technical specialists
- Subject-specific (within a discipline): maternal and child health, STD, vaccine preventable diseases, cancer, other chronic diseases
- Workplace basics: required of all personnel and includes literacy, writing and presentation skills and computer literacy

Limitations

The competencies listed are those known at the time of printing. The comprehensive search for related public health worker competencies included numerous global and site-specific web searches, list-serve queries, and personal contacts. Since the field of workforce development is evolving, many competency sets—be they produced by government, academic institutions, public health and professional organizations—are in development. Therefore, this list may not contain all available competency sets. Inclusion of any competency set in the table does not imply CDC endorsement.

How You Can Help

Please notify the CDC Office of Workforce Policy and Planning (PHPPO) of major omissions, corrections, and additions to this document, "A Collection of Competency Sets of Public Health-Related Occupations and Professions," updated for the Public Health Workforce Development Annual Meeting, January 21-23, 2003, Atlanta, GA, through our web site at www.phppo.cdc.gov/owpp or call 770 488 2480 (main office).

A COLLECTION OF COMPETENCY SETS OF
PUBLIC HEALTH-RELATED OCCUPATIONS AND PROFESSIONS

SOURCE: Public Health Practice Program Office, CDC (2003).

Updated for the Public Health Workforce Development Annual Meeting, January 21-23, 2003, Atlanta, GA

Competency Sets	Worker Level	Where to Find Them on the WWW
Core-Basic Public Health		
Council on Linkages: Core Competencies for Public Health Professionals, 2001	front-line, senior professional, supervisor, manager	Public Health Foundation (PHF), http://www.trainingfinder.org/competencies/list_nolevels.htm and http://trainingfinder.org/competencies/list_levels.htm
21 Competencies for the 21st Century, 1999 Commission, Dec. 1998, Chapter 4	professional	The 4th Report of the Pew Health Professions, http://www.futurehealth.ucsf.edu/pewcomm/competen.html
Competencies for Providing Essential Public Health Services, 1997	professional	*The Public Health Workforce: An Agenda for the 21st Century*, Public Health Functions Project, ODPHP, DHHS, http://www.health.gov/phfunctions/publhth.pdf essential services, www.apha.org/ppp/science/10ES.htm
Accounting		
Core Competency Framework for Entry into the Accounting Profession: Functional Competencies	entry-level professional	American Institute of Certified Public Accountants, (AICPA) http://www.aicpa.org/edu/func.htm
Competency Model for the New Finance Professional	professional, technical, support	American Institute of Certified Public Accountants (AICPA) tool being piloted, http://www.cpatoolbox.org

continued

Competency Sets	Worker Level	Where to Find Them on the WWW
Core Competencies (future of the CPA profession), 2001	professional, technical	Vision Project Team and State Societies, CPA Vision Project: 2001 and Beyond http://www.cpavision.org
Basic Life Skills *CASAS Competency List*	basic life skills	Secretary's Commission on Achieving Necessary Skills, DOL http://www.casas.org/01AboutCasas/01Competencies.html
High School Student Competencies and Indicators	high school graduates	National Occupational Information Coordinating Committee (NOICC), Academic Innovations http://www.academicinnovations.com/noicc.html
Behavioral Science (general) *Behavioral & Social Science Competencies*, draft 2001	professionals	School of Public Health Science and Research, CDC Corporate University, draft to be validated; Charlotte Wilson, HRMO CWilson@cdc.gov
Ethical Principles of Psychologists and Code of Conduct, December 1992	professionals	American Psychological Association (APA), "General Principles" http://www.apa.org/ethics/code.html
Biological Science *Biological Science Competencies*, draft 2001	professionals	School of Public Health Science and Research, CDC Corporate University, draft to be validated; Charlotte Wilson, HRMO CWilson@cdc.gov
Bioterrorism *Bio-terrorism*	All public health workers	Center for Disease Control, Bio-terrorism and related topics/including web casts http://www.cdc.gov/washington/reltopic/bioterro.htm

Bioterrorism and Emergency Readiness: Competencies for ALL Public Health Workers	all public health workers	Bioterrorism and Emergency Readiness: Competencies for ALL Public Health Workers, Center for Health Policy, http://www.nursing.hs.columbia.edu/institute-centers/chphsr/btcomps.html
Community-based Health		
Community Health Scholars Program: Goal and Competencies, June 1999	post-doctoral student	Community-Based Public Health (CBPH), University of Michigan School of Public Health, Kellogg sponsored, program competencies, http://www.sph.umich.edu/chsp/goal.html
Community Based Participatory Research (pending)		
Cultural Competency		
Providing Care to Diverse Populations State Strategies for Cultural Competency in Health Systems	all state, local health officials	Workshops sponsored by Agency for Health Care Policy and Research, http://www.ahcpr.gov/news/ulp/ulpcultr/htm
The provision of Culturally Competent Health Care	leader, professional, technical support	Amy Blue, PhD, Assistant Dean for Curriculum and Evaluation, Medical University of South Carolina College of medicine, http://www.musc.edu/deansclerkship/recultur.html
Courses/ training/online database/tools	health professionals	National Center for Cultural Competence, Georgetown University Center for Child and Human Development, University Center for Excellence in developmental Disabilities, http://www.georgetown.edu/research/gucdc/nccc
Learning Resources/Training Materials Cultural Competency Training	all healthcare professionals	Cultural Competency Training, Illinois Health Education Consortium: IHEC, http://www.ihec.org/f-pro3-3.html

continued

Competency Sets	Worker Level	Where to Find Them on the WWW
Dentistry		
Competency Statements for Dental Public Health, September 1997	professional	American Association of Public Health Dentistry (AAPHD), http://www.pitt.edu/~aaphd/dph.competency.html
Economics		
Nebraska Standards in Business Education Essential Leanings: Focus on Economics	student, public	EcEd Economics Education Web competencies and learning objectives, http://ecedweb.unomaha.edu/standards/home.htm
National and State Content Standards in Economics	student, public	Economics America, National Council on Economic Education (NCEE), 20 standards, learning objectives and performance benchmarks, http://www.economicsamerica.org
Emergency Preparedness		
Core Public Health Worker Competencies for Emergency Preparedness and Response, April 2001	leader, administrator, professional, technical, support	Center for Health Policy, Columbia University School of Nursing, http://cpmcnet.columbia.edu/dept/nursing/institute-centers/chphsr/COMPETENCIES.pdf (April 2001) and http://www.nursing.hs.columbia.edu/institute-centers/chphsr/btcomps.pdf (December 02)
Fire & Emergency Services Competency Module	technical	Industry-Specific Competency Modules, Knowledge Point, http://www.knowledgepoint.com/products/firecomp.html
Engineering		
Sample Elements and Tasks for Engineer, October 1999	professional	Headquarters Performance Management System, DOE, http://www.hr.doe.gov/hqpms/engineer.htm

Environmental Health

Environmental Health Competency Project: Recommendations for Core Competencies for Local Environmental Health Practitioners, May 2001	front-line, local-level professional	American Public Health Association (APHA) and National Center for Environmental Health (NCEH/CDC) with NEHA, NACCHO, ASTHO, FCA, AAS, NALBOH, final draft in clearance June 1, report due August 2001. Patrick Bohan, NCEH, PBohan@cdc.gov, http://www.apha.org/ppp/ehproject.htm
Environmental Health Competencies: Core Competencies for the Effective Practice of Environmental Health	professional	Funding Opportunity, Association of School of Public Health (ASPH), Developing Communities of Excellence in Environmental Health, http://www.asph.org/fac_document.cfm/69/69/5968
Registered Environmental Health Specialist/ Registered Sanitarian Examination	entry-level professional	National Environmental Health Association (NEHA), exam content outline; Ryan Rudolph, rrudolph@neha.org, http://www.neha.org

Epidemiology

Health Science and Epidemiology Competencies, 2001	professional	School of Public Health Science and Research, CDC Corporate University, draft to be validated; Charlotte Wilson, HRMO, CWilson@cdc.gov
Core Activities for Learning (CALS)	doctoral-level Epidemic Intelligence Officer	Epidemic Intelligence Service (EIS), CDC Jim Alexander, EPO/DAPHT, JAlexander1@cdc.gov
Evaluation of EIS Competency Domains: Epidemiologic Process, Communication, and Professionalism, 2001	doctoral-level Epidemic Intelligence Officer	Epidemic Intelligence Service (EIS), CDC Jim Alexander, EPO/DAPHT, JAlexander1@cdc.gov
Maternal and Child Health Epidemiology Fellowship Competency Guidelines	professional	Council of State and Territorial Epidemiologists (CSTE) with CDC, http://www.cste.org/MCHcompetencies.pdf

continued

Competency Sets	Worker Level	Where to Find Them on the WWW
Infection Control and Epidemiology: Professional and Practice Standards, 1998	professional	Association for Practitioners in Infection Control & Epidemiology (APIC) and Community and Hospital Infection Control Association, Canada (CHICA), http://www.apic.org/pdf/pracstnd.pdf
Ethics *Center for Ethics*	all health care professionals	Center for Ethics, Health Science Ethics. Health Care Ethics consortium of Georgia, Emory University, in development, http://www.emory.edu/ETHICS
Center for Bioethics and Health Law	MPH students/health care professionals	Center for Bioethics and Health Law, University of Pittsburgh, http://www.pitt.edu2-bioethic/
Evaluation/Program Analysis *Competencies for Public Health Analyst (GS-685)*, 2001	professional	School of Public Health Administration, CDC Corporate University, draft to be validated; Ronald Lake, HRMO RLake@cdc.gov, http://intranet.cdc.gov/hrmo/analyst.htm
Career Development: Core Competencies (Evaluation and Inspections), December 1999	manager, program analyst, team leader, administrator, technical support, secretary	Office of Evaluation and Inspections (OEI), Office of Inspector General (OIG), http://www.hhs.gov/oig/oei/evaluator/evaluator.html
Global Health Competency *Division of International Health, Core Competencies, CDC,*	International Health workers	Core Competencies and Outputs for Public Health Practitioners or Applied Epidemiologists, http://www.cdc.gov/epo/dih/core.html

Genomics

Genomics Competencies for the Public Health Workforce, May 2001	administrator, professional, all workers(clinicians, educators, environmental workers, epidemiologists, laboratorians), (technical, support)	Office of Genetics and Disease Prevention and Public Health Practice Program Office, CDC, http://www.cdc.gov/genetics/training/competencies/
Competencies in Public Health Genetics in the Content of Law, Ethics and Policy, June 1999	MPH, MS, PhD student	University of Washington, School of Public Health and Community Medicine (Training Collaboration CDC, HRSA funded), http://depts.washington.edu/phgen/DegreeTracks/competencies.html
Core Competencies in Genetics Essential for All Health Care Professionals, February 2000	all health care professional, student	National Coalition for Health Professional Education in Genetics (NCHPEG), (RWJ, DOE funded), http://www.nchpeg.org/news-box/corecompetencies000.html
Medical School Core Curriculum in Genetics, 1995	medical student	American Society of Human Genetics (ASHG), http://www.ashg.org/genetics/ashg/policy/rep-01.htm

Geographical Information Systems

Health Economics

Health Education

Responsibilities & Competencies for Health Educators, 1997	professional	National Commission for Health Education Credentialing (NCHEC), endorsed by Society for Public Health Education (SOPHE), American Association for Health Education (AAHE), Association of State and Territorial Directors of Health Promotion and Public Health Education (ASTDHPPHE), update due August 2001, http://www.nchec.org/competencies.htm

continued

Competency Sets	Worker Level	Where to Find Them on the WWW
Core Competencies/ "The Extension Educator"	professional	Department of Agriculture and Natural Resources Education and Communication Systems (ANRECS), Michigan State University, staff professional development, http://www.anrecs.msu.edu/extension/profdev/10areas.htm
Health Care Financing (resources only)		
Health Care Organization, Delivery and Financing Graduate Course offered by School of Public Health	graduate students	School of Public Health, Department of Health Policy, Management and Behavior, University of Albany, New York, http://www.albany.edu/courses
Health Insurance and Medical Services Financing, Financial Management of Healthcare Institutions	graduate students in health care administration track, MBA	Health Care Systems:/Wharton School of Business, University of Pennsylvania, http://www.wharton.upenn.edu
Information Resource/Government Financing of Healthcare	all healthcare and other professionals	Centers for Medicaid and Medicare Services, http://cms.hhs.gov/media/press
Human Resources		
Human Resource Competencies for the Year 2000: A Professionals' Toolkit for Professional Development	professional	Northeast Human Resources Association (NEHRA), www.nehra.com/about.php3, Society for Human Resource Management (SHRM) book, profiles of 31 competencies, http://shrm.org/competencies/home.htm
Human Resources Management Competencies, 2001	leader, manager, professional	School of Public Health Business Management, CDC Corporate University, draft to be validated; Jessi Stevens, HRMO, JStevens@cdc.gov
Directory of Competencies for the Human Resources Community in the Public Service of Canada, October 1998	professional	The Learning Centre, Public Service Commission, Canada, http://learnet.gc.ca/eng/lrncentr/index.htm

Human Resource Competency Model	manager	International Personnel Management Association (IPMA), 22 competencies, http://ipma-hr.org/public/training_template.cfm?ID=12
Informatics		
Public Health Informatics Competencies, 2001	professional	Northwest Center for Public Health Practice, University of Washington School of Public Health and Community Medicine, http://www.healthlinks.washington.edu/nwcphp/phi/comps/
Information Resources Management Competencies, 2001	professional, technical	School of Public Health Information Resources Management, CDC Corporate University, draft to be validated; Tonya Henderson, HRMO, TSHenderson@cdc.gov
Math and Statistical Competencies, 2001	professional, technical	School of Public Health Science & Research, CDC Corporate University, draft to be validated; Charlotte Wilson, HRMO, CWilson@cdc.gov
Recommendations of the International Medical Informatics Association (IMIA) on Education in Health and Medical Informatics, October 2000	physician, nurse, pharmacist, manager, record administrator, teacher, student	American Medical Informatics Association (AMIA), Health and Medical Informatics Education Workgroup, http://www.amia.org/ updated: introductory, intermediate, advanced levels, found at International Medical Informatics Association (IMIA), http://www.rzuser.uni-heidelberg.de/~d16/rec.htm
Registered Health Information Administrator (RHIA) and RHIT (technician) Examination Content: Domains, Sub domains and Tasks	administrator, technical	American Healthcare through Quality Information (AMIMA), http://www.ahima.org/certification/exam.html
Certified Coding Specialist (CCS) Coding Competencies	coder	American Healthcare through Quality Information (AMIMA), http://www.ahima.org/certification/exam.html

continued

Competency Sets	Worker Level	Where to Find Them on the WWW
Medical School Objectives Project: Medical Informatics Objectives, August 2000	MD student	Association of American Medical Colleges (AAMC), School Objectives Project, http://www.aamc.org/meded/msop/informat.htm
On-line Technology Competencies	undergraduate student	College of Education and Applied Professions, Western Carolina University, http://www.ceap.wcu.edu/Martin/Compdef.htm
Student Technology Competency Matrix	high school graduate	Millbury Public Schools, http://millbury.k12.ma.us/~hs/school/techplan/studentmatrix4.3B.html
Laboratory *Body of Knowledge*	laboratorian, specialist, phlebotomist, technician	American Society of Clinical Laboratory Science (ASCLS), book, competencies for CLS and CLT regardless of setting, http://www.ascls.org/index.htm
Leadership (Functional Area) *Public Health Leadership Competency Framework*, August 2000	health director, health officer	National Public Health Leadership Network (NLN), (graduates of the Public Health Leadership Institutes (CDC), http://www.slu.edu/organizations/nln/competency_framework.html
Leadership Competencies for Assistant Deputy Ministers and Senior Executives	senior executive	The Learning Centre, Public Service Commission of Canada, http://www.psc-cfp.gc.ca/aexdp/leaders_e.htm
Leadership Development Competencies: The Leadership Challenge	leader	Exploring Inspired Leadership, The Banff Center, http://www.banffmanagement.com
In development-leadership capacity for governmental and faith-based collaboration, October 2001–2004	leader	Institute for Public Health Faith Collaborations, Emory University, Interfaith Health Programs in development, http://ihpnet.org/4iphfc.htm

Library and Information Science

Information Literacy Competency Standards for Higher Education, January 2000	undergraduate student	Association of College and Research Libraries (ACRL), American Library Association (ALA), http://www.ala.org/acrl/ilcomstan.html
Competencies for Special Librarians of the 21st Century, 1998	entry-level professional	Special Libraries Association (SLA), supported by Association for Library and Information Science Education (ALISE) and Medical Library Association (MLA), http://www.sla.org/content/memberservice/researchforum/lisprograms/lisps.cfm
Students' Information Literacy Needs in the 21st Century: Competencies for Teacher-Librarians	teacher-librarian, high school student	Association for Teacher-Librarianship in Canada (ATLC), http://www.atlc.ca/Publications/competen.htm

Management

Core Competencies for Supervisors, Managers, and Executives, 2000	director, executive, team leader, program manager, supervisor	School of Public Health Leadership & Management Development, CDC Corporate University; Vicki Johnson, HRMO, VJohnson1@cdc.gov, http://intranet.cdc.gov/hrmo/masdevpl.htm
Supervisors' and Managers' Critical Elements, October 1999	supervisor, manager	Headquarters Performance Management System, DOE, http://www.hr.doe.gov/hqpms/supstan.htm
Management Academy for Public Health Competencies, March 1999	public & private sector manager	Management Academy for Public Health (MAPH), North Carolina Institute for Public Health (CDC, HRSA, Kellogg, RWJ funded), http://www.maph.unc.edu Stephen Orton, sorton@email.unc.edu
Competency Profile: Public Service Managers	middle managers	The Learning Centre, Profile for Leaders and Managers, Public Service Commission, Canada, http://learnet.gc.ca/eng/comcentr/manage/profile/auto.htm

continued

Competency Sets	Worker Level	Where to Find Them on the WWW
Public Health Prevention Service Competency Set, September 1997	MS-prepared entry-level manager	Public Health Prevention Service (PHPS) Fellowship, CDC (to be updated fall 2001) "perform", http://www.cdc.gov/epo/dapht/rfa.htm#perform
Competencies for Professional Development: Managing in the Middle, 1998	mid-level manager	Exploring Inspired Leadership, The Banff Center, http://www.banffmanagement.com
National Competency Standards-Public Administration, Competency Based Assessment and Training Handbook, 1999	mid-level administrator, clerical	Office of the Commissioner for Public Employment, Australia's Northern Territory Government, http://www.nt.gov.au/ocpe/documents/people-development/comp-standards
Mass Communications *Mass Communications and Public Health*	all public health practitioners	Course in Mass Communication and Public Health, Division of Epidemiology, School of Public Health, University of Minnesota, http://www.epi.umn.edu/epi_pages/syllabi/PubH5394.html
Public Health Education and Communication Competencies, August 2000	manager, public relations specialist, visual information specialist, technical writer, editor, audio-video technician	School of Public Health Education and Communication, CDC Corporate University; Christopher Stallard, HRMO, http://intranet.cdc.gov/hrmo/masdev2.htm
Maternal and Child Health *Maternal and Child Health Competencies,* February 2001	professional	Association of Teachers of Maternal and Child Health (ATMCH), http://www.atmch.org/mchcomps.pdf

Medicine

Competencies for Providing Public Health Services, 1998	medical student	C.W. Keck, "Core Competencies for the Synergistic Practice of Medicine & Public Health" Josiah Macy, Jr. Foundation Conference, 1998 http://www.josiahmacyfoundation.org/jmacy1.html
Preventive Medicine Residency (PMR) Competency Matrix, 2000-2001	MD-trained, Preventive Medicine Resident	Preventive Medicine Residency Program (PMR), CDC EPO/DAPHT, http://www.cdc.gov/epo/dapht/pmr.htm
Core Competencies and Performance Indicators for Preventive Medicine Residents, 1999	MD-trained, Preventive Medicine Resident	American College of Preventive Medicine (ACPM) with HRSA, http://www.acpm.org/corecomp.htm
Occupational and Environmental Medicine Competencies, January 1998	physician administrator, generalist, specialist	American College of Occupational and Environmental Medicine (ACOEM), http://www.acoem.org/paprguid/guides/comp.htm
An Inventory of Knowledge and Skills Relating to Disease Prevention and Health Promotion, 1989	MD student	Association of Teachers of Preventive Medicine (ATPM), http://www.atpm.org/library/inventory/inventory1.htm

Mental Health

Academic, Fellowship, Summer Institute Programs in Mental Health	public health professionals, MPH students.	Department of Mental Health, Baltimore Health and Mental Health Department, Johns Hopkins School of Public Health, http://commprojects.jhsph.edu/mh/training_programs.cfm
Workforce Development: Ensuring Competency in Public Mental Health	MPH students, clinicians/public health practitioners	Western Interstate Commission on Higher Education, http://www.wiche.edu/Mentalhealth/fyi/1001.htm

continued

Competency Sets	Worker Level	Where to Find Them on the WWW
Nursing		
Public Health Nursing Practice for the 21st Century, 2001	professional	Minnesota Department of Health, Division of Nursing and University of Minnesota, School of Nursing (HRSA-funded) draft tool for assessment, undergoing validation by the Association of Community Health Nurse Educator (ACHNE); Derryl Block, dblock@d.umn.edu
National Competency Standards for the Registered Nurse, 2000	registered nurse, student	Australian Nursing Council, Inc. (ANCI), http://www.anci.org.au/competencystandards.htm
Delivery of Occupational and Environmental Health Services, May 1998	nurse professional	American Association of Occupational Health Nursing (AAOHN), http://www.aaohn.org/servicedelivery_position.htm
Nutrition-Dietetics		
Core Competencies for the Supervised Practice Component of Entry-Level Dietician (Technician) Programs, 1997	dietitian student, dietetic technician student	Commission on Accreditation for Dietetics Education, "Accreditation Manual for Dietetics Education Programs, Revised 4th Edition," Catalog #6107, http://www.eatright.org/cade/standards.html
Standards of Professional Practice for Dietetics Professionals	dietitian	American Dietetics Association (ADA), http://www.eatright.org/qm/standardslist.html
Pharmacy		
Competency Statements: Disease State Management (DSM) Examinations	professional	National Association of Boards of Pharmacy (NABP), http://www.nabp.net/
Physical Activity		
Athletic Training Clinical Proficiencies, 1999	entry-level professional, student	National Athletic Trainer's Association (NATA), http://www.nata.org, clinical focus "Athletic Training Educational Competencies," http://www.cewl.com/

Physical Education for Lifelong Fitness, course	teacher, director, student	American Alliance for Health, Physical Education, Recreation & Dance (AAHPERD), http://www.aahperd.org curriculum book, http://americanfitness.net/Physical_Best/
Standards of Competence, August 2000	therapist	Federation of State Boards of Physical Therapy, http://www.fsbpt.org/news.htm
Public Health Advisor Series *Competencies for Public Health Advisors (GS-685), 2001*	professional	School of Public Health Administration, CDC Corporate University, intranet assessment of 1) foundation competencies and 2) occupational competencies; Ronald Lake, HRMO, RLake@cdc.gov
Public Health Law "*Core Legal Competencies for Public Health Practitioners*"	public health practitioners, lawyers, legislators, policy-makers, and others	Health Law, Center for Law and Public's Health, CDC Collaboration with Georgetown and Johns Hopkins Universities, http://www.publichealthlaw.net/index.html
Public Health Policy *Generic Policy Analyst Draft Competency Profile*	professional	The Learning Centre, Public Service Commission, Canada, http://learnet.gc.ca/eng/lrncentr/index.htm
Secretary-Support *Competencies for Secretary and Office Automation Clerk (GS-318, GS-326), 2000*	secretary, office automation clerk	School of Public Health Business Management, CDC Corporate University; Jessi Stevens, HRMO, JStevens@cdc.gov, http://intranet.cdc.gov/hrmo/crses.htm
Sample Elements and Tasks for Secretary	secretary	Headquarters Performance Management System, DOE, http://www.hr.doe.gov/hqpms.secy.htm

continued

Competency Sets	Worker Level	Where to Find Them on the WWW
National Competency Standards-Public Administration, Competency Based Assessment and Training Handbook, 1999	mid-level administrator, clerical	Office of the Commissioner for Public Employment, Australia's Northern Territory Government, http://www.nt.gov.au/ocpe/documents/people-development/comp-standards
Social Work *Description of the Doctoral Program: Educational Objectives*	PhD students	School of Social Work, University of North Carolina at Chapel Hill, learning objectives, http://www.sowo.unc.edu/doctoral/description/index.html
STD/HIV *Program Operations Guidelines for STD Prevention: Training and Professional Developments*	clinician, disease investigator, HIV counseling	Center for HIV, STD, and TB Prevention, CDC; Frankie Barnes, NCHSTP/DSTD, FBarnes@cdc.gov, http://www.cdc.gov/std/program/training.pdf
Veterinary Medicine *The Veterinary Clinical Skills Competencies*	all veterinarians	*Professional Competencies of Canadian Veterinarians: A Basis for Curriculum Development.* DVM 2000. Ontario Veterinary College, University of Guelph, 1996, http://www.ovcnet.uoguelph.ca/Services/College/DVM/DVM2000/compet.html

F

Data-Gathering Activities

Between July and November 2001, representatives of the Institute of Medicine Committee on Assuring the Health of the Public in the 21st Century conducted five site visits to two Turning Point projects and three Community Voices projects around the country. The goals of the site visits were to

• Collect qualitative and anecdotal information from community-based public health projects regarding lessons learned, best practices demonstrated, major issues and concerns, and input about the local and national governmental public health infrastructure;
• Witness community partnerships in action and communicate with stakeholders; and
• Conduct preliminary report dissemination by introducing the committee's charge and objectives

A timeline of the site visits with a summary of key facts is provided below.

TABLE F-1 Summary of Site Visits

Site	Host Organization	Focus/Mission, Goals, and Objectives	Public Health Department Role	Community Role and Level of Involvement	Other Partners
Community Voices project, Baltimore, MD (July 31, 2001), Sandtown-Winchester community	**Vision for Health** An unincorporated consortium of health care organizations, a health department, a community organization, a funder, and an academic institution	Health care access Community health promotion Basic community and individual needs	Integral, a primary partner	Moderate	Health care providers, academia, community organizations, media
Turning Point project, New Orleans, LA (August 27, 2001)	**Healthy New Orleans** A coalition consisting of the health department, health care providers, and a range of community representatives	Public health system change Community health improvement	Integral, a primary partner	High	County health department Community Organizations
Community Voices project, Denver, CO (September 26, 2001)	**Denver Health** An "integrated health delivery system" public–private health organization functioning both as a department of health and a major regional health care provider	Health care access Community health promotion	Administratively integrated into organization's functions and activities	Low to moderate	State and local government Foundations Local community college Local and statewide coalitions

Community Voices project, Oakland, CA (October 15, 2001)	Asian Health Center/La Clinica de la Raza Two federally qualified community health centers	Health care access Community health promotion	Supporter, partner	Moderate	County health consortium Health department Community organizations
Turning Point project, Franklin, NH, (November 5, 2001)	Caring Community Network of Twin Rivers	Community health promotion Public health system change	Community efforts to perform needed functions in the absence of a traditional health department	High	Community members with diverse skills

NOTE: This is a concise summary of key characteristics and activities identified during site visists.

BALTIMORE SITE VISIT
JULY 2001

About the Vision for Health Consortium

The Sandtown-Winchester community of Baltimore, Maryland, is a largely African-American, 72-block urban community of 10,500 people that has experienced significant rates of substance abuse, unemployment, and other problems. The Vision for Health (VFH) Consortium emerged from a "comprehensive neighborhood transformation program" begun in 1990 by the Community Building in Partnership, Inc., a partnership among Sandtown-Winchester residents, the mayor, and the city government, with funding from the Enterprise Foundation and a neighborhood block grant from the city. At the end of a 2-year process of planning, assessing, and discussing community needs, health (particularly substance abuse issues, children's health, chronic disease, HIV/AIDS, and homicide) emerged as an area of high community priority, second only to education.

VFH's founding partners include Community Building in Partnership, Inc., which is the organizational representative for the citizenry of Sandtown-Winchester, as well as the Baltimore City Health Department, the Bon Secours Baltimore Health System, the Enterprise Foundation, Total Health Care, the University of Maryland Medical System, and the University of Maryland School of Nursing. In addition to these formal partners, VFH has informal partners, such as the *Baltimore Times*, a local newspaper that has been a supporter and facilitator of the community health improvement initiative from the beginning. Previously, several of these partners had been competitors, providing health care services within the same territory. Coming together, they agreed to collaborate in the creation of an integrated system of care that would reach out to uninsured or underinsured individuals and respond to the community's need for health improvement. These partners signed a community compact at the beginning of their collaboration, agreeing upon basic principles for their work together. For example, the compact outlined goals and objectives, agreements for financial and administrative collaboration and accountability, and most importantly, reflected commitment to addressing the needs of the community.

In 1998, VFH received funding from the W. K. Kellogg Foundation as part of a national initiative at 13 sites, called Community Voices: Health Care for the Underserved. The Community Voices project administered by VFH mainly targets Sandtown-Winchester and some Baltimore residents—including recently released ex-offenders—least likely to be reached by other social services programs.

VFH help to maintain its accountability to the community by employing a resident advisor—a community resident who serves as a liaison to the community and who is involved in all decision-making and planning processes.

VFH's Mission, Values/Principles, and Goals

VFH's mission is "to work with the neighborhood transformation efforts of Community Building in Partnership, Inc., to create a community-driven health system in Sandtown-Winchester with the goal of improving the community's overall health status. This will be accomplished by promoting early intervention, prevention, and access to quality health care regardless of ability to pay" (VFH, 1997: 9).

The project's values and principles include a focus on quality and service excellence, on being community driven, having respect and compassion for the community, assuring relationships of integrity between and among partner institutions, and promoting innovation as an integral part of the community transformation process.

The goals of the Community Building in Partnership, Inc., initiative were to transform a range of community systems that seemed inadequate or ineffective in addressing major community problems such as unemployment, crime, and poor housing. This wide-ranging perspective on community well-being appears to have formed the foundation of the VFH Consortium's profound understanding of how social and environmental factors can affect health outcomes and the importance of the individual's and the community's roles in improving health. Based on priorities identified by the community, the VFH Consortium describes five goals: (1) adult primary care and health promotion, (2) community outreach, (3) school-based children's health services, (4) substance abuse treatment, and (5) violence prevention.

VFH Activities and Accomplishments

In keeping with the spirit of the Community Voices, the residents of the Sandtown-Winchester community have always been an integral part of the VFH Consortium and the process of transforming the health and human services systems in the area. Approximately 500 residents were active in the initial planning process, with community members participating on planning work groups and identifying top neighborhood health priorities. In addition to the resident advisor to the VFH Consortium, several community members work as outreach workers in the community, linking people to needed health promotion and health care services. VFH and its partners continue to conduct community forums and gatherings, where residents engage with administrators and providers in dialogue about the community's health, its needs, and its accomplishments.

The activities of VFH involve no overhead costs, because consortium members take turns providing administrative and other resources. VFH staff members are employees of Bon Secours health system, whereas Men's Health Clinic staff are city health department employees. The Enterprise Foundation takes the lead financial role by receiving funding and reimbursing consortium members as appropriate. For instance, the comprehensive services provided by the neighborhood's elementary school health centers (fine-tuned through meetings between school principals and VFH staff) are a direct response to the community's expressed needs for child health care that is more than just "Band-Aids and shots." The University of Maryland School of Nursing manages the school-based clinics that provide comprehensive preventive primary health care as well as mental and oral health care services. Asthma management and mental health services are some of the extras available in school-based clinics. Baltimore Health Department funds for school health centers go to the Enterprise Foundation, which then reimburses the School of Nursing for services rendered. In other areas, partner agencies donate or otherwise contribute certain services to help support the continuum of care envisioned by the collaborative and the community. For instance, men with substance abuse or mental health needs who receive services at the Men's Health Clinic (discussed below) are referred to Bon Secours for follow-up care or to the University of Maryland medical system for psychiatric urgent care.

Research and evaluation are relatively new areas for the VFH Consortium. They received assistance with needs assessment surveys from the Baltimore Health Department and some evaluation support from a local university.

In June 2000, VFH opened the Men's Health Center, the first component of an integrated health care delivery system for uninsured men. The need for a men's health care center was identified through community assessments which showed that many women in need of health care lacked a medical home, but had some access to the health care safety net through family planning and prenatal (Healthy Start) services. Men, however, had much less access. This problem was compounded by the men's reported feelings of discomfort with clinical settings that seemed primarily attuned to women's health care needs and their concerns about not being able to take care of their own health, let alone their families' health. Acknowledging these issues, as well as the important roles men can play in maintaining healthy families and neighborhoods, VFH sought to use the Men's Health Center as a way of both providing care and "building families . . . one man at a time." The Men's Health Center currently provides quality primary health care, as well as referrals to substance abuse services and dental care. Through the social workers and community outreach workers on staff, men can also access job training and social services, participate in weekly support/discussion groups, and even get registered to vote. Additionally, there are plans to develop similar comprehensive, high-quality health care services to uninsured women. Other VFH plans include expanding the activities of Women Against Violence, a community group that is currently exploring the various effects of neighborhood violence on the family structure and considering future opportunities to partner with churches and organizations on issues related to fatherhood.

VFH's outreach component involves creating bridges between community residents and local agencies and services. Outreach is essential to connecting people who mistrust government programs or systems to the services they badly need. The project employs two types of outreach workers: VFH workers, who conduct general community outreach and education about access to services and related matters, and Men's Clinic workers, who perform the dedicated role of linking uninsured men to health care services, following up with them when needed and referring them to other human services.

In addition to activities specific to the Sandtown-Winchester neighborhood, VFH has been a partner in broader community health improvement efforts. For instance, VFH has participated in and contributed funding for the Maryland Citizen's Health Initiative, a statewide grassroots effort working to attain universal health coverage. VFH has also been involved in Phases I and II of the National Community Care Network Program, which is part of the Maryland Health Improvement Plan 2000–2010. VFH is also a charter sponsor of the Maryland Citizens Health Initiative Education Fund (MCHIEF), which operates under the banner of "Health Care for All." VFH has further played a convening role, holding a large symposium for outreach workers and emphasizing the importance of outreach (a state bill passed in recent years mandates an outreach component as part of all managed care organizations).

As a result of VFH's efforts, the rate of childhood immunization, which was about 68 percent in 1994, increased to 100 percent and has remained at that level for several years.

Site Visit Discussion

In July 2001, representatives of the Institute of Medicine Committee on Assuring the Health of the Public in the 21st Century engaged in a daylong dialogue with staff and partners from VFH.

VFH approaches community health improvement primarily from a health care emphasis. More specifically, the consensus among community and institutional partners holds that health care is an essential determinant to good individual and community health, and the fact that many people in the community lack access to adequate and high-quality care affects their total lives, including their ability to get physicals required for new jobs and to get treatment for health conditions that impair their quality of life and ability to function.

The consortium appears to include substantial community input, from assessment to planning to implementation. VFH staff members, many of whom are themselves residents of the Sandtown-Winchester community, reported that members of the community feel that they own the initiative and that they have a part in what gets accomplished. However, this relationship between the "public" and the public health enterprise is fraught with complexity, and VFH partners described some of the challenges they experienced in thinking about and addressing it. The Men's Health Center is clearly a product of collaboration between the local public health agency and health care expertise and resources, on the one hand, and community members' cultural knowledge and social experiences, on the other. On an organizational level, the Men's Health Center is located in a health department facility, yet it is a separate entity. However, there were initial concerns on the part of community clinics that perceived the center as a sign that the health department was overstepping its bounds and expanding its provision of direct services. VFH partners noted that the role of the health department is to facilitate, support, bring resources to the table, and look at the community in a way that affirms assets, motivation and power for change rather than focusing on the "empty half of the glass," that is, needs and deficiencies.

The local newspaper has been a noteworthy informal partner to Sandtown-Winchester's health improvement efforts. The newspaper is a trusted and respected source of information in the neighborhood, and it was able to successfully organize and publicize community health events such as an annual health walk, a mall-based health fair, and events targeting both women's and men's health issues. In addition to creating several forums for community education (including educating local ministers on health issues) and a gateway for people's management of their own health, the paper also provides regular health education messages, including special health publications. The *Baltimore Times* has also formed a new alliance with the health department. In the past, the newspaper's leadership, committed to community empowerment and education, felt compelled to act as a community advocate in light of what it perceived as the health department's insufficient regard for the community's awareness of its own health needs as well as its assets and resources. Over time and through ongoing dialogue, the relationship between the newspaper and the health department has become one of mutual support—the health department even provides copy to the newspaper.

As different community needs have been identified, new opportunities for partnership have emerged. For example, the correctional system is often the only link to primary care for adult men who had not previously qualified for or accessed other health care and social services. The VFH Consortium recently started a collaboration with the local police department to help newly released former inmates returning to their community make the links to care that may include sexually transmitted disease/HIV prevention and treatment, substance abuse treatment, counseling, and mental health care services.

For more information about the Vision for Health Consortium, visit www.communityvoices.org/LL-Baltimore.asp.

DENVER SITE VISIT
NOVEMBER 2001

About Denver Health and Its Community Voices Project

Denver Health is both a nonprofit health care system that integrates safety net services and a public-private public health enterprise. Denver Health received funding from the W. K. Kellogg Foundation to establish a Community Voices: Healthcare for the Underserved community outreach program in 1998. Denver Health has five goals that provide for a unique integration of personal health care and public health services and "take care of the special needs of all populations and the needs of special populations" (Gabow, 2001). These goals include:

• Provide access to quality preventive, acute, and chronic health care for all citizens in Denver regardless of ability to pay.
• Provide expert emergency medical services to Denver and the Rocky Mountain.
• Fulfill public health functions as dictated by the charter and the needs of citizens.
• Conduct health education of patients and education of health care professionals.
• Conduct research that addresses patient needs as well as the educational needs of health care professionals in training.

The position of Denver Health in the local public health system is unique. The organization performs some of the functions of a governmental public health agency, but others, such as environmental health, are under the purview of the local county/city government's Environmental Health agency.

Denver Health Community Voices Mission and Goals

The 5-year Community Voices initiative has two goals, namely (1) "to improve the health of Denver's medically underserved through innovations in community outreach, enrollment in publicly funded health insurance and small employment health plans, and intensive community-based case management" and (2) "to change public policy at the state and federal level for health program funding and reduce barriers to enrollment in publicly funded health insurance."

Program Activities and Accomplishments

The Community Voices initiative fits smoothly into the operations of Denver Health. Its main activities include: community outreach to enhance access to health care, provide health education and health promotion services, and engage communities in health improvement; facilitating enrollment to link eligible individuals to publicly sponsored health insurance programs; and case management, providing personalized care and services to vulnerable patients.

In conformity with the initiative name, Denver Health Community Voices involves community perspectives and partners in health improvement. The initiative's community outreach component is guided by a multicultural steering committee and includes community health advisors who are staff members drawn from the community and community partners that include schools, local businesses, organizations, religious congregations, and neighborhood groups. Community partners help publicize information about Denver Health and access to health care, and provide opportunities and/or support for community health promotion events. Community health advisors facilitate communication between Denver health and the community about community needs, and help to reduce the impact of cultural and other barriers to access. The advisors also provide health promotion and disease prevention education and some informal counseling and support to individuals and groups in the community.

At the state level, Denver Health is involved with the Colorado Coalition for the Medically Underserved and Colorado Access, a safety-net health maintenance organization and Medicaid managed care entity for the Denver area that also includes two local hospitals (one children's), a physicians' group, and the network of federally qualified health centers.

More information about Denver Health Community Voices is available at http://www.communityvoices.org/LL-Denver.asp.

More information about Denver Health is available online at http://www.denverhealth.org/.

NEW HAMPSHIRE SITE VISIT
NOVEMBER 2001

About Caring Community Network of the Twin Rivers

Caring Community Network of the Twin Rivers (CCNTR) is a nonprofit organization established in 1996. The Network is active in a tricounty area that includes 12 towns in central New Hampshire. CCNTR member agencies include a wide range of local social services organizations (ranging from shelters, to elder care, drug abuse, and the Women with Infants and Children Program), a regional hospital, the chamber of commerce, a regional nursing association, a mental health service provider, schools, an affordable housing provider, a visiting nurse association, and a clergy association. The CCNTR board consists of 24 members; half of the members are community representatives, and the remainder represent different agencies.

CCNTR's Mission, Goals, and Objectives

CCNTR has been a participant in the Turning Point Program, which is funded by the W. K. Kellogg and Robert Wood Johnson Foundations, and directed by the National Association of County and City Health Officials with assistance from the University of Washington School of Public Health. CCNTR is one of three Turning Point project sites in the state of New Hampshire, but it is somewhat unique compared with the other projects in the state and projects in other states, as it works on the creation of local public health capacity in an area with limited public health staffing and infrastructure.

CCNTR has six main objectives, including: (1) improving access to health and mental health care; (2) establishing programs to lower youth risk behaviors related to substance abuse and other issues; (3) health promotion and disease prevention; (4) community/public health improvement; (5) increasing social capital, engagement in community health, and development; and (6) supporting the basic needs of individuals and families. There has been some progress in both planning and implementing activities in most areas. In 1998, for instance, CCNTR conducted a large-scale community needs assessment that revealed youth risk behaviors as a major issue, especially because teens do not have many available activities or opportunities for after-school and extracurricular entertainment. As a result, the community and CCNTR developed three strategies for addressing risk behaviors. The first two, which have already been funded and initiated in several communities, include school-based prevention curricula and structured after-school (3:00 to 7:00 p.m.) programs. The third strategy, not yet funded at the time of the site visit, is the alignment of community attitudes to enable recognition of risk and the involvement of adults in community wide prevention activities.

Public Health Infrastructure: Existing and Needed Capacity

As in most states, the public health infrastructure in New Hampshire has experienced certain difficulties. In New Hampshire, these stem from fragmentation, a lack of coordination between the state and local levels, limited resources, and other factors (Rhein et al., 2001). This means that effective communication, sharing of information, and the standardization of functions, services, and roles can be difficult to accomplish. Local public health entities function under separate and often dissimilar town ordinances. There is one public health laboratory for the entire state, and surveillance functions are covered by individual hospitals, at least in the Twin Rivers area. Unlike localities where there are health departments, a public health infrastructure, adequate facilities, and many public health workers to help facilitate and support community health improvement efforts, the Twin Rivers area does not have an easily visible public health presence. There is no official agency building, and the health officers (one in each town) are mostly semivolunteers who have other full-time jobs (e.g., a firefighter, a plumber, and a city legislator) in addition to their public health responsibilities. The services provided across the region are thus fragmented and reactive, as well as lacking in uniformity, because of local differences in policies and procedures. The collection of public health information, such as the collection of data by the state, has been recognized as one of the areas in need of improvement. For example, people at the local level have charged that the data collected by the state may skew or entirely miss the needs of small, heterogeneous local communities.

CCNTR used the state Turning Point project grant to assist local health officers in ensuring the three core public health functions are performed, and to join existing public health efforts with community resources to accomplish more in improving and assuring the health of the population in the area. CCNTR is working on the development of a public health system of governance that would help to shape local public health policy, interface with the state about policy and service delivery issues, and deliver and assure public health services (such as assessment and surveillance). The Caring Community Network has been conducting assessment of a range of basic health indicators, such as adolescent pregnancy, immunization levels, and school-based administration of Behavioral Risk Factor Surveillance System questionnaires. Furthermore, CCNTR carries out formal and informal community needs assessment activities, identifies local strengths and assets that can be used to respond to the identified needs, and also maintains a "big picture" of state policy and other issues that have impact on the local level. CCNTR has also worked with the state to change state policies about data collection (e.g. going beyond county data and collecting data in a way that recognizes the heterogeneity of health data across towns) and means for making data available to local levels (e.g., through the Internet). CCNTR's mission is to work with communities to plan and develop an integrated health and human service delivery system that optimally addresses regional social and health problems, such as an underfunded and fragmented public health system, barriers to accessing services, high-risk behaviors, and many unmet basic needs (e.g., for shelter, food, and transportation).

CCNTR embraces a broad and inclusive definition of public health that includes attention to social issues from a low level of community engagement in collective development and change to the mental health and the social needs of youth. The point, according to a CCNTR partner, is to include "things we all do for work and play" in order to engage "as many people as possible in improving community health." As a result of a perspective that is expansive, flexible, and truly interested in the community's expressed needs, CCNTR supported the community's first area of priority: the development of a multipurpose trails/greenways system that could provide a place for recreational activities and that could provide a safe and environmentally friendly alternative for pedestrian and bike traffic. Being responsive to community needs also ensured the interest and involvement of a wide cross-section of community members who felt that they could rally around an issue critical to them rather than being obliged to accept an issue determined by outside "experts." Other accomplishments of CCNTR have included the redevelopment of the old city hall/opera house in recognition of the economic and social potential of cultural education and the importance of the arts to nurturing the community and developing creative and artistic skills in young people. An important dimension of CCNTR's work has been its consistent emphasis on communicating with and providing feedback to the community.

Site Visit Discussion

Because of the limited nature of the public health infrastructure of the Twin Rivers area, CCNTR, local health officers, and the community have creatively assembled a public health system that draws on the locally available public health expertise that is available but also capitalizes on community resources and skills. The committee heard about the potential implications posed by this specific scenario to national-level attempts to standardize local public health infrastructures and credentialing public health workers. Although the Twin Rivers community leaders present at the site visit expressed a clear vision of quality public health services, they expressed some concern that credentialing and other efforts to formalize local public health services may impair rather than help local work. Although not having a "real" health department may be perceived as a problem in some ways, one participant in the site visit stated that they consider themselves "lucky" that they have no existing infrastructure to "undo" to make it correspond to actual community needs. Workers and community representatives at the site visit noted that they have a great deal of flexibility and the ability to respond to needs in a manner that is unencumbered by the potential rigidity and resistance to change of more formal, highly bureaucratic structures.

CCNTR members further stated that they would prefer something more basic than credentialing to ensure standardization and quality. Having standards for health officers is important, they noted, but a formal credential may not be a good idea given their local situation and the already diverse professional backgrounds of existing health officers. Site visit participants would also like to see continuing education available in areas where the infrastructure is underdeveloped and more focus on Internet-based tools. This highlights the potential of distance education and other emerging technologies for the purpose of continuing education and capacity building. Even so, there are some local limitations in terms of technical capacity (e.g., the low level of availability of T1 or DSL connections to the Internet), as well as logistical issues, such as the absence of a central office where public health officers may check in regularly.

For more information about Caring Community Network of Twin Rivers, visit http://www.naccho.org/files/other/nh3.html and http://www.ccntr.org/.

NEW ORLEANS SITE VISIT
AUGUST 2001

About Healthy New Orleans

The Healthy New Orleans (HNO) Partnership was formed in 1997 and received a Turning Point project grant from the Robert Wood Johnson and W. K. Kellogg Foundations. It is one of three local Turning Point project partnerships funded in the state of Louisiana. Like other Turning Point partnerships, HNO, formally known as *Healthy New Orleans, the City That Cares*, emerged to address problems in the public health system that contributed to poor community health outcomes, as well as fragmented and inadequate services. The total grant funding is $20,000 for 3 years. HNO's diverse membership includes representatives of local community organizations, the state and local health departments, academia, faith-based organizations, non-profit health care providers, and community residents of various ages and of various backgrounds.

In August 2001, representatives of the committee participated in a dialogue with some of the membership of HNO about their objectives, accomplishments, and lessons learned.

Healthy New Orleans Vision, Mission, Goals, and Objectives

HNO developed its vision in partnership with the community through a consensus-seeking process and in answer to the question "What will *Healthy New Orleans: the City that Cares* have in place by 2050?" The "shared practical vision" that emerged is a complex of nine components needed to achieve community wellness. These components were visually arranged by the groups as a pyramid with the vision of community wellness at its heart and with community involvement at its apex. The components of the vision include state-of-the-art diagnostic approaches, emphasis on prevention, expanded view of public health, an electronically linked delivery system, community-based health centers, comprehensive consumer information, community-driven (public health) governance, protective public health policy, and varied funding. HNO developed six objectives to be accomplished in three phases: (1) partnership development, (2) assessment of resources and needs, (3) development of a public health improvement plan, (4) the availability of communications and information systems to serve the community, (5) broad ownership by expanding the vision to nontraditional stakeholders, and (6) accountability in terms of evaluation and feedback to the community. The first phase of HNO's work, partnership development, was conducted between January 1998 and March 1999. This phase included work on establishing and deepening partner relationships and interorganizational linkages and, most importantly, on defining a partnership structure and partnership objectives in a manner congruent with the resources and needs identified by community members.

During the second phase, HNO conducted a strategic planning process in coordination with the state public health entity, resulting in the development of a Community Public Health System Improvement Plan (considered a road map to influence health outcomes in New Orleans) that includes a conceptual framework centered around achieving community wellness by transforming public systems, personal health, and health systems. The third phase involves implementation of the planning process, with particular attention to 17 recommendations for action developed through community workshops. The recommendations with the highest priority ratings included establishment of the Center for Empowered Decision-Making, development of community health networks, and expansion of the definition of public health to include quality-of-life indicators.

Accomplishments of HNO

From the beginning of its work to transform the way in which public health is done in New Orleans, HNO used a broad definition of public health that encompassed social and environmental issues such as poverty, housing, and green spaces. HNO is further distinguished by its attention to the human and social elements involved in making partnerships and coalitions work. Collaborative planning has been the centerpiece of HNO's activities both in terms of establishing a workable representative coalition that "owns" the process and the products and in terms of planning community health improvement in a detailed and strategic way. HNO recognized the assets and resources that the community and other partners had to contribute. However, the group also identified what it termed "underlying contradictions" or areas of conflict, such as a lack of community empowerment, systemic resistance to change, and other barriers to progress (Healthy New Orleans Partnership, 2001). "The community means everyone," stated one participant during the site visit, and others commented on the need to end the separation between "public" and "health" in public health. Furthermore, when discussing where the public health enterprise begins and ends, HNO partners emphasized that public health agencies are part of the community and should act as "amoebas," adapting to circumstances, being responsive to community needs, and focusing on the psychosocioeconomic determinants of health. Participants also acknowledged a prevalent misconception about public health as being "for the poor" and suggested that public health be equated to community wellness. Subsequently, they noted, public health funding must be aligned with community definitions and needs rather than categorically linked to a predetermined framework. When asked about the role of public health departments, HNO participants remarked on the unique position of public health practitioners as keepers and communicators of data and people who "get" the holistic view of health, unlike some providers and funders.

HNO has had some influence on its partners, for instance, helping to facilitate changes in state-level data collection and reporting to increase its usefulness and accessibility to the local level. HNO has also taken steps to implement several of the recommendations that emerged from the community health improvement planning process. For instance, three of eight New Orleans neighborhoods, Carollton, Bienville/Tulane, and St. Bernard/Gentilly, have received small HNO grants to conduct some collaborative planning activities in their communities. Their visions and goals focused on specifics such as creating a multipurpose community center, improving and developing neighborhoods, and addressing violent crime. A fourth neighborhood is beginning its own process of grassroots collaborative planning.

HNO has been involved in a slow, thoughtful process of facilitating change; members of the partnership stated that there is no "quick fix," that achieving something lasting takes time, sensitivity, valuing equity, and civic engagement. There was also agreement that public health education should change to fit the times (that is, there is a need for outreach and community-based public health) and should be extended to the private sector, health care providers, and others. Some attendees expressed concerns about the limitations on funding that addresses the root causes of health problems (e.g., determinants of health), as well as frustration with the dichotomy between community knowledge and scientific expertise. Although HNO participants articulated a desire to evaluate their work in a scientifically valid way, a question lingered: "What will it take before communities can be heard without first having to get the Ivory Tower Seal of Approval?"

It is apparent that the community members and organizations involved in HNO have become profoundly engaged in the process of collaborative planning and have begun to achieve objectives on their way to transforming the local public health system. Further efforts to research and evaluate community-level outcomes will help guide the initiative. The ultimate sustainability of the process, although a stated goal of the grant and foremost in the minds of the facilitators of the project, is not clear at this time.

For more information about Healthy New Orleans, visit http://www.naccho.org/files/other/la1.html.

OAKLAND SITE VISIT
OCTOBER 2001

About Asian Health Services and La Clinica de la Raza

The committee visited the Oakland Community Voices for Immigrant Health project site in October 2001. The Community Voices project in the city of Oakland, California, is administered by the Asian Health Services and La Clinica de la Raza, two multisite, nonprofit, community-based, federally funded clinics in Oakland. The partnership among these two health care services providers, the Alameda County Health Department, and other community organizations like the Alameda Health Consortium has been fruitful and effective in addressing several of the complex and interrelated issues facing area communities, ranging from a lack of health insurance to tobacco use among minority, disadvantaged populations.

Both La Clinica and Asian Health Services have an impressive history of community engagement. La Clinica de la Raza was founded in 1971 by a group of students, health professionals, and community activists and was organized under a board consisting of patients, community members, and professionals elected in annual elections. La Clinica employs approximately 350 staff at four locations in Alameda County and at a medical and dental clinic in a neighboring county. The services provided include primary medical care; dental, mental, and eye care; clinic- and community-based health education; nutrition services; social services; and off-site inpatient care. Asian Health Services has been serving the community since 1974 at three locations and with 120 staff. Its services include clinical services like maternal and child health; HIV testing, counseling, and care; adolescent, adult, and elderly care; and urgent care. It provides health education services on topics ranging from family planning to disease prevention (cancer and HIV/AIDS) and women's health.

Mission, Values/Principles, and Goals of the Oakland Community Voices Project

In 1998, Oakland became 1 of 13 sites in the nation funded by the W. K. Kellogg Foundation's Community Voices initiative to address the problem of uninsurance in local communities. The Community Voices project has been advocating on behalf of Alameda County's 130,000 to 140,000 uninsured individuals and aiming to develop policy, organize the community to support policy change, inform the community about access to health care, and develop a new insurance model. The project's primary goal is to create "an integrated community health system of care for the working poor and uninsured immigrants." Its objectives include:

• educating and informing immigrant communities about insurance and health coverage;
• expanding immigrants' eligibility for health programs;
• facilitating the inclusion of social services in health coverage;
• developing alternative models for financing affordable health coverage;
• documenting effective strategies for outreach and health coverage enrollment in immigrant communities; and
• collecting in-depth information about uninsured immigrants for continuing advocacy.

Activities and Accomplishments of Oakland Community Voices

Noteworthy features of the project include a profound level of community involvement and representation in the process; a partnership among community clinics, community organizations, and the local health department; and exceptional attentiveness to cultural competency. Providing health promotion and health care services in a culturally and linguistically appropriate manner is a routine part of "doing business" among these Oakland partners rather than a minor "tag-on" to the services that they provide. Asian Health Services even includes a Language and Cultural Access Program that provides translation services and interpreter training in a total of seven languages. Another aspect of the relationship with the community is both La Clinica's and Asian Health Services' use of community outreach workers as well as *promotoras* (female health promoters) to serve as links to the community, in addition to conducting community-based health education and health promotion. La Clinica has also developed a curriculum for training *promotoras* on a range of health topics. The promotoras are paid through stipends and gift certificates.

Asian Health Services conducts specialized, strategic outreach to the various populations that it serves, for instance, to Korean groups at churches and to Vietnamese groups at street festivals. Outreach to diverse audiences also implies a need for awareness of and sensitivity to the sociocultural issues of new immigrants and other underserved populations.

The County of Alameda Uninsured Survey was conducted by Community Voices in 2000 (Ponce et al., 2001). The random-probability telephone survey of more than 11,000 households resulted in 1,673 core questionnaires completed by adults 18 and older in English and six other languages (over 40 percent of respondents). The main findings were as follows:

- More than 70 percent of uninsured adults in the county are people of color.
- More than half of the uninsured adults in the county are immigrants.
- The county's uninsured rate of 16 percent is lower than California's rate of 25 percent.

The objectives of the Oakland Community Voices program are implemented in part through the linked enrollment and outreach activities of community health specialists and community outreach workers based at La Clinica and Asian Health Services. In addition to their educational and health promotion activities, these community workers have made it a priority to discuss issues of health access and health insurance with their communities and to help facilitate linkage to medical homes for any families and individuals who lack coverage.

Through the efforts of a strategic collaborative, Oakland Community Voices has participated in the creation of a new health insurance product called Family Care, administered by Alameda Alliance for Health, the local nonprofit managed care plan

The Alameda County Health Department has transformed its goals and services to become more community based and has increased staff capacity to work with the community. For instance, field staff have been organized into 11 community health teams to strengthen the relationship with the public, increase responsiveness and visibility, and decrease duplication of effort through expanded collaboration with community organizations, such as the Asian Health Services. The health department has also developed a 5-year strategic plan based on the 10 essential public health services. The department's collaborative efforts include sharing the California tobacco settlement money with community partners.

REFERENCES

Gabow P. 2001. Denver Health: a health system integrating safety net services. Presentation to the IOM Committee on Assuring the Health of the Public in the 21st Century, September 26, 2001.

Healthy New Orleans Partnership. 2001. Annual Progress Report. Funded by National Association of County and City Health Officials.

Ponce N, Conner T, Barrera BP, Suh D. 2001. Advancing universal health insurance coverage in Alameda County: results of the County of Alameda uninsured survey. UCLA Center for Health Policy Research and Community Voices Project Oakland. Los Angeles: Regents of the University of California.

Rhein M, Lafronza V, Bhandari E, Hawes J, Hofrichter R. 2001. Advancing Community Public Health Systems: Emerging Strategies and Innovations from the Turning Point Experience. Washington, DC: National Association of County and City Health Officials.

Vision for Health Consortium. 1997. 1994-1996 Annual Report. Baltimore, MD: Vision for Health Consortium

G

Agendas for
Public Committee Meetings

FIRST MEETING

February 21, 2001
National Academies Building, Washington, D.C.

Welcome and Introductions

IOM Committee
Liaison Panel
Other guests

Presentation of the charge to the committee by sponsoring agencies

Claude Earl Fox, M.D.
Administrator, Health Resources and Services Administration

Edward L. Baker, M.D., M.P.H.
Assistant Surgeon General, Director, Public Health Practice Program Office, Centers for Disease Control and Prevention

William F. Raub, Ph.D.
Acting Principal Deputy, Assistant Secretary for Planning and Evaluation, Department of Health and Human Services

Joseph H. Autry III, M.D.
Acting Administrator, Substance Abuse and Mental Health Services Administration

Steve Kaler, M.D., M.P.H.
Deputy Associate Director for Disease Prevention, Office of Disease Prevention, National Institutes of Health

Arthur J. Lawrence, Ph.D.
Acting Assistant Secretary, Department of Health and Human Services

Remarks from Public Health Partners

Tom Milne
Executive Director, National Association of County and City Health Officials (NACCHO)

Patricia A. Nolan, M.D., M.P.H.
Commissioner, Rhode Island Department of Health, Immediate Past President, Association of State and Territorial Health Officials (ASTHO)

Richard Levinson, M.D.
Associate Executive Director for Policy, American Public Health Association (APHA)

Harrison Spencer, M.D., M.P.H.
President, Association of Schools of Public Health (ASPH)

Question-and-Answer Period

SECOND MEETING

April 4, 2001
The Beckman Center, Irvine, California

Welcome and Introductions

IOM Committee
Liaison Panel
Other guests

Presentations by guest speakers and committee members on special topics in public health

Public Health Infrastructure in DHHS and Federal Government
Jo Ivey Boufford

Legal and Constitutional Basis of Public Health
Lawrence Gostin

Structure and Function of State Health Departments
John Lumpkin

Structure and Function of Local Health Departments
George Flores

Models of Health Determinants
Lisa Berkman

Local Public Health: the LA Story
Jonathan Fielding

Question-and-Answer Period

THIRD MEETING

June 5, 2001
National Academies Building, Washington, D.C.

Welcome and Introductions

IOM Committee
Liaison Panel
Other guests

Public Health Perspectives

Panel Presentation

Business Perspectives on Population Health

Robert S. Galvin
Director, Health Care, General Electric, Inc.

Education Perspectives on Population Health

Michael Feuer
Director, Center for Education, National Research Council

Question-and-Answer Period

FOURTH MEETING

July 31, 2001
National Academies Building, Washington, D.C.

Welcome and Introductions

IOM Committee
Liaison Panel
Other guests

Challenges and Opportunities for Strengthening Public Health

Dr. Edward L. Baker, Jr.
Director, Public Health Practice Program Office
Centers for Disease Control and Prevention

Question-and-Answer Period

H

Committee Biographies

Jo Ivey Boufford, M.D. *(Co-chair)*, is professor of health policy and public service at the Robert F. Wagner Graduate School of Public Service at New York University, where she served as dean between June 1, 1997, and December 31, 2002. Before that she served as principal deputy assistant secretary for health in the Department of Health and Human Services (DHHS) from November 1993 to January 1997 and as acting assistant secretary from January 1997 to May 1997. While at DHHS she served as the U.S. representative on the Executive Board of the World Health Organization (WHO) from 1994 to 1997 and was reappointed to this position in May 1998. From May 1991 to September 1993, Dr. Boufford served as director of the King's Fund College, London, England. She served as president of the New York City Health and Hospitals Corporation (HHC), the largest municipal health system in the United States, from December 1985 to October 1989. She was elected to membership in the Institute of Medicine in 1992. She is currently a member of the National Advisory Council on Graduate Medical Education and the National Advisory Council for the Agency for Healthcare Research and Quality. She received a B.A. (psychology) magna cum laude from the University of Michigan and an M.D. with distinction from the University of Michigan Medical School. She is board certified in pediatrics.

Christine K. Cassel, M.D. *(Co-chair)*, is dean of the School of Medicine, Oregon Health and Science University. Previously, she was the chairman of the Henry L. Schwarz Department of Geriatrics and Adult Development, professor of geriatrics and internal medicine at the Mount Sinai School of Medicine, and director of the Geriatric Research, Education, and Clinical Center at the Bronx Veterans Affairs Medical Center. She joined Mount Sinai in 1995 after 10 years as chief of general internal medicine at the University of Chicago, where she was also professor of medicine and public policy studies, chief of the Section on General Internal Medicine, director of the Center for Health Policy Research, and George M. Eisenberg Professor in Geriatrics, Health, and Society. Dr. Cassel's numerous publications include the textbooks *Geriatric Medicine: Principles and Practice* (Springer, New York, 2003) and *Ethical Dimensions in the Health Professions* (Saunders, Philadelphia, 1981). Dr. Cassel is a member of the Institute of Medicine (IOM) of the National Academy of Sciences, past president of the American College of Physicians, and past chair of the American Board of Internal Medicine. She chairs the boards of trustees of the American Board of Internal Medicine, The Greenwall Foundation, and the Ethics Advisory Panel for the Kaiser Permanente Health System. She is a trustee of the Russell Sage Foundation. Dr. Cassel has served on several IOM committees: as the chair of the Committee on Care at the End of Life, as the chair of the Committee on Non-Heart Beating Organ Donation, and as a member of the Committee on Quality of Care in America.

Kaye W. Bender, Ph.D., R.N., F.A.A.N. (Mississippi Department of Health), was appointed deputy state health officer for the Mississippi State Department of Health in October 1998. As deputy, Dr. Bender is second in command of the statewide public health system. Before accepting this position, Dr. Bender served for 10 years as the chief of staff of the state health officer at the Mississippi State Department of Health. Her responsibilities included directing the Offices of Policy and Planning, Public Health Nursing, Field Services, and Primary Care Development, among others. Over her professional career, Dr. Bender has served in leadership positions as director of public health nursing, field services nurse consultant, District V supervising nurse, and maternal-child health nurse consultant with the Mississippi State Department of Health. Dr. Bender is active in the American Nurses Association, the Mississippi Nurses Association, the American Public Health Association, and the Association of Community Health Nursing Educators.

Lisa Berkman, Ph.D. (Harvard School of Public Health), is a social epidemiologist whose work focuses extensively on psychosocial influences on health outcomes. Her research has centered on understanding social inequalities in health related to socioeconomic status, different racial and ethnic groups, and social networks, support, and social isolation. The majority of her work is devoted to identifying the role of social networks and support in predicting declines in physical and cognitive functioning, onset of disease, and mortality, especially related to cardiovascular or cerebrovascular disease. The primary studies in which Dr. Berkman is involved are large prospective cohort studies, like the Established Populations for the Epidemiologic Study of the Elderly Studies and the MacArthur Foundation Research Network on Successful Aging longitudinal studies in communities. She is also involved with a secondary set of studies that consist of clinical trials to test the effects of psychosocial interventions in improving the prognosis in people with cerebrovascular or cardiovascular disease.

JudyAnn Bigby, M.D. (Harvard Medical School), is a graduate of Wellesley College and Harvard Medical School. She completed a primary care internal medicine residency at the University of Washington Affiliated Hospitals in Seattle and was a Henry J. Kaiser Fellow in General Internal Medicine at Harvard Medical School and Brigham and Women's Hospital. Currently, Dr. Bigby is the medical director of community health programs at Brigham and Women's Hospital and associate professor of medicine at Harvard Medical School. Dr. Bigby has devoted her career to addressing the health care needs of disadvantaged and vulnerable populations. Currently, Dr. Bigby's work focuses on the health care of low-income and minority women. She is working on integrated primary care and public health models for care of disadvantaged women to identify ways to overcome barriers to care and to address racial disparities in health status and health access, particularly in breast and cervical cancer and infant mortality. Dr. Bigby serves on many boards, including the Public Health Commission for the City of Boston, the Women's Education and Industrial Union, the Medical Foundation, and the Center for Community Health, Education, Research and Service. She has also served on national committees including the Council on Graduate Medical Education.

Thomas A. Burke, Ph.D., M.P.H. (Johns Hopkins University), is an associate professor at the Department of Health Policy and Management of the Johns Hopkins University School of Public Health, with joint appointments in the Department of Environmental Health Sciences and the Department of Oncology, School of Medicine. He is also codirector of the Johns Hopkins Risk Sciences and Public Policy Institute. His research interests include environmental epidemiology, the evaluation of community exposures to environmental pollutants, the assessment and communication of environmental risks, and the application of epidemiology and health risk assessment to public policy. He is a principal investigator for the Pew Environmental Health Commission aimed at revitalizing the national infrastructure for environmental health. Dr. Burke is the chair of the Advisory Committee to the National Center for Environmental Health of the Centers for Disease Control and Prevention and a member of the National Research Council

Board on Environmental Studies and Toxicology. He is particularly interested in health and environment in the cities. Before his appointment at Johns Hopkins, Dr. Burke was deputy commissioner of health for the state of New Jersey. He has also served as assistant commissioner for occupational and environmental health at the New Jersey Department of Health and as director of the Office of Science and Research in the New Jersey Department of Environmental Protection. Dr. Burke received a Ph.D. in epidemiology from the University of Pennsylvania, an M.P.H. from the University of Texas, and a B.S. from Saint Peter's College.

Mark Finucane (Ernst & Young, LLP) is Principal, Leadership Development Solutions, Ernst & Young Health Sciences Advisory Services. Formerly, Mr. Finucane served as director of the Los Angeles County Department of Health Services (DHS), where for 5 years (until July 2001) leading the second largest public health system in the nation. The Department provides over 85 percent of all uncompensated medical care in Los Angeles County, which is home to the largest concentration of uninsured (more than 2.5 million) in the country. Under Mr. Finucane's leadership, DHS increased its ambulatory care visits by 800,000, resulting in substantial cost savings and decreases in inappropriate emergency room use. During Mr. Finucane's tenure, the department created the Office of Women's Health, the Diversity Program, and the multiagency Health Authority Law Enforcement Task Force. In June 2000, Mr. Finucane successfully led negotiations with the federal and state governments to secure a 5-year extension of the Medicaid Demonstration Project that will allow DHS to continue its restructuring efforts with an influx of approximately $2 billion in funding from county, state, and federal governments. Before accepting his position with the Los Angeles DHS, Mr. Finucane was the director of the Contra Costa County Health Services Department from 1984 to 1996 and held a series of senior executive positions at the San Francisco Department of Health and San Francisco General Hospital from 1977 to 1984.

George R. Flores, M.D., M.P.H. (California Endowment) is a public health policy and program consultant. Until May 2002, Dr. Flores was health officer and director of public health for the San Diego County Health and Human Services Agency in California. His present work focuses on health disparities, social justice, access to care, and migrant and border health issues. Recent work includes public health/bioterrorism preparedness and public health system performance assessment. Dr. Flores has also served as a health officer in Sonoma County, California; program director for Project HOPE in Guatemala; deputy health officer, Santa Barbara County, California; and clinical faculty, University of California, San Francisco, School of Medicine. He presently serves on the Public Health Advisory Committee to

California's Little Hoover Commission and the Board of Directors of the Latino Coalition for a Healthy California and is a former member of the Department of Education's Committee on Foreign Medical Education and Accreditation. He is an alumnus of the University of Utah College of Medicine, Harvard School of Public Health, the Kennedy School of Government, and the Public Health Leadership Institute.

Lawrence O. Gostin, J.D. (Georgetown University Law Center), is a professor at the Georgetown University Law Center, a professor of law and public health at the Johns Hopkins School of Hygiene and Public Health, and a fellow of the Kennedy Institute of Ethics. He is also director of the Center for Law and the Public's Health at Johns Hopkins and Georgetown Universities and health law and ethics editor of the *Journal of the American Medical Association*. Previously, he served as executive director of the American Society of Law, Medicine, and Ethics and as an adjunct professor at the Harvard Law School and the Harvard School of Public Health. He was also consulting legislative counsel to the U.S. Senate Labor and Human Resources Committee, chaired by Senator Edward Kennedy, and a member of the President's Task Force on National Health Care Reform. He also serves as a consultant or advisory committee member for the World Health Organization, the Centers for Disease Control and Prevention, the National Institutes of Health, and the National Academies. From 1974 to 1985, Mr. Gostin was the head of the National Council of Civil Liberties, legal director of the National Association of Mental Health, and a faculty member at Oxford University in Great Britain. He received the Rosemary Delbridge Memorial Award from the National Consumer Council (United Kingdom) for the person "who has most influenced Parliament and government to act for the welfare of society." His latest book is *Public Health Law: Power, Duty, Restraint* (University of California Press and the Milbank Memorial Fund, 2001). Mr. Gostin was elected to the Institute of Medicine in 2000.

Pablo Hernandez, M.D. (Wyoming Mental Health Division), has been the hospital administrator at the Wyoming State Hospital since 1995. On June 1, 1997, he was appointed as the Behavioral Health Division Administrator (now known as the Mental Health Division) for the Wyoming Department of Health, which encompasses the State Hospital and the state's community programs. Dr. Hernandez received a medical degree from the Salamanca Medical School in Salamanca, Spain. His clinical career began in 1968 in the state of Virginia, where he was director of gerontological services. He moved on to the state of Mississippi, where he spent the next 14 years establishing community-based service programs as well as active psychiatric treatment modalities and substance abuse services. He also served as the director of the East Mississippi State Hospital and the Las Vegas Medical

Center in Las Vegas, Nevada. Dr. Hernandez has served on multiple state and national committees addressing issues of persons with persistent mental illness, mental health service system changes, as well as cultural perspectives to mental health services. He has served as a consultant to the Substance Abuse and Mental Health Administration reviewing service system designs and as a reviewer of federal grants to states. He is an active member of the National Alliance of the Mentally Ill and the National Latino Behavioral Group.

Judith R. Lave, Ph.D. (University of Pittsburgh), is a professor of health economics at the Graduate School of Public Health and codirector of the Center for Research on Health Care at the University of Pittsburgh. She holds secondary appointments in the Graduate School of Public Health, the Katz Graduate School of Business, the Department of Economics, and the Department of Psychiatry. She received her undergraduate training at Queen's University in Canada (from which she received an honorary doctorate in 1994) and a Ph.D. in economics from Harvard University. She has been a faculty member at Carnegie-Mellon University; director of the Division of Economic and Quantitative Analysis, Office of the Deputy Assistant Secretary, Department of Health and Human Services; and director of the Office of Research in the Health Care Financing Administration. She was a charter member of the federal government's Senior Executive Service. Dr. Lave has published widely. Her main interests are in the cost, utilization, and financing of health care services, and she has conducted cost-effectiveness studies and cost–benefit analyses. Her recent interest has focused on selected issues related to managed care. Dr. Lave has served as a consultant to private and public agencies in the United States and Canada. She is a member of the Institute of Medicine and the National Academy for Social Insurance and is a distinguished fellow of the Academy for Health Services Research. She is past president of the Association (now Academy) for Health Services Research. She is currently on the Steering Committee for the National Academy of Social Insurance's project on Restructuring Medicare for the Long Term and on the Technical Advisory Group for the Pennsylvania Health Care Cost Containment Council.

John R. Lumpkin, M.D., M.P.H. (Illinois Department of Public Health), was appointed director of the Illinois Department of Public Health in January 1991, after serving as acting director since September 1990 and previously as associate director of the Department's Office of Health Care Regulation. Before joining the state health department, Dr. Lumpkin served as an emergency physician at several Chicago hospitals. He teaches public health information systems and performance measurement at the University of Illinois at Chicago School of Public Health. He is also a leading expert on injury prevention and has provided technical assistance to Egypt's Ministry of Health on behalf of the U.S. Public Health Service. He has served on a number of national advisory committees and currently serves as chair of the National Committee on Vital and Health Statistics (NCVHS) and is member of the NCVHS Executive Subcommittee and Workgroup on National Health Information Infrastructure. Dr. Lumpkin received a medical degree in 1974 from Northwestern University Medical School, where he continues to serve as assistant professor in emergency medicine. He trained in emergency medicine at the University of Chicago and earned an M.P.H. from the University of Illinois at Chicago School of Public Health. Dr. Lumpkin is past president of the Association of State and Territorial Health Officials, a former member of the Board of Trustees of the Foundation for Accountability, a former commissioner of the Pew Commission on Environmental Health, a board member of the National Forum for Health Care Quality Measurement and Reporting, a past board member of the American College of Emergency Physicians, and past president of the Society of Teachers of Emergency Medicine.

Patricia A. Peyser, Ph.D. (University of Michigan), is professor of epidemiology at the University of Michigan School of Public Health, where she founded the Public Health Genetics Interdepartmental Concentration. She is also a faculty member in the Center for Statistical Genetics and is on the executive committee for the Genome Sciences Training Grant, which is funded by the National Institutes of Health (NIH). She has served on the editorial board of the *American Journal of Epidemiology* and is currently on the editorial board of *Human Genome Epidemiology*. Her research interests for the past 20 years have focused primarily on the genetic basis of common chronic diseases and their risk factors. She is a coinvestigator in the National Heart Blood and Lung Institute's Family Blood Pressure Program in the project Genetic Determinants of High Blood Pressure in Three Racial Groups. She is also principal investigator in the National Heart Lung and Blood Institute-funded study Epidemiology of Coronary Artery Calcification, a cohort study that focuses on the genetic and environmental determinants of coronary artery calcification. Dr. Peyser serves on an NIH advisory committee for the Family Heart Study. Most recently, she served as a member of the Program Planning Committee for the September 2000 3rd National Conference on Genetics and Public Health, sponsored by the Centers for Disease Control and Prevention, the Health Resources and Service Administration, the National Human Genome Research Institute, the University of Michigan Department of Community Health, and the Association of State and Territorial Health Officials. Dr. Peyser received a Ph.D. in ecology and evolution from the State University of New York at Stony Brook and a B.A. in mathematics from the University of Vermont.

George Strait, M.S. (MedComm Inc.) is a recognized media expert in health and science and chief executive officer of MedComm Inc. His most recent position was managing editor with the Kaisernetwork.org. Previously, he was the senior vice-president for media and distribution for The Dr. Spock Co., a media company. From 1977 until 2000 he was ABC News's primary correspondent for medical and health news and was named senior medical correspondent in 1983. In that capacity, he contributed to World News Tonight with Peter Jennings and Nightline on such issues as health care reform, the medical and ethical concerns regarding new technologies, and AIDS. Mr. Strait was the first U.S. network correspondent allowed to enter The Democratic Republic of Congo (formerly Zaire) to report on the AIDS epidemic in Africa. He also reported in depth on the former Soviet Union's health care system. In 1995, for the second time, Mr. Strait received the broadcast news industry's highest award, the Alfred I. DuPont Award, for his groundbreaking series on the disparity in health care between men and women. In addition, Mr. Strait received a Gold Medal Award from the National Association of Black Journalists and a Blakesely Award from the American Heart Association. He was cofounder of the National Association of Black Journalists. Mr. Strait writes and lectures frequently about quality-of-care issues in the changing medical environment. In 1986, Mr. Strait was in residence at the Harvard School of Public Health on an annual fellowship for science writers and has been a member of Directors of the Council of the Advancement of Science Writing. Mr. Strait currently serves as the chair of the Henry J. Kaiser Family Foundation. A native of Boston, Mr. Strait graduated from Boston University with an A.B. in biology in 1967. He also completed an M.S. program in biochemical genetics at Atlanta University in 1969. In 1995, he received Boston University's Distinguished Alumnus Award for his career in journalism.

Thomas W. Valente, Ph.D. (University of Southern California) is the director of the Master of Public Health program and an associate professor in the Department of Preventive Medicine at the University of Southern California School of Medicine. He is newly arrived from the Johns Hopkins University School of Public Health, where he spent 9 years conducting research and teaching health communication, program evaluation, and network analysis. His main research interest is understanding health-related behavior through mathematical and network models using empirical studies and computer simulations. Dr. Valente conducts research on substance abuse prevention and treatment programs and is also interested in the evaluation of communication programs designed to promote health-related behavior. He is also the author of *Network Models of the Diffusion of Innovations* (Hampton Press, 1995) and *Evaluating Health Communication Campaigns* (Oxford University Press, 2003). He received a B.S. in mathematics from Mary Washington College, an M.S. in mass communication from San Diego State University, and a Ph.D. from the Annenberg School for Communication at the University of Southern California.

Patricia W. Wahl, Ph.D. (University of Washington). Since 1971, Dr. Wahl has been a professor of biostatistics at the University of Washington and was associate dean of the School of Public Health and Community Medicine from 1985 to 1997. She also served as the acting chair of the Department of Pathobiology and acting dean before becoming dean of the school in 1999. Dr. Wahl currently participates in three collaborative research projects: the Cardiovascular Health Study, a longitudinal study of cardiovascular disease in elderly men and women; the Multi-Ethnic Study of Atherosclerosis, a longitudinal study of subclinical cardiovascular disease in multiethnic groups; and the Japanese American Community Diabetes (JACD) study, a longitudinal investigation of type II diabetes in a local Japanese-American community. In 1999 Dr. Wahl received the American Public Health Association's Statistics Section Award for outstanding contributions to the field of statistics and public health in administration, research, and training.

Index

Q